T0369601

STEM-H for Mental Health Clinicians

STEM-H for Mental Health Clinicians

MARILYN WEAVER LEWIS, PHD
LIYUN WU, PHD, AND
ZACHARY ALLAN HAGEN, MD

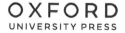

OXFORD
UNIVERSITY PRESS

Oxford University Press is a department of the University of Oxford. It furthers
the University's objective of excellence in research, scholarship, and education
by publishing worldwide. Oxford is a registered trade mark of Oxford University
Press in the UK and certain other countries.

Published in the United States of America by Oxford University Press
198 Madison Avenue, New York, NY 10016, United States of America.

Library of Congress Cataloging-in-Publication Data
Names: Lewis, Marilyn Weaver, editor. | Wu, Liyun, editor. | Hagen, Zachary Allan, editor.
Title: STEM-H for Mental Health Clinicians / Marilyn Weaver Lewis, Liyun Wu, Zachary Allan Hagen.
Description: New York, NY : Oxford University Press, [2023] |
Includes bibliographical references and index.
Identifiers: LCCN 2022037326 (print) | LCCN 2022037327 (ebook) |
ISBN 9780197638514 (hardback) | ISBN 9780197638521 (epub) |
ISBN 9780197638545
Subjects: LCSH: Medical care—Technological innovations. |
Medicine—Practice—Technological innovations. |
Medical technology—Management.
Classification: LCC R855.3 .S746 2023 (print) | LCC R855.3 (ebook) |
DDC 610 .285—dc23/eng/20221020
LC record available at https://lccn.loc.gov/2022037326
LC ebook record available at https://lccn.loc.gov/2022037327

DOI: 10.1093/oso/9780197638514.001.0001

1 3 5 7 9 8 6 4 2

Printed by Integrated Books International, United States of America

Dr. Marilyn Weaver Lewis dedicates this text to her children, Kathryn and Hilary, and her grandchildren, Haley and Marshall, as well as her students in the master's social work program at Norfolk State University. Remember, you can do anything you put your mind to.

Dr. Liyun Wu dedicates this book to her parents, uncle, siblings, and her only child for their encouragement and support.

Dr. Zachary Allan Hagen dedicates this book to his patients in Baltimore for the endless lessons in community and resilience.

Contents

Foreword

Written by Dr. E. Delores Dungee-Anderson
STEM-H for Mental Health Clinicians
(Lewis, M.W, Wu, L., & Hagen, Z.)

As widely understood in academic areas of study, STEM is the commonly recognized abbreviation for four intricately connected fields of academic study: *science, technology, engineering,* and *mathematics.* These fields are frequently associated because they share similarities in both theory and practice. Each field is dependent on sensical conceptual inputs for positive and logical outcomes in all areas of discipline practices.

This text, *STEM-H forMental Health Clinicians,* is both a relevant and exciting work. It is a long-awaited, clearly written, and significantly informative resource, primarily designed for clinical practitioners in the social sciences, clinical students, and faculty who teach and train students in the social science disciplines of social work, psychology, and counseling. However, the clarity of the content readily serves as an invitation to all who are seeking to enhance their understanding of cellular level and systems functioning and the related health and disease processes that frequently are identified as underlying factors of health and mental health concerns.

The authors include an intricate, detailed, and broad overview of STEM-Health content. Their treatment of STEM and identification of the important relationship of STEM to overall health provide salient connections to the understanding and identification of disease processes and related conditions for social science faculty who teach, train, and supervise students in each discipline—and for students enrolled in graduate programs and required internships. The focus of the authors on STEM and STEM connections to health suggests that primary audiences for this text are (1) graduate students who elect social science majors and train as clinical counselors and psychotherapists for professional roles in the employment marketplace and (2) social science majors previously employed in positions in other areas of their disciplines but who desire to further study and train as clinical practitioners. The health content provided in this text offers both a formal and an informal opportunity to study STEM and health for its relevance to clinical practice and successful outcomes.

Although the disciplines of social work, psychology, and counseling each offer multiple theories of human development and behavior and environmental and/

or social determinants of health and mental health that frequently include differential and diagnostic assessments of sociobehavioral challenges, this book very
clearly provides a broader scope of requisite clinical and neuroclinical content in
its detailed treatment of STEM and health and related disease processes. It serves
to fulfill a missing emphasis in clinical curricula in the social sciences. The text
is a well-positioned and essential work that clearly highlights the importance of
genetics and its major contributions to the identified aspects of the social and environmental determinants of health and mental health!

The authors include basic and requisite neuroscience content, such as a comprehensive treatment of neuroanatomy (e.g., the structure and functioning of the
brain and body systems). They identify and describe related disease processes
and include technological interventions that address physical health treatments
for these disease processes, which ultimately and significantly impact health
and mental health. Importantly, this work serves as a necessary bridge between
the biological sciences and the social sciences for clinical practitioners. Such
explicated health content is important for all counseling disciplines but is especially useful and necessary for social science academic curricula, which may not
include a STEM health focus that extends to sociobehavioral and mental health
concerns in the social science counseling professions.

The authors also add important clarifying features in the text, such as
glossaries, detailed illustrations and illustrative definitions, chapter summary
content, and chapter integration so that the chapter material is clearly affiliated.
Each chapter builds on and/or relates to the previous chapter. Additionally, individual chapters are rich with references and connect to research-based content
and relevant data, including website addresses that lead the reader to additional
information and/or original sources of support.

In conclusion, this text is an exciting contribution and a welcome addition to
the social sciences literature and disciplines! It is an especially exciting work for
the connected social sciences and health-related disciplines. The authors bring
together, and highlight in depth, the often unexplored and unexpressed intricate
connections between STEM and health and the significance such connections
occupy in the everyday work of clinical practitioners in the social sciences.
The addition of such extensive discipline content provided by this text is both
energizing and timely and deserves a place in social sciences literature, curricula,
and the libraries of all social science clinicians!

E. Delores Dungee-Anderson, PhD, LCSW, Certified Trauma Specialist Trainer
Professor
Ethelyn R. Strong School of Social Work
Norfolk State University
Norfolk, Virginia

Acknowledgments

We would like to acknowledge David Follmer, president of the Follmer Group, who has provided encouragement and advice for the life of this text; Dana Bliss, executive editor, Oxford University Press; Sarah Ebel, project editor, Social and Behavioral Sciences, Oxford University Press; and Sujitha Logaganesan (She/her), production editor, Newgen KnowledgeWorks Pvt Ltd. Without them, this book would never have seen the light of day.

List of Figures

1
How Understanding Genetics Can Benefit Mental Health Clinicians

Introduction

Research-informed practice and its counterpart practice-informed research are critical to clinical work and are mandated by the accrediting bodies of social work (Council of Social Work Education [CSWE], 2015), psychology (American Psychological Association [APA], 2017), and counseling (American Counseling Association [ACA], 2014). This text is designed to teach clinicians who aim to enter a medically oriented field, or who have private or community practice clients who suffer from illnesses, how to apply concepts of science, technology, engineering, and mathematics to health (STEM-H).

STEM-H Principles Underlying Genetics

(S) Mental health clinicians can benefit from understanding the science underlying genetics

For STEM-H (STEM principles as applied to health), explaining the genetic contribution may be the first place to start when working with an individual or family because many diseases have a genetic component that causes a person to have, carry, or express a trait. Explaining how genetic influences can interact with the environment and thereby exacerbate or ameliorate the illness is an important function. Understanding is the first step to changing variables that contribute to social determinants of health.

Structure
Beginning in 1990 and lasting until 2003, the Human Genome Project (HGP) mapped each of the three billion chemical base pairs of deoxyribonucleic acid (DNA) in the human body. This was an incredible feat and a critically important contribution to science because the human genome contains all of the individual's approximately 20,500 genes in human DNA and is responsible for the structure and function of all bodily systems (U.S. Department of Energy,

STEM-H for Mental Health Clinicians. Marilyn Weaver Lewis, Liyun Wu, and Zachary Allan Hagen, Oxford University Press.
© Oxford University Press 2023. DOI: 10.1093/oso/9780197638514.003.0001

DNA double helix

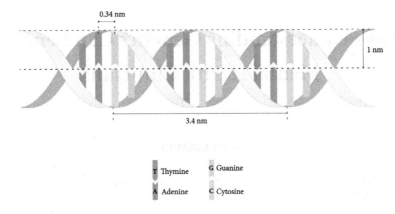

Figure 1.1 Double helix.

From https://www.istockphoto.com/vector/structure-of-dna-double-helix-deoxyribonucleic-acids-nitrogenous-base-and-sugar-gm1385627024-444281529?clarity=false#.

2019). As can be seen in Figure 1.1, each chromosome is a ladder-like structure with rungs made from base pairs of amino acids that are always adenine (A), thymine (T), cytosine (C), and guanine (G) and are normally arranged with the A pairing with T, and the C pairing with G (National Human Genome Research Institute [NHGRI], 2020). DNA itself is actually millions of these base pairs connected in long strands, which then form the characteristic double helix of DNA. These DNA strands are then tightly packaged by many proteins and cellular machinery to form chromosomes.

Chromosomes are the form of DNA that may be replicated and passed on to newly formed cells or, in the case of sexual reproduction, zygotes (embryo precursors). The first aim of the HGP was to identify the order, or sequence, of all the base pairs that constitute the DNA of each gene (NHGRI, 2020) because knowing the sequencing of genes allows researchers to identify mutations in the pairings. As is shown in Figure 1.2, abnormalities can take several forms, including chromosomal deletions, or translocations, where part of one chromosome migrates to another chromosome.

The importance of identifying sections on the chromosomes is important because where one gene is located in relation to the others influences which genes will be inherited together when cells divide during replication (NHGRI, 2019). For example, let us say that we are interested in Gene A, which is close to Gene B on the chromosome. During reproduction, when the cells divide, the individual may inherit two genes that are close together, in this case, both A and B. This

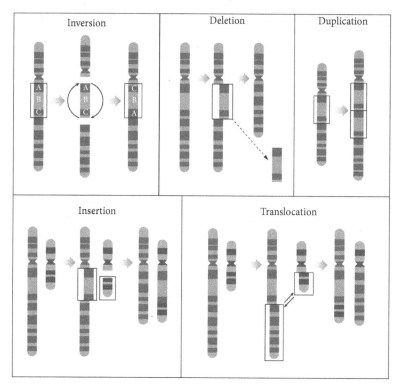

Figure 1.2 Chromosomal abnormalities.

From https://www.istockphoto.com/vector/chromosome-mutation-is-the-process-of-change-that-results-in-rearranged-chromosome-gm1334659652-416698904?clarity=false#.

is called gene linkage because two neighboring genes are often "linked" and inherited together. But let us suppose that we are also interested in Gene Z, which is far away from Gene A. When the cells divide, A and Z probably will not be inherited together because they are "unlinked." The third objective of the project was to create linkage maps to show where genes interact over several generations by mapping the position of the genome from an identified patient (proband) with the disease to that individual's genome with family members without the disease.

Function

There have been two types of classic studies that looked at the impact of genes on drinking behavior. To test the influence of genetic makeup on drinking problems, identical (monozygotic, MZ) twins were compared to fraternal (dizygotic, DZ) twins. Whether the rate of alcoholism was higher among the identical twins was examined. Theoretically, identical twins should be more likely to both have similar alcohol use compared to fraternal twins because they share 100% of their genetic material. However, Hrubec and Omenn (1981) found that while genetics did contribute to alcoholism, something else was going on to predict the twins' drinking rates—more than likely, environment.

In another classic study, Goodwin and colleagues (1974) compared drinking among grown children of alcoholic parents. One group remained in the alcoholic home as children versus the other group that had been adopted as infants and reared in non-alcoholic, non-kin, homes. Goodwin and colleagues found that the odds of developing drinking problems occurred among the male children of alcoholic parents, whether they were reared in non-alcoholic homes or in the original alcoholic home (OR = 3.6 vs. 3.4). Thus, the stronger predictor of whether the child developed an alcohol use disorder was "nature" (their genetic pedigree), not "nurture" (the environment).

Illness. The Collaborative Study on the Genetics of Alcoholism (COGA) project examined the genetic component of alcoholism (National Institute on Alcohol Abuse and Alcoholism [NIAAA], 2016) and has explored the gene–environment relationship of first-, second-, and third-degree biological relatives of over 2,255 families (17,702 individuals) (Begleiter et al., 1995). The project has identified genes that protect a family member from alcoholism, differences in symptoms of alcohol use disorders, and identified which specific chromosomal regions certain psychiatric symptoms are located (Agrawal et al., 2008). These findings can identify an individual's genetic susceptibility or predisposition (Turnpenny et al., 2022). The COGA project's findings are that complex behaviors like alcoholism and psychiatric symptoms are influenced by multiple genes as well as the environment (Lewis, 2016).

Injuries. A mutated gene is a gene that has experienced damage to its genetic material. According to Campbell (2011), embryos are especially at risk for injury if they are subjected to radiation during early gestation when the cells are rapidly dividing. Ozasa (2016) found that effects from radiation exposure from the explosion of the atomic bomb were related to cancer risk depending on distance from the epicenter of the explosions plus shielding conditions.

Chromosomal breakage may also occur during radiation treatment (Bryant et al., 2010), which is correlated to onset of leukemia (Thys et al., 2015). Carcinogens from smoking (Jin et al., 2017) and other environmental hazards (Barnes et al., 2018) cause cancer by randomly damaging DNA within normal cells. Some inhaled carcinogens have been more strongly linked to lung disease.

(T) <u>Mental health</u> clinicians can benefit from understanding the technology used to treat genetic anomalies

There are three types of telemedicine methods: "store and forward," "remote monitoring," and "real-time interactive services," which differ in several ways, one of which is the length of time it takes information to get from the patient to the clinician. The physician may use all three types of technologies when working with patients. The first is store and forward, an example of asynchronous communication that does not happen in real time and is achieved using imaging, such as a mammogram or sonogram. For example, a woman who is being evaluated for breast cancer will meet with a radiology technician who will send images from a procedure to the physician, who will determine if there are tumors or other abnormalities in the area of concern. This store-and-forward process can take hours or days.

A second type of telemedicine, remote patient monitoring, is used if the physician needs more detailed information on an ongoing basis. The patient wears a monitor that sends information to their physician from a variety of biomeasures, including their heart rate, glucose level, and sleep apnea scores. This type of telemedicine is correlated with fewer high-risk pregnancy visits and fewer exposures to potential viral infection. Cardiology also heavily utilizes remote monitoring to evaluate patients for irregularities in the patient's heartbeats over the course of days to months.

The third type of telemedicine is the real-time interactive service, an example of synchronous communication that transmits information in real time using video chats with social media apps (e.g., Zoom, FaceTime, Skype). Dialogue with the patient will allow the clinician to assess and treat the client when the client cannot come to the office. Video chats can also provide opportunities for clinicians to interact with interdisciplinary team members who will follow the patient. While each method of telemedicine is important, video chats provide direct contact between the patient and the team members and are popular methods during periods of time when face-to-face sessions are risky because the patient's immunity is compromised.

Another area where telehealth is used is "contact tracing," where public health officials seek to identify acquaintances of an individual who has become infected with a disease. For many years, contact tracing has been employed when an individual tests positive for syphilis; more recently, this involved the novel SARS-CoV-2 (severe acute respiratory syndrome coronavirus 2) (COVID-19; 2019-nCoV) (Centers for Disease Control and Prevention [CDC], 2021). In contact tracing, the public health technician identifies immediate persons with whom the patient has come in contact and then identifies secondary persons with whom the contacts have come in contact, resulting in an extensive network map of potentially infected persons.

(E) Mental health clinicians can benefit from understanding the biomedical engineering of medications

As the name implies, biomedical engineering is the development of products, including medicines that were developed using engineering methods. Side effects, along with the therapeutic dosage and efficacy of a drug, are all discovered during the multistage engineering of the medication. For example, after a drug used in chemotherapy is constructed or discovered in a laboratory, it may undergo testing on laboratory systems or animals. If these tests are promising, the medication will move to a multiphase human trial pathway. These trials start by testing for adverse outcomes on healthy participants without cancer, followed by testing to determine if the drug works as a proposed treatment for a small number of patients with cancer. Then the trial may move on to large-scale testing to discover the efficacy of treatment outcomes among a population and to find rare side effects. Finally, the new drug will be tested against the current drugs being used to treat the same disease to ensure that it offers an improvement over currently available treatments.

Adhering to the research protocol protects the public from unanticipated side effects and ineffective outcomes. Today, because of the current pandemic and expected pandemics in the future, manufacturing vaccine's safety is paramount. Ensuring the public's confidence is necessary for there to be enough buy-in among members of society for an adequate number of individuals to take the medication in order to result in widespread immunity. Clinicians will be called on to process patients' fears and reluctance to become inoculated.

(M) Mental health clinicians can benefit from understanding the mathematics underlying heritability

Mathematics explain epidemiological concepts, such as heritability, which is the proportion of the way a person looks or behaves (phenotype) that can be explained by the person's genetic makeup, or DNA (Hesselbrock et al., 2013). Understanding the concepts of epidemiology is important because they address the distribution of health conditions in society. To understand these health conditions, epidemiologists examine the following: who contracts or does not contract the illness; what variant they contract; why they contract the illness or are immune to it; when they contract the illness; and where they contract it

(Carneiro, 2017). One branch of epidemiology is genetic epidemiology, which is the study of how persons inherit diseases. It includes examining how risks for the disease were inherited and how the environment contributed to the expression of the disease. To understand the person-in-environment, we can benefit from determining the gene–environment interaction.

An example of a genetic contribution to alcohol use can be found among the Asian population. Normally when someone drinks alcohol, the liver enzyme breaks it down and it is excreted from the body (Suddendorf, 1989). Many individuals of East Asian descent have a mutated gene that decreases the amount of the hormone that breaks alcohol down (Chen et al., 2021) and the Asian flushing reaction (AFR) occurs. AFR is an uncomfortable flushing on the chest and up the neck that can be accompanied by nausea, sweating, headache, racing heart, and dizziness (Oh et al., 2019). While this is a common phenomenon, other individuals of Asian descent have the enzyme that allows alcohol to be metabolized, and they do not report the unpleasant side effects of drinking. The population estimate of individuals of East Asian descent with the mutated gene is estimated to be 36% (Brooks et al., 2009). Because the accumulation of non-metabolized alcohol among people who do not have the enzyme is noxious, a medication that blocks the enzyme that breaks down alcohol has been used to medically treat alcoholics who are having a difficult time becoming abstinent; therefore, drinking alcohol after taking the medication Antabuse causes unpleasant reactions.

(H) Mental health clinicians can benefit from applying principles of STEM to health

Dr. Michie Hesselbrock maintained that clinicians should contribute their expertise to interdisciplinary research because they are trained to evaluate the impact of the environment using a person-in-environment model (Lewis, 2016) and stated that contemporary clinicians are poised to engage in translational science, which is known as the "bench-side to bedside" practice, to evaluate phenotypes (behaviors) and their concordance with the genotype (Hesselbrock et al., 2013). When applying the STEM model to health, Waites suggested that the abbreviation STEM-H may be more appropriate than merely STEM (Lewis, 2016).

Learning that the fetus is carrying a mutated gene can result in the grief reaction called "ambiguous loss" (Boss, 1999). For example, Down syndrome is associated with the baby inheriting an extra chromosome 21 (Trisomy 21) in addition to the two inherited from the parents. On learning this news, the family may grieve the loss of their ideal child and their aspirations for it. This ambiguous loss can result in what Boss called a loss characterized by a "Goodbye, without

Leaving." In this case, the family feels ambivalence about the child who is simultaneously inside and outside of the family. According to Boss, as the ambivalence persists, conflict grows within the family, and clinicians may be called on to help the family accept the loss of their idealized child.

Another phenomenon the family may experience is "stigmatized grief" (Goffman, 1963), which is characterized by feeling embarrassed because the fetus is not perfect. For example, if the family decides to carry to term a fetus that demonstrates Trisomy 21, the child will show limitations in cognitive development that, if severe, may result in an extensive burden for the family and perhaps the government. According to Goffman, a stigma is something that turns others away from the individual because of a difference that is "an undesired attribute of our stereotype of what a given type of individual should be" (Goffman, 1963).

On the other hand, women who learn that they carry certain genetic mutations that are linked to breast cancer will be advised that the mutation is related to different levels of lifetime risk. Depending on the patient's prognosis and personal risk tolerance, she may choose one of many options to address her genetic predisposition. A patient with very high-risk mutations may decide to undergo prophylactic double mastectomy before the age that the cancer generally develops. Alternatively, another patient with the same risk profile may choose a breast cancer screening schedule that starts earlier in life and prescribes more frequent mammograms than is recommended for the general population. However the patient chooses to address her new diagnosis, clinicians have a unique opportunity to discuss the medical options with her and explore her priorities. If the patient elects to have a double mastectomy as a preventive measure, clinicians will work with the woman to help process her grief, much like she would experience with any major loss. For the clinician to be effective, they must understand the body and be able to listen to the patient process her doctor's advice.

An important aspect of STEM-H work is supporting family members who are often the primary caregivers for their loved ones after they are discharged, many times with complicated technological apparatuses. The patient–family dyad often becomes the focus of the clinical intervention as the family's ability to function as individuals and as a unit is critical for the optimal well-being of the patient. Educating clinical professionals about STEM-H principles is germane to understanding the patient through a biopsychosocial, person-in-environment lens.

Conclusion

Chapter 1 has introduced the concept of STEM principles when applied to health (STEM-H) as introduced by Hesselbrock (Lewis, 2016) in an interview on the intersection of genetics and social work. Genetics were introduced using information from the HGP and the COGA project. Studies of alcoholism that compared children of alcoholics adopted out of, or raised in, the alcoholic home were used to explain the gene–environment relationship of alcoholism. The technology of telehealth devices and protocols were discussed, as was information about the process of drug approval by the Food and Drug Administration. This chapter applied science, technology, engineering, and mathematics to clinical work regarding health and introduced concepts of ambiguous loss and stigmatized grief. Organizing this chapter using a STEM-H format provides clinicians a useful method by which to examine genetics and the injuries and illnesses that are commonly found as the result of genetic mutations and to organize this information in a cohesive way.

Glossary

Amino acids   Basic building block of proteins[*]
Chromosome   Present in the cell nucleus, carries genetic material DNA
Dizygotic   Twins that develop from two ova, as in the case of fraternal twins
Genome   Complete set of genes on each chromosome of each cell in an individual
Monozygotic   Twins that develop from one ovum, as in the case of identical twins
Nucleotide bases   Building blocks of nucleic acid

Websites

American Counseling Association: https://www.counseling.org/
American Psychological Association: https://www.APA.org
Council on Social Work Education: https://www.cswe.org

---

[*] The glossaries in this book are from Sell, R., Rothenberg, M. A., & Chapman, C. F. (2018), *Barron's Dictionary of Medical Terms* (7th ed.), Kaplan, unless otherwise noted.

2

How Understanding the Nervous System Can Benefit Mental Health Clinicians

Introduction

This chapter covers the structure and function of the central (CNS) and peripheral (PNS) nervous systems in regard to STEM-H (science, technology, engineering, and mathematics as applied to health). Traumatic brain injury (TBI), the signature injury among military veterans, is covered and special attention is given to technology associated with treatment. Biomedical and pharmaceutical engineering explain the mechanisms of action of medications and nonmedical treatments that are prescribed to avoid secondary damage after brain trauma. This chapter introduces common principles of prevalence and incidence. Finally, principles of clinical practice with families experiencing caregiver burden are introduced.

STEM-H Principles Underlying the Nervous System

(S) Mental health clinicians can benefit from understanding the science of the nervous system

The nervous system is the foundation of all bodily systems and affects behaviors, emotions, and cognitions. Regardless of one's area of clinical practice, it is important to know the terminology and understand the concepts.

Structure

The CNS develops during embryonic life. The first area to form is the neural tube, which is a cylindrical structure developing after embryonic cells fold in on themselves (Molnar & Collins, 2021). The cells at the end of the tube eventually develop into the brainstem, cerebellum, pons, and medulla oblongata (Advokat et al., 2019). The cells in the middle develop into the midbrain, which contains nerve fibers that travel from the hindbrain to the forebrain (Chhetri & Das, 2020). The cells at the front, or cranial end, of the neural tube migrate to areas that develop into the forebrain. These later become the cortex, which contains

STEM-H for Mental Health Clinicians. Marilyn Weaver Lewis, Liyun Wu, and Zachary Allan Hagen, Oxford University Press.
© Oxford University Press 2023. DOI: 10.1093/oso/9780197638514.003.0002

the limbic system, thalamus, and hypothalamus (Advokat et al., 2019). The adult brain consists of gray matter, which derives its color from the neuronal cell bodies, and white matter, which is the deeper layer and derives its color from the myelin on the axons that travel down from the cell bodies (Mercadante & Tadi, 2020). The structure of a neuron contains the cell body and dendrites, which resemble twigs from a tree. These dendrites connect with axon terminals of adjoining neurons, forming a neural network that connects to billions of other cells in the brain, each of which is attached to other neurons (Colbert et al., 2020). As Figure 2.1 shows, the axon is a long structure covered by a myelin sheath, which breaks it into separate sections that allow electrical messages from the cell body to jump from section to section on the axon, decreasing the time it takes to reach the axon terminals (Advokat et al., 2019).

Because the adult cerebral cortex contains approximately 90 billion cells (Advokat et al., 2019), the skull is too small to house a brain large enough to house all those cells. To accommodate the smaller size of the skull, the developing brain folds in on itself to create the sulci (grooves) and gyri (ridges) to increase the space for more cells to reside. These grooves divide the cortex into frontal, temporal, parietal, and occipital lobes (Advokat et al., 2019). While there is no clear demarcation between the lobes, each is associated with a different function: the occipital lobe with vision; the temporal lobe with memories; the parietal lobe with sensory and perception; and the frontal lobe with thought (Advokat et al., 2019). In addition to different lobes, a deep groove develops lengthwise down the center of the cortex, which essentially divides the brain into two hemispheres. These hemispheres are connected by a bundle of threads called the corpus

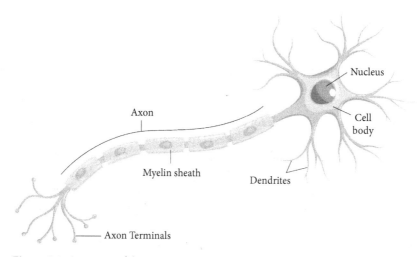

Figure 2.1 Anatomy of the neuron.

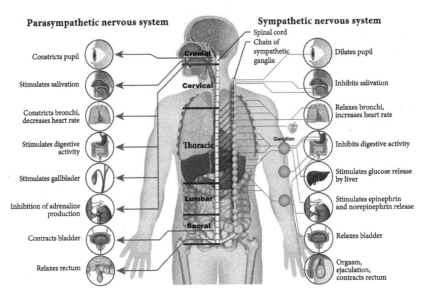

Figure 2.2 The autonomic nervous system.

callosum, which allows communication between the two hemispheres (Catani & Zilles, 2021).

As shown in Figure 2.2, the CNS consists of the brain and the spinal column. The brainstem begins at the base of the head and extends from the skull to become the spinal cord, which travels down the back. The spine has 33 hollow vertebrae that are stacked, one on top of another, and are cushioned by discs that act as shock absorbers to protect them from rubbing against each other (Cleveland Clinic, n.d.). The hollow vertebrae house nerves that run the length of the spine while branching out from the cord (Baron & Solanki, 2021). The autonomic nervous system (ANS) comprises the sympathetic and the parasympathetic systems, which enervate organs of the body.

Function

While the brain is responsible for controlling cognition, feelings, and memories, the spinal, or vertebral, column provides (1) protection of the nerves of the spine, (2) structural support that allows the individual to stand and sit, and (3) flexibility, which allows the body to bend forward, backward, and sideways (Colbert et al., 2020). The spinal cord is responsible for controlling voluntary and involuntary movements and receiving information about the external environment and sending it to the brain (Baron & Solanki, 2021). The nerves in the PNS go to different areas of the body and then carry sensory information from the environment back to the brain, which interprets that information and then sends directions to the appropriate organs and muscles (Advokat et al., 2019).

The functions of the hindbrain. The functions of the hindbrain are necessary for survival. This area includes the cerebellum, or the "little brain" (Northern Brain Injury Association [NBIA], 2020), the brainstem, the pons, and the medulla oblongata, as can be seen in Figure 2.3. Each has functions that are life sustaining: The cerebellum is responsible for movement and balance (Jimsheleishvili & Dididze, 2021). The brainstem controls cardiac functions and respiration (Medicine Libre/Texts, 2020). The pons bridges the cerebral cortex and the cerebellum and affects sleep regulation and respiration. The midbrain links the hindbrain and the forebrain and facilitates functioning of the auditory and visual systems (NBIA, 2020). The medulla oblongata is the last structure in the hindbrain and is associated with breathing, swallowing, and maintaining the heart's rate and joins the brain and the spinal cord (NBIA, 2020).

The function of the brainstem. The brainstem contains fibers that travel up to the cerebral cortex, passing through the amygdala and hypothalamus (Advokat et al., 2019). These fibers contain neurotransmitters, which are released during the "fight-or-flight" reaction to stress. The cerebellum coordinates movement and reflexes and is associated with motor memory (Schmahmann, 2021). According to Schmahmann, the cerebellum communicates with the thalamus, which is in the forebrain, and functions as a relay center that carries information

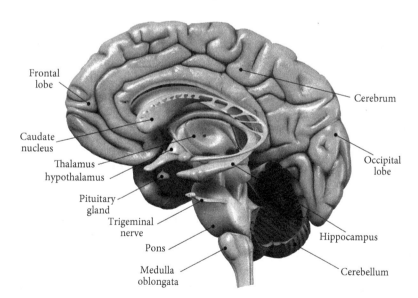

Figure 2.3 Structures of the human brain.

from the environment to the CNS, coordinates reflexes, and is associated with motor memory.

The function of the midbrain. The midbrain is located above the hindbrain and below the forebrain. It is a more primitive site than the cerebral cortex and functions as a relay center for visual and auditory information (NBIA, 2020). It houses the limbic system, which includes structures that regulate rage and fear and is involved in determining fairness and empathy (Advokat et al., 2019). It is known as the "emotional brain" (NBIA, 2020). The midbrain also contains the hippocampus, which is intricately linked to the spatial environment (Advokat et al., 2019).

The midbrain also houses the thalamus and the area under the thalamus, the hypothalamus; these areas are essential for recognizing hunger and thirst, sexual behavior, feeling satisfied, maintaining body temperature control, and breathing (Colbert et al., 2020). The hippocampus, also in the midbrain, is responsible for forming, storing, and retrieving memories, as well as linking emotions and senses to memories (Seladi-Schulman, 2019). It is linked with the pituitary gland, which is associated with growth, sexual development, reproduction, and endocrine functions (Advokat et al., 2019). The thalamus plays an important role in maintaining consciousness and memory and relays information from every sensory area (except the olfactory system) to the cerebral cortex (Advokat et al., 2019). Even though the hypothalamus is a small area, it is critical to maintaining life as it is responsible for many essential functions, including eating, drinking, and temperature (Colbert et al., 2020).

The functions of the cerebral cortex. The cortex has many functions but its most important one is that of the sense of consciousness. Its other higher order functions include executive functioning and cognitive decision-making, including planning and making judgments. Specific areas work together to form the individual's internal sensations and experiences of the environment (Catani & Zilles, 2021). It is divided into lobes. The frontal lobe is associated with not only executive functioning but also self-regulation of behavior and spontaneity (NBIA, 2020). According to the NBIA, the parietal lobe integrates sensory information and is associated with self-awareness and insight. The occipital cortex is associated with the perception of body language, while the temporal lobe is associated with autobiographical memories (NBIA, 2020).

The function of the autonomic nervous system. The PNS contains the ANS, which regulates the bodily systems, including the most basic: breathing, sleeping, temperature regulation, sexual responses, and hunger or thirst (Crossman & Catani, 2021). The ANS comprises one branch, that of the sympathetic and the parasympathetic nervous systems (Colbert et al., 2020). These nervous systems work in unison to maintain balance, or homeostasis. When the sympathetic system is stimulated pupils dilate, salivation slows, and heart rate increases. After the stimulation has passed, the parasympathetic system takes over: The pupils constrict, salivation resumes, and the heart rate slows (Crossman & Catani, 2021). This interchange causes homeostasis to be maintained (Colbert et al., 2020). In colloquial terms, the sympathetic nervous system is responsible for fight or flight, while the parasympathetic nervous system is responsible for the "rest-and-digest" response (Crossman & Catani, 2021). Sustained stimulation, due to either drugs (Advokat et al., 2019) or trauma, results in a complicated reaction that maintains the aroused state, inhibiting a return to the resting state, resulting in chronic physical and emotional problems.

The function of neurotransmitters. There are several neurotransmitters, including dopamine, serotonin, norepinephrine, acetylcholine, endocannabinoids, γ-gamma aminobutyric acid (GABA), and endorphins/enkephalins. According to Figures 2.4 and 2.5 (respectively), serotonin and dopamine have specific neurochemical pathways that innervate the brain. The neurotransmitter is created in the neuron and stored in the synaptic vesicles, where it waits to be released (Advokat et al., 2019). When the brain needs the neurotransmitter, it directs the storage vesicles to release the neurotransmitter into the space between the vesicle and the receptor of the adjoining synapse, or synaptic cleft (Advokat et al., 2019). After neurotransmitters are released, they cross the synaptic cleft to stimulate the dendrite of the postsynaptic receptor, the adjoining cell's dendrites, its cell body, or other axon terminals (Advokat et al., 2019). After it has stimulated the postsynaptic cell, it is either taken back up into the presynaptic cell in a process called reuptake. On the other hand, if reuptake is inhibited (e.g., by a selective serotonergic reuptake inhibitor), the transmitter continues to stimulate the postsynaptic receptors until it is degraded. However, when the neurotransmitter is taken back into the presynaptic nerve cell, it is sent back to the synaptic vesicles and becomes ready to be released again (Advokat et al., 2019).

Illnesses

The brain and spinal cord are protected by three membranes. The meninges includes (1) the dura mater, which is the outside of the brain that lies directly below the skull; (2) the arachnoid layer, which is the middle layer that separates the dura mater from the layer closest to brain tissue; and (3) the pia mater, the area closest to brain tissue (Bhangoo et al., 2021). One of the functions of the meninges is to protect the nervous system from pathogens (McGill et al., 2018), but occasionally viruses, bacteria, or fungi enter the nervous system through the cerebrospinal fluid or through the blood–brain barrier (Koelman et al., 2019).

Meningitis can be contracted from viruses (chickenpox, shingles) or bacteria (*Streptococcus pneumoniae*, *Haemophilus influenza type b*, and *Neisseria meningitis* [meningococcus]) (Schiess et al., 2021). According to McGill and colleagues (2018), meningitis is most often caused by a virus. It may go undetected because

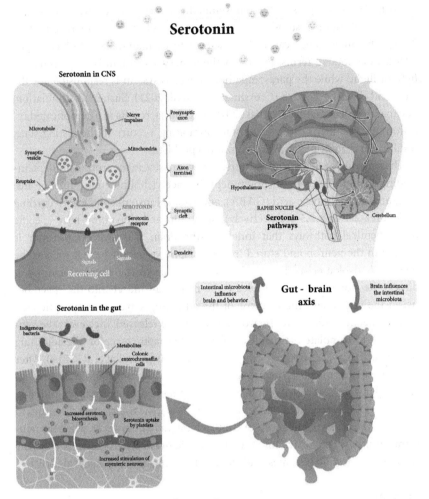

Figure 2.4 Neurotransmission of serotonin.

the symptoms may be mild, and individuals may spontaneously recover (Logan & MacMahon, 2008), although untreated bacterial meningitis can be deadly (Hoffman & Weber, 2009) or may result in a deteriorated mental state. Thus, it is important to identify persons who have contracted the illness. McGill and colleagues (2018) reported findings from September 30, 2011, to September 30, 2014, and found that among the 638 patients in the United Kingdom with meningitis (57%), 36% of the cases were viral, 16% were bacterial, 42% had unknown causes, and 6% had other causes. Of the patients with viral meningitis, 55% contracted it from enteroviruses, while other causes were *Herpes simplex*

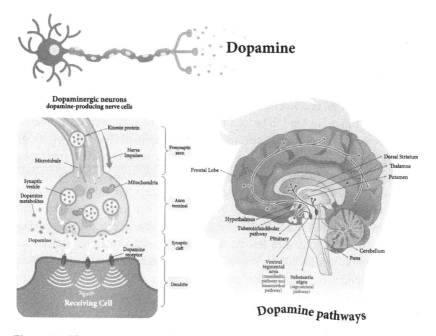

Figure 2.5 Neurotransmission of dopamine.

virus types 1 and *2* (44%). *Streptococcus pneumoniae* accounted for 54% of bacterial cases.

The United Kingdom is classified as a high-income country, which is important to know when determining morbidity and mortality because they are affected by poverty. Correlates of poverty include poor health, malnutrition (Schiess et al., 2021), and lack of accessible and responsive healthcare. The accessibility of healthcare that is equipped to diagnose meningitis is important because there is a wide range of symptoms, from mild and flu-like to severe, which may result in death. Acute symptoms of either viral or bacterial meningitis can include severe headache, high fever, sensitivity to light, stiff neck, and nausea and vomiting (Logan & MacMahon, 2008). While viral meningitis can resolve without medical treatment, bacterial cases can deteriorate quickly and cause long-term damage. Because the choice of treatment depends on the diagnosis, prompt identification is of the essence. If the pathogen is bacterial, it is amenable to antibiotic treatment (Hoffman & Weber, 2009) but not if it is viral (Meningitis Research Foundation, n.d.).

Injuries

Because of functional properties of brain areas, lesions to different structures are related to corresponding injuries (Human Origin Project, n.d.). For example, because of the involvement of the hypothalamus with the limbic system, lesions can disrupt production and release of hormones associated with bonding that are released from the mother's brain after giving birth (Colbert et al., 2020), and lesions to the area of the locus coeruleus can affect the sleep–wake cycle and impact attentiveness (Campbell, 2011). Interestingly, localized lesions in the right and left hemispheres can cause specific deficits, indicating that certain functions tend to be localized in different areas, although state-of-the-art research indicated that this may be oversimplified (Pirau & Lui, 2020). Findings indicated that lesions to both (bilateral) hemispheres of the prefrontal cortex can result in the "frontal lobe syndrome," which is characterized by profound changes in one's personality, and a loss of executive functions, such as reason and insight (Pirau & Lui, 2020). On the other hand, a lesion in only one hemisphere does not usually result in major changes to the personality, although some persons with lesions to the right hemisphere also experience loss of empathy (Hillis, 2014). When a person experiences brain trauma from a primary injury, the brain injury may range from mild to severe. While the trauma may injure a specific location of the brain, it can also have global effects (Teasdale & Jennett, 1974).

Traumatic brain injury is one of the signature injuries among military personnel (Hodge et al., 2008). Because today's conflicts are fought in unconventional ways where there are no distinct battle lines, each soldier is essentially at the front line. The preferred weapon during modern wars has been the improvised explosive device (IED), which often injures rather than kills. Many of the injuries result in brain trauma from flying shrapnel or the force of the explosion. Medicine's understanding of brain trauma in particular has progressed significantly due to the incidents of TBI among service members who served during recent wars. Lessons learned from treating TBIs among military personnel have translated to the treatment of civilians who have sustained brain injuries (Applebee, 2020).

(T) <u>Mental health</u> clinicians can benefit from understanding technology when working with TBIs

Detonation of an improvised explosive device (IED) can result in brain injuries from its direct impact, shrapnel or flying debris, or shock waves from the blast. Secondary brain injury can occur when the brain swells in response to the explosion (Centers for Disease Control and Prevention [CDC], 2020). According to Algattas and Huang (2013), immediate assessment of brain function is the best way to prevent secondary injury. Two types of imaging tests are used to assess the extent of the individual's injury (Mayo Foundation for Medical Education & Research [MFMER], 2020): The first is the computerized tomographic (CT) scan, which provides a series of x-rays that create detailed views of damaged bone, swollen tissue, blood clots, and hemorrhages, is considered the gold standard when assessing TBIs, especially if there is the possibility of metal shrapnel in the head (Lee & Newberg, 2005). According to Lee and Newberg, after a TBI, repeated CT scans should be done to identify the location of a potential hemorrhage when there is swelling that could cause a stroke. According to Haselsberger and colleagues (1988), CT scans are preferable to magnetic resonance images (MRIs) after severe head trauma in order to assess bleeding outside the brain tissue and if there is a possibility of postoperative complications (Haselsberger et al., 1988). This is critical as the authors found a mortality rate of 80% among patients who did not have surgery within two hours of the injury.

The second type of imaging is the functional MRI (fMRI) test, which provides a detailed map of the brain in real time to detect brain lesions that cannot be identified with a CT scan (Lee & Newberg, 2005). Because of the level of detail in the images, the physician can identify if there are individual brain lesions that are treatable (Lee & Newberg, 2005). This is important because increased oxygen reduces the amount of energy the body must use in order to access enough oxygen. Using hyperbaric oxygen treatment (HBOT) to facilitate healing involves administering 100% oxygen through a facial mask while the patient is in a compression chamber (Mayo Clinic, 2020). Increasing oxygen in the chamber increases the amount of oxygen in the blood (saturation) and makes it more available to tissues that have been damaged during brain trauma. Huang and Obenaus (2011) reported that patients' clinical outcomes from HBOT showed greater improvement than outcomes of patients who received oxygen treatment at regular atmospheric pressure, as well as patients who did not receive any oxygenated therapy.

The immediate objective after receiving a TBI is to limit swelling by increasing the level of oxygen to the tissues (Lin et al., 2008). This reduces the amount of energy the body must use to access enough oxygen. Reducing brain temperature is another treatment to alleviate swelling and restricted blood flow after a TBI (Sinclair & Andrews, 2010). Hypothermia can be achieved from cooling the external temperature of the body or the core bodily temperature. Chen and colleagues (2019) found that hypothermia was related to reduced mortality among persons if the treatment was begun within 24 hours of an incident. Andresen and colleagues (2015) reported that the target temperature should be between 89.6°F and 93.2°F (32°C and 34°C) for more than 48 hours, while Sokhi and Reddy (2019) recommended maintaining a core temperature of less than 95.9°F (35.5°C).

(E) Mental health clinicians can benefit from understanding the biomedical engineering of medication

After brain trauma the most important goal is to reduce the brain's pressure against the skull (intracranial pressure). Diuretics, or water pills, are typically prescribed to reduce the amount of sodium and water in the body to reduce swelling.

There are two methods of achieving hypothermia, pharmacological and nonpharmacological (Sokhi & Reddy, 2019). Of the pharmacological methods, Andresen and colleagues warned that because the body attempts to warm itself by shivering during the cooling process it can lengthen the amount of time it takes to lower the body's temperature to the preferred level. They suggested using internal cooling techniques with an external blanket plus low doses of an analgesic or anxiolytic to counteract the body's reactions to the cooling process. Among the pharmacological methods to manage hypothermia, according to Sokhi and Reddy (2019), Tylenol' is preferred because, in addition to its pain-relieving and fever-reducing effects, it has temperature-reducing effects, and antiseizure medication has been prescribed to reduce incidence of early seizures (Thompson et al., 2015). The third type of medication is coma-inducing medication to allow the brain to reduce the amount of oxygen it requires and to reduce the work it needs to function while the swelling goes down.

(M) Mental health clinicians can benefit from understanding mathematics to learn disease frequency

There are several important terms that epidemiologists and persons in the field of public health use to understand the frequency of injuries and diseases. "Population at risk" refers to a segment of the population that is susceptible to a particular disease. For example, Figure 2.6 shows the mathematical trend in TBI-related deaths from 2006 to the end of 2014. In 2006, there were 54,433 TBI-related deaths reported, compared to 52,667 in 2009 and 56,800 in 2014 (CDC, 2019).

Another important concept, public health surveillance, refers to "ongoing, systematic collection, analysis, and interpretation of health-related data" (CDC, 2018). There are two major types of public health surveillance: active surveillance and passive. Active surveillance requires health departments to make contact and solicit reports from all health providers and institutions on a regular basis to retrieve mathematical data regarding total number of patients examined with certain diseases (CDC, 2017). Despite its high cost, this method can ensure more complete and comprehensive reporting of the total number of patients examined

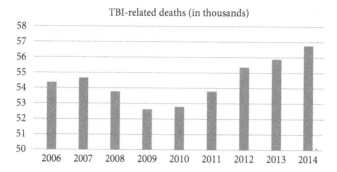

Figure 2.6 Deaths related to traumatic brain injury (TBI), United States, 2006–2014.

Note: Data are expressed in thousands.

Data source: Centers for Disease Control and Prevention. (2019). *Surveillance report of traumatic brain injury-related emergency department visits, hospitalizations, and deaths—United States, 2014.* https://stacks.cdc.gov/view/cdc/78062. Chart created by Dr. Liyun Wu.

with certain diseases. In contrast, passive surveillance follows the opposite data collection method, which allows healthcare providers to directly report diseases. Despite its low cost and simple process, this method is subject to incomplete reporting and variability of data quality from different sources of information. Public health often determines the distribution of disease using graphs.

(H) Mental health clinicians can benefit from applying principles of STEM to the health of patients with TBI

Family members often struggle with the patient's long-term, chronic deficits that impact their own quality of life as caregivers. Family members of patients who sustained moderate or severe TBI stated that they were overburdened with responsibilities, felt their life was interrupted or lost, grieved the loss of the person, and felt anger, guilt, anxiety, and sadness (Kratz et al., 2017). Koehmstedt and colleagues (2018) found that three main themes emerged in a qualitative study in which participants reported what would improve their feeling of well-being: increased personalized medical plan; having an advocate or point person; and help adjusting to the chronic nature of the effects of the TBI. Clinicians can coordinate health and social services, provide the family with more information about a specific injury, and discuss the medical information in less technical language. Clinicians can also provide coordinated access to community support and professional in-home help. Koehmstedt and colleagues (2018) found that both patients and caregivers lamented the loss of pre-TBI function, and the best way to intervene would be to offer around-the-clock support. Thus, coordinating clinical work with the caregiver is critical to allay caregiver burden. As stated previously, lesions to the prefrontal cortex can result in profound personality changes that make it difficult for the caregiver to care for the patient, and clinicians may need to support family members whose loved one has experienced a personality change. Working with the family who is managing heightened irritability, anxiety, and suspiciousness will be challenging, and the clinician may need to access resources for support groups for additional support. Families may experience additional burden based on discharge decisions.

Schumacher and colleagues (2016) reported that severity of trauma; preexisting conditions (e.g., alcohol or drug use, misuse, or dependency; psychiatric disorders); and conditions the patient experienced before they were transferred to the hospital (e.g., lack of oxygen [hypoxemia] and low blood pressure [hypotension] that were identified by emergency medical technologists) were correlated with discharge dispositions after controlling for confounding variables. Schumacher and colleagues also found that age and gender predicted the level and type of postacute care, and that, typically, older and female patients were referred to less intensive rehabilitation compared to younger men, who received specialized neurorehabilitation. While this bodes well for members of the Armed Forces, further studies need to be conducted to avoid bias in discharge decisions.

Conclusion

In conclusion, knowing STEM-H principles as they pertain to the human nervous system will increase a clinician's ability to understand the diagnosis of TBI, work with a medical team, and contribute to the treatment process. In addition, recognizing and understanding technical terminology increases a clinician's ability to support the patient and family. Students who master this chapter will be prepared to add this material when working with their private clients or if they join a medical team in a hospital or outpatient clinic or rehabilitation center.

Glossary

Analgesic   Pain-relieving substance
Anxiolytic   Anxiety-relieving substance
Catecholamines   Produced by the medulla of the adrenal gland, function in response to stress
Forebrain   Area of fetal brain that develops into the cortex

Gyri   Ridges in brain that occurred during gestation

Hindbrain   Area of fetal brain that develops into the cerebellum

Hypoxemia   Oxygen in blood that is below normal

Intracranial pressure   Pressure inside the brain

Limbic area   Brain area known as the area associated with emotions

Meninges   Three-layer membrane covering and protecting the brain

Midbrain   Area of the brain developing into the limbic area

Parasympathetic system   System responsible for reducing the fight-or-flight response

Sulci   Grooves in brain tissue that occurred during gestation

Sympathetic system   System responsible for eliciting the fight-or-flight response

Websites

Brain Injury Association of America: https://www.biausa.org/

Concussion Alliance for Veterans: https://www.concussionalliance.org/veterans

Defense and Veterans Brain Injury Center: https://dvbic.dcoe.mil/

3

How Understanding the Endocrine System Can Benefit Mental Health Clinicians

Introduction

There are two types of glands. One type is the exocrine gland, which secretes hormones outside the body via a duct (e.g., sweat, milk, salivary) (Campbell, 2011). The second type of gland is the endocrine gland, so named because *endo-* means within or inside. The endocrine gland releases the hormone, or a chemical messenger, directly into the bloodstream inside the body (Colbert et al., 2020). While the endocrine glands are small, they have a mighty impact on one's metabolism, growth, and development, as well as reproductive function, and one's mood (National Institute of Diabetes and Digestive and Kidney Diseases [NIDDK], n.d.). This chapter deals with the endocrine system in regard to STEM-H (science, technology, engineering, and mathematics as applied to health).

STEM-H Principles Underlying the Endocrine System

(S) Mental health clinicians can benefit from understanding science pertaining to the endocrine system

This segment covers the structure and function of the system. Glands make chemical messengers, or hormones, and secrete them into the bloodstream, where they find a target receptor (Campbell, 2011) that has a specific shape that accommodates the specific shape of the hormonal chemical, rather like a key in a lock. When the hormone meets the target, it binds to the receptor of that organ, causing it to react. According to Campbell (2011), neither the hormone nor the target receptor can carry out their function without the other.

Structure

As Figure 3.1 shows, endocrine cells are dispersed and occur in clusters, cords, or hollow structures (Wigley, 2021). They vary in size, shape, and makeup, and their location approximates a straight line that travels from the brain to the

STEM-H for Mental Health Clinicians. Marilyn Weaver Lewis, Liyun Wu, and Zachary Allan Hagen, Oxford University Press.
© Oxford University Press 2023. DOI: 10.1093/oso/9780197638514.003.0003

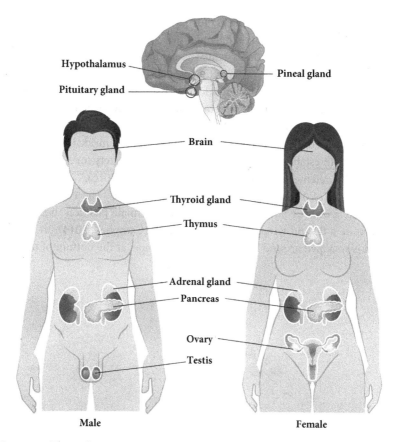

Figure 3.1 The endocrine system.

reproductive organs. The hormonal system and the nervous system are the only two systems that direct organs via chemicals (Campbell, 2011). The nervous system communicates via neurotransmitters, and the hormonal system operates using neurohormones (Colbert et al., 2020). Their relationship is even more intricate as one of the two pituitary lobes comprises neurological tissue from the hypothalamus. Exocrine glands have ducts that may have several branches, or trees, ending in small bulbs or tubes (Wigley, 2021). These ducts travel to the skin and interact with the environment by secreting substances to the outside of the body and potentially taking in secretions from outside the body. On the other hand, endocrine glands are ductless. They secrete their hormones into the connective tissue's interstitial fluid, which targets cells in the blood to tell the body to respond to physiological stimuli (Campbell, 2011).

The structure of the pituitary gland. As can be seen in Figure 3.2, the pituitary is attached to the hypothalamus by a stalk of tissue. There are two components: the posterior lobe, which is actually part of the hypothalamus gland; and the anterior lobe, which is the front part and is a true endocrine gland (Colbert et al., 2020). At the posterior lobe, two hormones, oxytocin and the antidiuretic hormone (ADH), are secreted. Each is actually made in the hypothalamus structure of the brain.

The structure of the pineal gland. The pineal gland is inside the brain and is associated with establishing one's sleep–wake cycle (Society for Endocrinology [SFE]), 2021) and melanin production (United Nations, 2016).

The structures of the thyroid and parathyroid glands. The thyroid gland is shaped like a bow-tie and is located in the approximate position that it would be if it were a tie and wrapped around the neck (Campbell, 2014). In fact, the thyroid is wrapped around the trachea, or windpipe, at the bottom of the neck

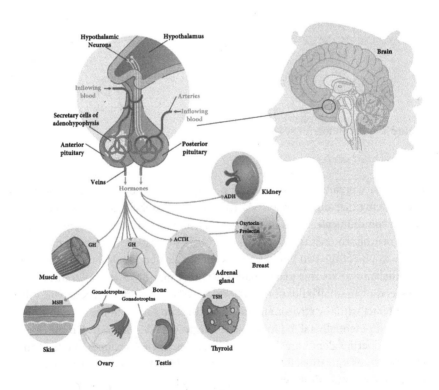

Figure 3.2 The pituitary gland.

and above the collarbone (Taylor, 2020). The parathyroid gland comprises four circles of specialized tissue that are on the back side of the thyroid, one circle in each of the two "wings," or lobes, of the bow-tie (Sell et al., 2018).

The **structure of the thymus gland.** The thymus is a small gland that is centrally located in the body, behind the breastbone and below the collarbone. It protects the individual from hypertension. If the individual suffers from malnutrition, the thymus gland shrinks and is ineffective (Rytter et al., 2017) but can be revived and increase in size with improved nutrition. The thymus gland is also considered part of the lymphatic system because it manufactures white blood cells, which fight infections (Figueiredo et al., 2020) and differentiate foreign invaders from one's own cells (Geenen, 2021).

The **structure of the adrenal gland.** There are two triangular-shaped adrenal glands, one on top of each kidney. The adrenal cortex covers the medulla and contains three layers of cells that secrete steroid hormones. The center of the adrenal gland, the medulla, secretes catecholamines (adrenaline/epinephrine and noradrenaline/norepinephrine) and Substance P (involved in pain management).

The **structure of the pancreas.** There are five areas of the pancreas: the hook, head, neck, body, and tail. It sits in front of the kidneys and points to the left at a 90° angle. The pancreas differs from other glands because it is made of both endocrine and exocrine tissue (Taylor, 2020). Because exocrine tissues secrete hormones outside the body, only the endocrine tissues are part of the endocrine gland, and only the islet cells of the pancreas are considered part of the endocrine gland because they secrete their hormones, insulin and glucagon, directly into the bloodstream (Conrad, 2021).

Function

The main function of the endocrine system is to manufacture hormones that control activity of glands that produce and secrete hormones that control important bodily reactions (Miller, 2019). Another primary function is to manufacture and distribute hormones to target organs. The hormones include pituitary hormones (growth hormone (GH); antidiuretic hormone (ADH); prolactin (PRL); follicle-stimulating hormone (FSH); luteinizing hormone (LH); and oxytocin. Other endocrine glands include the pineal gland (melanocyte-stimulating hormone, MSH); thyroid gland (thyroid-stimulating hormone, TSH); adrenal glands (adrenocorticotropic hormone [corticotropin], ACTH); and the pancreas (insulin and glucagon) (Colbert et al., 2020).

The **function of the pituitary gland.** The pituitary is called the "master gland" because it secretes many hormones (Colbert et al., 2020). Those released by the anterior lobe of the pituitary gland include (1) ACTH, which causes the outer layer of the adrenal gland to release cortisol or aldosterone (National Institute of Child Health & Human Development, n.d.); (2) TSH, which stimulates the thyroid gland to produce triiodothyronine (T_3) and thyroxine (T_4) (Rhys, 2013); (3) GH, which controls growth of muscles and bones; and (4) MSH, which controls melanin in the body and affects sleep, inflammation, and hunger (Colbert et al., 2020).

The function of the thyroid and parathyroid glands. Thyroid hormones are essential for normal brain development and intelligence (Schroeder & Privalsky, 2014), such that severely low levels in utero, or during the first few days following birth, can result in mental retardation as well as deafness and ataxia. If thyroid hormones are depleted, symptoms can include weight gain, fatigue, mental and physical lethargy, deepening of one's voice, hair loss, and depression (ThyroidUK, 2021). On the other hand, an overactive thyroid results in increased heart rate and palpitations, nervousness, and irritability, as well as an increased appetite with weight loss (Bancos, 2018). The third hormone that is released by the thyroid is calcitonin, which lowers the level of calcium circulating in the blood. The parathyroid glands also contribute to the absorption of calcium (Colbert et al., 2020) by secreting parathyroid tissue hormones (PTHs) when the levels of calcium in the blood drop to low levels (Campbell, 2011).

The function of the adrenal gland. Two adrenal glands are located on top of the kidneys and release the stress hormone, cortisol (Colbert et al., 2020). The glands' hormones, adrenaline and noradrenaline, along with cortisol, regulate the "flight-or-fight" stress response (National Institute of Child Health & Human Development [NICHD], n.d.) and maintain homeostasis of the immune system and suppress inflammation (Johns Hopkins Medicine, n.d.).

Davis and colleagues (2011) found that exposure to elevated levels of cortisol during the third trimester of pregnancy predicted the newborn's exaggerated response to the "heel-stick procedure." Although extremely high levels of prenatal cortisol are toxic, normally elevated levels of intrauterine cortisol have a positive function and enhance brain development and cognitive performance (Davis et al., 2011). On the other hand, the extreme levels of cortisol are related to poor cognitive developmental outcomes.

The function of the pancreas. The islet cells of the pancreas control one's blood sugar (Miller, 2019). These cells are differentiated into two types: alpha and the beta cells. The alpha cells manufacture glucagon, while the beta cells manufacture insulin (Taylor, 2020). If there is not enough glucose, the alpha islet cells manufacture glucagon, which tells the muscle and liver to release glucose into the bloodstream. On the other hand, if there is too much glucose in the blood, the beta islet cells release insulin to send the glucose in the blood to cells, which are then stored with glycogen (Taylor, 2020) and secreted when more energy is needed (Taylor et al., 2002). According to Watson (2021), extra glucose is stored in the liver, muscles, and fat to be available when blood glucose becomes depleted. When this occurs, the pancreas releases glucagon to metabolize the stored sugar into glycogen to be released back into the blood (Watson, 2021).

The function of the pineal gland. The pineal gland is triggered by ultraviolet (UV) light. People tend to have light skin, hair, and eyes if they live in countries in the far northern hemisphere, where the amount of light received is very low. People in areas of the world that receive stronger light for more hours of the day and more months of the year have more melanin and darker skin tones than people who are exposed to less light. When the individual's pineal gland does not secrete melanocyte-stimulating hormones (MSH), melatonin is not manufactured (Aulinas, 2019), and these individuals lack pigmentation and are at higher risk for skin cancer (SFE, 2021). A second important function of the pineal gland is to establish circadian rhythms, which regulate one's diurnal, sleep–wake cycle in response to daytime versus nighttime light (SFE, 2021). According to Taylor (2020), the body produces melanin in low light or darkness, causing people to feel drowsy during nighttime hours.

Illness

This section of the chapter covers one of the signature illnesses of the pancreas, pancreatitis. Pancreatitis is an inflammation of the pancreas that can be acute or chronic and is potentially fatal (Herreros-Villanueva et al., 2013). According to Herreros-Villanueva and colleagues, it is associated with heavy drinking even though most heavy drinkers do not develop bouts of acute pancreatitis. Clinically, the patient presents with abdominal pain, which Tang and Anand (2021) described as "dull, boring, and steady"; nausea; fever among 76% of the patients; irregular heartbeat among 65%; and distended stomach. In addition to heavy alcohol use, chronic pancreatitis has been associated with recent invasive procedures, penetrating injuries, and some medications (Tang & Anand, 2021). Infrequently, pancreatitis has been caused by viral infections, including hepatitis, measles, rubella, and mumps (Tang & Anand, 2021), but not COVID-19 (coronavirus 2019) (Bulthuis et al., 2021). Bacterial infections that are associated with pancreatitis include salmonella, pneumonia, and tuberculosis. The parasitic *Ascaris* worm has also been identified as causing pancreatitis because it invades the pancreas (Khuroo et al., 2016).

Acute pancreatitis is characterized by damage to the veins and arteries or death to tissue from white blood cells devouring damaged cells. It is also characterized by three levels of severity, while the newer system evaluates severity of predictors of mortality: mild, moderate, severe, and critical acute pancreatitis. Acute pancreatitis is the most common cause of hospitalization for a gastrointestinal disease in the United States (Afghani et al., 2015; Yadav & Lowenfelds, 2013) and is related to excessive drinking: 2.5% to 3.0% of heavy drinkers develop pancreatitis, compared to 1.3% of nondrinkers (Herreros-Villanueva et al., 2013).

According to Herreros-Villanueva and colleagues, 70% individuals with chronic pancreatitis were heavy drinkers.

Injury

Blunt force trauma to the brain can injure the pituitary gland through sports-related head injuries, placing youth and adults at risk. There are approximately 170,000 sport-related traumatic brain injuries (TBIs) among children and adolescents annually (Sahler & Greenwald, 2012), with injuries ranging from a bump on the head to a brain hemorrhage and coma. According to the Centers for Disease Control and Prevention (CDC, 2011), sports activities are responsible for more than 21% of all TBIs among U.S. children and youth. The pituitary gland is an outgrowth of the brain that dangles on a stalk (Colbert et al., 2020), and sports-related accidents can cause the brain to shake back and forth so forcefully that it causes the pituitary stalk to rip from the brain (Javed et al., 2015).

There are several levels of TBI, and the Glasgow Coma Scale (GCS) is used frequently to evaluate TBIs. First, the evaluator determines whether the person is unconscious, how long they have been unconscious, and how well they can understand and communicate when they become conscious. According to Blythe and Bazarian (2010), mild traumatic brain injury (mTBI), or concussion, is characterized by a period of unconsciousness lasting for fewer than 30 minutes, amnesia lasting less than 1 day, and normal brain images. Moderate TBI is characterized by loss of consciousness from 30 minutes to 24 hours, amnesia from 1 to 7 days, and brain scans that can show either normal or abnormal images. Severe TBI is characterized by loss of consciousness longer than 24 hours, amnesia lasting longer than 1 week, and either normal or abnormal brain images. Cognitive symptoms associated with TBI include headaches, dizziness, and seizures, as well as poor memory and concentration, slow decision-making, impulsivity, and lack of motivation (Bullock, 2018).

(T) Mental health clinicians can benefit from understanding technology to treat illnesses of the endocrine system

Diabetes is the signature illness of the endocrine system. Controlling the relationship of insulin and blood glucose is the goal in diabetes management. Glucose levels must be assessed regularly to prevent acute (e.g., shakiness, confusion, labored or rapid breathing) or chronic (e.g., kidney failure, heart disease) life-threatening problems (Nazario, 2004). According to Nazario, when beta cells in the pancreas stop functioning, blood glucose becomes elevated, and the patient needs to take in insulin to supplement the inadequate amount.

Subcutaneous injections of insulin below the skin, in response to the level of blood glucose, has been the treatment of choice for many years. Certain side effects limit success of this method. The first and most important drawback to success is patient noncompliance because of pain, difficulty loading the syringe, and cost. The technological advancement, the insulin pump is a solution to several problems inherent in injections, most notably by providing a steady stream of insulin directly into the body without the need for patients to inject themselves several times during the day in response to meals or exercise (Cleveland Clinic, 2021). The pump contains an electronic computer that is programmed to recognize glucose and insulin levels, has a reservoir that holds insulin, and is attached to a long, thin tube, or cannula, that delivers the insulin to the body (MedTronic, 2021).

There are two types of insulin pumps on the market: One type delivers a sustained dose in response to the patient's background insulin rate (MedTronic, 2021); the other type delivers a bolus, or concentrated amount, of rapid-acting insulin when it is needed (e.g., before eating) (Sell et al., 2018). These rates are programmed into a monitor, which is approximately the size of a small cell phone, and are visible on the screen. The patient must revise the data and re-enter data to give themselves a rapid-acting insulin infusion in cases where the meal may be late or their exercise was more extensive than usual. These two methods require replacement every 2 to 3 days (Cleveland Clinic, 2021).

Regardless of the apparatus, the Cleveland Clinic reported that the patient's glucose level must be checked at least four times each day unless the patient is fitted with a glucose monitor (Mount Sinai, n.d.). The monitor checks the glucose level on an ongoing basis and transmits that information in real time back to the patient. The most important information is the glucose level in the blood so the pump will release the appropriate amount of insulin (Mount Sinai, n.d.). The insulin pump's function is to keep the body's glucose–insulin level in homeostasis. In anticipation of glucose rising following a meal, the pump is programmed to inject, before the meal, an appropriate amount into the body that is required based on the patient's height, weight, and metabolic or basal rate. This allows insulin, which the body would normally make, to lower the glucose level, thus maintaining homeostasis.

(E) Mental health clinicians can benefit from understanding biomedical engineering to develop medication

Acromegaly, or giantism, is often caused by a tumor on the pituitary gland (Mayo Clinic, 2021a). The incidence of the disease is approximately three to four people per million annually, resulting in a prevalence of 60 people per million

(Ayuk & Sheppard, 2006). It is rarely observed today because it is successfully treated with surgery or medication that decrease excessive growth hormones. The main symptoms are excessive longitudinal growth of the torso, face, and hands (Ayuk & Sheppard, 2006). Other symptoms can include more increased mass and strength, coarse oily skin, joint pain, sleep apnea, and vision problems (Mayo Clinic 2021b); unpleasant body odor, deep voice, headache (Chanson & Salenave, 2008); and other illnesses, such as Type 2 diabetes, cardiac problems, and enlarged thyroid (Mayo Clinic, 2021a).

Treatment often includes surgical removal of the tumor followed by medication (Mayo Clinic, 2021a). Because the tumor results in release of excessive growth hormones, and medications, including somatostatin, which tricks the pituitary gland into thinking that there is more growth hormone in the brain than there is (Chanson & Salenave, 2008) thereby reducing its production. According to Ayuk and Sheppard, other medications that may be prescribed lower levels of the growth hormone. One medication, a dopamine agonist, reduces secretion of growth hormones because dopamine cell bodies are in the midbrain, which is linked with the pituitary gland and associated with growth (Advokat et al., 2019). A third medication that is used to treat acromegaly is an antagonist. It works against the neurotransmitter and prevents it from achieving its end result by blocking the action of the growth hormone after it is secreted (unlike somatostatin, which blocks secretion).

(M) Mental health clinicians can benefit from understanding mathematics underlying pancreatic cancer

The most recent estimates released by the American Cancer Society in January 2022 reported that 62,210 Americans (32,970 men and 29,240 women) will be diagnosed with pancreatic cancer during 2022. The American Cancer Society (2022) also reported the estimated deaths from pancreatic cancer in 2022 will be approximately 25,970 men and 23,860 women.

The following figures utilized data from the Surveillance, Epidemiology, and End Results (SEER) Program of the National Cancer Institute (2021). Figure 3.3 displays the incidence of pancreatic cancer from 1975 to 2018, measured by total number of new cases per 100,000 persons. During the period 1975–2004, the incidence fluctuated within the range of 11 to 12 cases per 100,000 persons. However, during the recent period 2005–2018, new cases witnessed a sharp increase, reaching 13.3 cases per 100,000 persons in 2018.

Figure 3.4 reports the incidence of deaths from pancreatic cancer by race/ethnicity and gender during the period 2014–2018. According to the SEER program

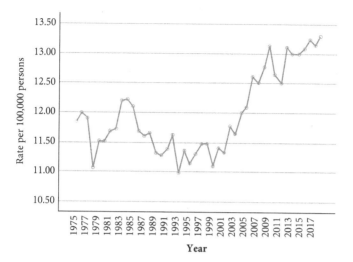

Figure 3.3 The incidence rate of pancreatic cancer per 100,000 persons, 1975–2018.
Note: Data are expressed per hundred thousand persons.
Data source: National Cancer Institute. (2021). *Cancer Stat Facts: Pancreatic cancer*. https://seer.can cer.gov/statfacts/html/pancreas.html. Graph created by Dr. Liyun Wu.

(2021), regardless of race/ethnicity, the incidence of pancreatic cancer per 100,000 individuals is more common among men than women: 15.0 cases versus 11.8, respectively. However, the incidence of pancreatic cancer per 100,000 persons also varied by race/ethnicity and gender. Among Caucasians, there were 15.2 new cases among males versus 11.7 cases among females. Among persons of African descent, there were 17.0 cases among males versus 14.3 cases among females. For the Asian/Pacific Islander population, there were 10.9 cases among males versus 9.3 cases among females. For the American Indian/and Alaska Native population, there were 13.4 cases among males versus 8.2 cases among females. For the Hispanic population, there were 12.8 cases among males versus 11.1 cases among females. Last, there were 15.4 cases among non-Hispanic males versus 11.8 cases among non-Hispanic females.

Figure 3.5 reveals the death rate from pancreatic cancer by age during the period 2014–2018. During this period, the newly diagnosed cases were distributed among eight groups: 0.1% of newly diagnosed cases were found among people aged younger than 20; 0.6% among people 20–34 years; 1.8% among people 35–44 years; 7.8% among people 45–54 years; 21.7% among people 55–64 years; 30.6% among people 65–74 year; 24.4% among people 75–84 years; and 12.9% among people 85 and older. As shown in this graph, people aged 65–74 had the highest rate of diagnosis (National Cancer Institute, 2021).

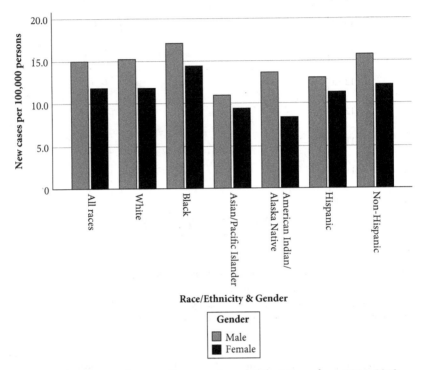

Figure 3.4 New cases of pancreatic cancer by race/ethnicity and sex, 2014–2018.
Note: Data are expressed per 100,000 persons.
Data source: National Cancer Institute. (2021). *Cancer Stat Facts: Pancreatic cancer*. https://seer.can
cer.gov/statfacts/html/pancreas.html. Chart created by Dr. Liyun Wu.

(H) Mental health clinicians can benefit from understanding how to apply STEM to health using contingency management–prize reinforcement

Parents often need support to manage their child's treatment regimen for Type 1 diabetes. Managing Type 1 diabetes is a complicated process. On a daily basis, if the patient relies on multiple daily injections, it can involve painful finger pricking and then painful insulin injections. On the other hand, for patients whose treatment involves an insulin pump the parent must monitor the glucose levels frequently, manually adjust the program in order to increase rapid-acting insulin when warranted (e.g., exercise level, stress) (MedTronic, 2021), and exchange the pump and the tubing every few days. Young diabetic children may develop a fear of the procedures and distrust the parent's attempt to have physical contact with them because of painful injections and finger pricking. Older

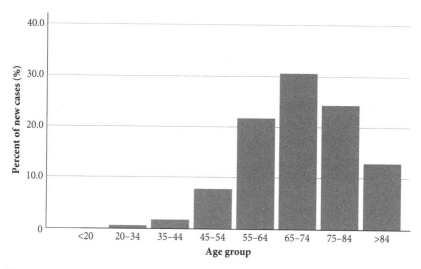

Figure 3.5 New cases of pancreatic cancer by age group, 2014–2018.

Note: Data are expressed per 100,000 persons.

Data source: National Cancer Institute. (2021). *Cancer Stat Facts: Pancreatic cancer*. https://seer.can cer.gov/statfacts/html/pancreas.html. Chart created by Dr. Liyun Wu.

children may resent having to care for themselves with more deliberation than their peers and to be unable to eat popular foods.

One type of behavioral therapy that can be useful to elicit cooperation from the child is contingency management–prize reinforcement (CM-PR) (Petry et al., 2000). CM-PR is a behavioral modification system that rewards the child with drawing from a fishbowl for tokens that can be exchanged for prizes after they allow the procedure to be administered. In the CM-PR method, the child draws a token from a fishbowl that has been designated as representing a small, medium, large, and jumbo prize. They can immediately "buy" a comparable prize from cabinet that is accessible. The magnitude of the prize value can range from small (e.g., plastic ring, hair barrette, toy watch, stuffed toy); medium (e.g., harmonica, art supplies); large (e.g., toy train, DVD of favorite movie); or jumbo (e.g., Xbox). Prizes for older children may range from small (e.g., $5); medium (e.g., iTunes gift cards); large (e.g., access to online games, movie voucher); and jumbo (e.g., gaming console, PlayStation).

The clinician will need to help the parent set up the reinforcement schedule that determines the number of designated tokens in the fishbowl. Younger children will need the opportunity to win prizes each time they draw from the fishbowl, thus many small prizes must be available, followed by fewer medium prizes, still fewer large prizes, and one jumbo prize. For example, the fishbowl might contain a total of 25 tokens, with 12 designated as small, 8 designated as medium, 4 as large, and 1 designated as jumbo. Older children will need the opportunity to earn more medium-size prizes, and the parent may designate the total number of tokens at 50, with 27 designated as small prizes, 15 as medium prizes, 7 as large, and 1 as the jumbo prize. The goal is to strike a balance between affordability for the parent and motivation for the child. In order to do the latter, the reinforcement schedule must increase when the child habituates to the protocol. The child must win something desirable each time they submit to a procedure in order for them to remain motivated, thus choosing desirable motivators will change over time.

A schedule for a child who must submit to a procedure several times a day would include several opportunities for reinforcement every day, rather than weekly. Each day would begin with the child earning one draw for the finger prick and one for the injection, at the second glucose testing the child would earn two draws for the finger prick and two for the injection, for the third procedure of the day the child would receive three draws for the finger prick and three for the injection. Day 2 would reset the number of draws back to one draw. Limiting the reinforcement by resetting the schedule, however, may interfere with the child's motivation. In that case, the parent may find it necessary to increase the desirability of the prizes instead of the number of draws from the fishbowl. The clinician can support the parent to carry out this protocol, which requires that desirable prizes be available at all times to strengthen the child's motivation. While it is cumbersome, the consequences are paramount to the child's health.

Because there are several methods of treatment (insulin injections, insulin pen, insulin pump), the child's treatment protocols will differ. The parent will need to determine which behaviors to reinforce. Perhaps the child refuses to eat. Reinforcing health-related behaviors is important, and the treatment schedule could include earning draws from the fishbowl for finishing the allotted meal. Older children may inject themselves and change their cartridges in their pens. Demonstrating completion of those health-related behaviors would result in drawing one or more times from the fishbowl. The clinician can work with the parent and the child to support management of this illness.

Conclusion

The endocrine system directs the manufacture and distribution of hormones, which are necessary for survival. This chapter has introduced these important hormones and explained their function. Because their effects are widespread, the clinician may have occasion to work with clients and families who have illnesses or injuries pertaining to these systems. Much creative work has gone into the research and development of biomedical and technological apparatuses and medications to treat these illnesses and injuries. Specific information was introduced pertaining to CM-PR behavioral treatment for children with diabetes. In conclusion, a student who has mastered the information in this chapter will be prepared to work with team members, or independently, to treat clients with endocrine disorders.

Glossary

Adrenocorticotropic hormone (ACTH)   Referred to as the "corticotropin hormone"; secreted by the anterior pituitary gland in response to stress or trauma

Aldosterone   Hormone released by the adrenal gland to regulate sodium and potassium

Alpha islet cells   Cells in the pancreas that release glucagon

Antidiuretic hormone (ADH)   Secreted by the hypothalamus and stored and released by the pituitary gland; limits production of urine by increasing reabsorption of water by the kidney

Beta islet cells   Cells in the pancreas that release insulin

Follicle-stimulating hormone (FSH)   A reproductive hormone secreted by the anterior lobe of the pituitary

Glucocorticoids   Secreted by the adrenal gland; have anti-inflammatory effect; released during stress and fatigue

Islet cells   Cells within the pancreas that are categorized as alpha or beta cells and release glucagon or insulin, respectively

Luteinizing hormone (LH) A reproductive hormone secreted by the anterior lobe of the pituitary

Melanocyte-stimulating hormone (MSH)   Secreted by the anterior pituitary gland and contributes to pigmentation

Norepinephrine   Released by the adrenal gland to increase heart rate and blood pressure by constricting blood vessels; also acts as a neurotransmitter

Parathyroid   Four distinct round areas of tissue on back side of the thyroid gland; maintains the level of calcium

Pineal gland   Secretes melatonin

Pituitary gland   Two-lobe endocrine gland attached to the hypothalamus

Prolactin (PRL)   A reproductive hormone secreted by the anterior lobe of the pituitary

Thyroid-stimulating hormone (TSH)   Secreted by the anterior lobe of the pituitary; controls the release of thyroid hormones

Websites

Juvenile Diabetes Research Foundation (JDRF) Network for Pancreatic Organ Donors with Diabetes (nPOD): https://www.jdrfnpod.org/

National Institute of Diabetes and Digestive and Kidney Diseases (NIDDK): https://www.niddk.nih.gov/

4

How Understanding the Lymphatic System Can Benefit Mental Health Clinicians

Introduction

This chapter covers the structure and function of the lymphatic system in regard to STEM-H (science, technology, engineering, and mathematics as applied to health). The signature illnesses covered in this chapter are human immunodeficiency virus positivity (HIV⁺) and acquired immune deficiency syndrome (AIDS). The injury we discuss is damage to one of the small organs, the spleen, a component of the lymphatic system. Special attention is given to the technology associated with prevention of HIV⁺ and AIDS using female condoms. Biomedical and pharmaceutical engineering explain the action of highly active antiretroviral therapy (HAART) medication that is prescribed for HIV⁺ and AIDS. This chapter introduces epidemiological data for prevalence and incidence rates of the HIV diagnosis. Harm reduction is discussed.

STEM-H Principles Underlying the Lymphatic System

(S) Mental health clinicians can benefit from understanding science pertaining to the lymphatic system

There are basic facts one needs to know to understand the action of the lymphatic system. First, any molecule that causes the immune system to react is called an antigen and can create an allergic response (Campbell, 2011a). Second, a pathogen is a virus or bacteria that causes an infection. Third, all pathogens have antigens on their surface. And fourth, when pathogens get past the natural barriers of the body, the lymphatic system's function is to identify them as dangerous and kill them (Campbell, 2011b). However, it's just as important to keep in mind that not all antigens are pathogens. On the one hand, pollen and pet dander may activate an individual's immune system, but not be a threat, even though they initiate an allergic reaction. On the other hand, an antigen can be a deadly pathogen like the HIV or COVID-19 (coronavirus 2019) virus, and the body's reaction is warranted.

STEM-H for Mental Health Clinicians. Marilyn Weaver Lewis, Liyun Wu, and Zachary Allan Hagen, Oxford University Press.
© Oxford University Press 2023. DOI: 10.1093/oso/9780197638514.003.0004

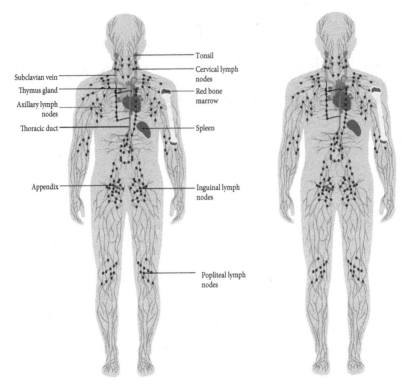

Figure 4.1 The lymphatic system.

Structure

As can be seen in Figure 4.1, there are many lymph nodes that dot the body and work in concert with organs that are part of the lymphatic system. These small structures that are part of the lymphatic system do double duty and are also part of the immune system. The glands and organs include the thymus and the spleen. The thymus is a two-lobe gland that sits close to the collarbone and produces white blood cells (WBCs) called T lymphocytes, which are essential for detecting and destroying pathogens (Ward, 2021). The spleen is also a critical component of the lymphatic system and is located in the abdomen under the ribs. According to Colbert and colleagues (2020), the nodes are clusters of lymphatic tissue that form in the areas where infections often enter the body (e.g., the gut and the groin). The tissue consists of collagen/protein strands that create a sieve to catch and dispose of bacterial cells to keep them from spreading throughout the body.

Function

Every day, the lymphatic system reacts to stimuli coming from the environment. On most occasions, the body's natural defense barriers prevent pathogens from entering the body. For example, the skin provides two types of barriers: a physical barrier to keep pathogens from entering the body and a chemical barrier that disarms the pathogens if they do slip by (Campbell, 2014). According to Campbell (2011a), when a pathogen slips through the barriers and enters the body, the function of the lymphatic system is to defend against the pathogens that are introduced from the environment. In its pivotal role in protecting the body, the lymphatic system carries out several functions. First, when the lymphatic system reacts to stimuli from the environment (the pathogen), its function is to divert the interstitial fluids to the lymph nodes, where pathogens are filtered and sterilized, causing the fluid to become harmless (Colbert et al., 2020). According to Colbert and colleagues, the second function is to destroy pathogens in the blood and filter out the remaining debris after they are killed, which causes the blood to become sterile. At the end of this process the sterile blood plasma can safely enter the heart. In addition to the lymph nodes, the thymus removes damaged red blood cells and debris left in the lymph nodes after the bacteria or viruses are destroyed by the T lymphocytes (Colbert et al., 2020).

The overall objective of the immune component in the lymphatic system is to reduce infection. After an antigen is introduced to the system, WBCs proliferate, and the system makes proteins containing antibodies to kill the infections. It accomplishes this by recognizing the antigen and initiating an immune response to destroy it (Campbell, 2011b). For example, when an individual is wounded, antigens are able to enter the circulatory system through the skin and infect the blood. This response causes the immune system to release components that start a chain reaction of immunological responses.

First, it's important to know that every cell in the human body has special receptors on its surface that allow the immune system to recognize its own cells by a process known as self-recognition (Colbert et al., 2020). Likewise, when an antigen enters the individual's circulatory system, the immune system identifies it as an outside invader by the process known as non–self-recognition. In the healthy body, antibodies are released and attach to the invading antigen and destroy it. But, if the individual has an autoimmune disease, such as HIV+ or AIDS, the receptors that normally recognize their own cells respond to them as invading cells and attack them (Campbell, 2011b).

There are two types of immunity: innate immunity and adaptive/acquired immunity. Innate immunity is the type of immunity that the healthy human gets from their mother during gestation. It exists in fetal DNA and is genetically hardwired into their system (Colbert et al., 2020). The purpose of innate immunity is to prevent, or rapidly recognize and destroy, an infection. It is less specific than adaptive immunity, and because it cannot recognize specific infections, it sometimes kills good cells along with the bad (Alberts et al., 2002). According to Alberts and colleagues (2002), innate immunity has no memory and therefore cannot remember or recognize that a specific pathogen had already disrupted the system. This is a problem because the system does not react more rapidly the second time the pathogen enters the body. Ultimately, however, innate immunity succeeds in weakening the pathogens, making it easier for the adaptive immune system to destroy them (Colbert et al., 2020).

Adaptive immunity differs from innate immunity because it is acquired through vaccinations or previous exposure to the pathogen (Alberts et al., 2002). It is not innate. A baby gets some adaptive protection from their mother's antibodies, but it goes away, and their body must begin creating its own immunity from interactions with the environment (Colbert et al., 2020). The first exposure to the antigen initiates an immunological response that prevents or eliminates an infection. Because the cells in the adaptive immune system have memory, every time the body is exposed to the antigen it eliminates new infections faster. One of the advantages of adaptive immunity is that it can remember specific pathogens that it had disarmed in the past. This allows the immune system to get better at recognizing and destroying pathogens every time they reoccur. Adaptive immunity also differs from acquired immunity in that it can target specific pathogens. According to Alberts and colleagues (2002), the adaptive immune system can fine-tune its response to the point that it can differentiate between very similar antigens. This exquisite specificity protects our "good" cells from being destroyed along with the "bad" cells and is not found with innate immunity, where the system may be unable to differentiate beneficial from detrimental cells.

In the case of adaptive immunity, when an antigen enters the body (e.g., the flu virus) it causes the body to send antibodies to attack and destroy it (Colbert et al., 2020). The second time the flu virus enters that individual's body, the antibodies recognize it, attack it, and destroy it faster than they did the first time. According to Colbert and colleagues, the innate and acquired immune responses may differ in how they achieve it, but ultimately, their goal is the same: to destroy the invading pathogen. They do this by first recognizing the antigen, second binding to the surface of its membrane, and third killing it (Campbell, 2011a).

As shown in Figure 4.2, there are several types of leukocytes, or WBCs, in the immune system. The largest group is the neutrophils, comprising approximately 50% to 70% and with a very specific and important role to play (Leliefeld et al., 2016). First, they engulf the pathogen, then incorporate themselves into and fuse with the cell, and then release toxic enzymes to kill it (Blumenreich, 1990). Other WBCs include mast cells, basophils, dendritic cells, eosinophils, macrophages, and natural killer (NK) cells, which are also designed to fight off infection by

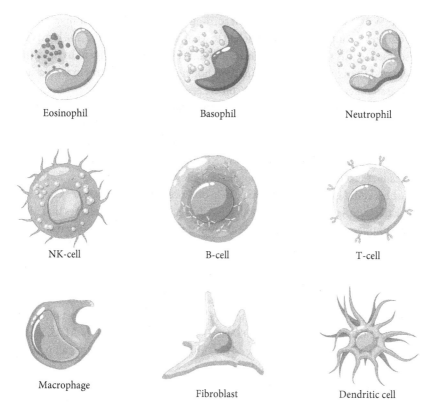

Eosinophil   Basophil   Neutrophil

NK-cell   B-cell   T-cell

Macrophage   Fibroblast   Dendritic cell

Figure 4.2 Cells of the immune system.

immobilizing or killing pathogens (Campbell, 2014). According to Campbell, another WBC that kills a type of bacteria, the phagocyte, does so by secreting an enzyme that fuses with the bacteria, making it desirable to eat.

As can be seen in Figure 4.2, there are many types of WBCs, but they have the same goal: to kill or render harmless the invading cells (Colbert et al., 2020). They typically accomplish it in violent ways. For example, eosinophils comprise only a few of the WBCs and are primarily responsible for killing parasites (Blumenreich, 1990) and making allergies and infections harmless. According to Campbell (2011b), basophils are also WBCs in the innate immunity system. They also kill parasitic infections but differ in how they accomplish this: They make allergic reactions harmless and prevent blood clotting. Still another kind of cell is the mast cell, which is unique in that it is part of both the innate and the adaptive immune responses. Mast cells are found in the mucous membranes and connective tissue. They help heal wounds and provide histamines to defend against allergic reactions (Campbell, 2011a). One of the most interesting of the WBCs is the macrophage. According to Campbell, after a macrophage recognizes an antibody that is attached to a pathogen, it may eat it. The last WBC discussed in this section is the dendritic cell. These cells kill antigens by detecting them and then luring them over to lymphocytes, which cover them with a substance so other cells will eat them (Colbert et al., 2020).

Other lymphocytes that are a part of the adaptive immune system include B and T cells. T cells are synthesized in bone marrow and reside in the thymus gland and lymph nodes (Brennan, 2021), where they provide cellular immunity and destroy pathogens (George & Kishore, 2021). As stated by Alberts and colleagues (2002), T cells are unique in that they can detect pathogens hiding inside host cells and either kill them or help other cells to kill them. For example, in the latter case, some T cells are helper T cells that recruit macrophages that identify pathogens and eat them. If T cells are not functioning, immunity decreases, and an immunodeficiency develops.

Illness

The HIV$^+$ is a viral infection that is transmitted through blood found in bodily fluids, including saliva, urine, and tears (Campbell, 2011b). It is important to differentiate between HIV$^+$ and AIDS. HIV$^+$ is the virus that causes AIDS, which is the end result of an uncontrolled HIV$^+$ infection. This means that all patients with AIDS are HIV$^+$, but not all HIV$^+$ patients have developed AIDS. According to Campbell (2011a), when someone is infected with HIV$^+$, they will go into an incubation period and will not feel any symptoms. Their blood will test negative for approximately 2 months. While they will not have physical symptoms, viral cells will begin to multiply within their body, resulting in an increased viral load that leads to seroconversion. During seroconversion, the viral cell's genetic material will enter the healthy cells and infect its T helper cells (Campbell, 2011b). According to Campbell, when the helper T cells become infected, they die, causing a decrease in their antibodies, which allows an increase in infection.

After seroconversion, the individual's blood will test positive for the antibodies, showing that they are positive for the virus, but they will enter a latency period lasting from 7 to 10 years before becoming symptomatic (Campbell, 2011b). Unfortunately, as so often happens, the individual can infect many people during this long latency period when they are asymptomatic. The physician is able to diagnose AIDS if the individual tests positive for the antibodies in their blood, has an elevated viral load, and has a low CD4 T helper cell count below 200 cells/mm^3 (Naif, 2013). When symptoms appear, they may be in the form of opportunistic infections that have taken advantage of the individual's weakened immune system or in the form of full-blown AIDS.

HIV$^+$ and AIDS have been in existence a very long time. Worobey and colleagues (2016) reported that the virus had been in the United States throughout the 1970s and was in the Caribbean earlier. Other researchers pre-dated the emergence of the HIV⁺ virus to 1931 (95% confidence interval = 1915–1941) (Korber et al., 2000), but maintained that it didn't reach epidemic proportions because infected individuals were not living in crowded cities. Campbell (2011b) identified HIV-1, the precursor to HIV⁺, as having jumped over to humans from chimpanzee meat in 1931 and again to meat from monkeys in 1940. Definitively identifying HIV has been difficult until the modern era because it mutates rapidly (Worobey et al., 2016). This rapidity has also made it difficult to eradicate the disease because medications developed to kill earlier variants became rapidly ineffective with the newer strains of the virus (Naif, 2013).

While some scientists were working on treating AIDS, others were working on preventing AIDS. Early in the AIDS crisis, it became apparent that young homosexual men were more likely to contract the virus than individuals from other groups; eventually, it became clear that one of the mechanisms that caused the AIDS epidemic was infected bodily fluids from sexual intercourse (Centers for Disease Control and Prevention [CDC], 1981). Later, cases emerged that could trace their initial contact with the HIV⁺ infection to blood transfusions (CDC, 1982) or shared needles used for intravenous drug use (CDC, 1989). Because researchers learned that HIV⁺ was transmitted through bodily fluids, including blood and semen, the CDC cautioned the public to take precautions when having sexual intercourse. They urged condom use, and rates of infection began to fall after it became clear that the virus was transmitted by behaviors that could be changed. However, when their findings fell on deaf ears, clinicians encouraged HIV⁺ testing and counseling (World Health Organization [WHO], 2008).

Ultimately, it became clear that many individuals were failing to take precautions and were spreading and contracting HIV⁺. Individuals may not seem ill if their viral load is low and their CD4 T helper cell count is high. But if HIV⁺ killed their helper cells, the individual became at risk for opportunistic infections (Campbell, 2011b), The most common of these are esophageal candidiasis, Kaposi's sarcoma, non-Hodgkin lymphoma, and pneumonia (Buchacz et al., 2010), each of which can be fatal if they are not successfully treated.

In addition to the T helper cells, a second family of T cells, called Killer Cells, directly kill specific invading cells in an ingenious way. They create a pore in the membrane of the viral cells to allow antibodies to flow in to destroy them (Malmquist & Prescott, n.d.). A third group of T cells, the NK cells, kills invading cells by the ones that have been coated with an antibody, attaching themselves to them, secreting a protein that perforates the cell's membrane and kills it. In addition to T cells, when another type of lymphocyte, the B cell, recognizes antigen-specific antibodies, the lymphocytes trick pathogens to migrate over to cells that will digest them (George & Kishore, 2021). So, as you can see, when the doctor says the patient is "fighting an infection" they are actually describing the activity of the immune system.

While there is no cure to date, and no vaccine to inoculate individuals to protect them from contracting the illness, physicians urged members of at-risk groups to take precautions to avoid contracting the illness. If individuals contract HIV$^+$, then they are counseled to take HAART medication to reduce the concentration of the virus in the blood, which is called the viral load. HAART is a combination of three antiretroviral drugs that decrease viral replication (Campbell, 2011b). According to the Joint United Nations Program on HIV/AIDS (UNAIDS) data from 2017 (UNAIDS, 2018), the number of deaths per year due to AIDS has decreased from 1.8 million in 2004, at its peak, to 940,000 in 2017. This decrease is primarily attributed to the use of HAART and a reduction of high-risk behaviors.

Because of HAART's efficacy, contracting HIV$^+$ and developing AIDS are no longer death sentences. HIV$^+$ patients may live normal healthy lives with treatment, but if a patient with uncontrolled HIV$^+$ develops AIDS, they usually have a relatively poor prognosis. The key clinically is to decrease the number of people developing AIDS from their HIV$^+$ infection. Because it is a chronic illness, and medication has reduced the number of deaths, the prevalence of cases of persons living with HIV$^+$ has increased. While HAART has decreased the death rate significantly and transformed AIDS to a chronic disease, the immediate threat of death has been reduced, and individuals have become more casual about protecting themselves and their partners from the infection. This has resulted in an upsurge in new cases among intravenous drug users (IVDUs), adolescents, and men who have sex with men, especially among young African American men (Volkov, 2012). Infection among gay and bisexual men in the United States dropped 44% from 2014 to 2018, except among Native Hawaiians and Native Americans/Alaskan Natives, where it increased 78% and 15%, respectively (CDC, 2020a). According to the CDC, new cases of HIV diagnosis have decreased by 9% among heterosexual women and 13% among heterosexual men, but the proportion of new cases of HIV among IVDUs increased 9% (CDC, 2020a).

Injury

The spleen is a small organ in the body, but the largest organ in the lymphatic system (Festa, 2021). It is located in the upper left of the abdomen above the stomach and sits under the ribs, which protect it from injury (Newman, 2018). It has two components: the white pulp, which primarily houses immune cells, and red pulp, which contains blood from veins and connective tissues containing red blood cells and WBCs. The spleen has a variety of important functions, including making WBCs to fight infections and supporting healthy red blood cells. According to Zarzaur and Rozycki (2017), the spleen filters the bacteria that haven't been processed well enough and creates antibodies that can make the bacteria desirable to be eaten by phagocytes. According to Festa (2021), the spleen directs lymph through the immune system and stores blood for emergencies. The spleen filters the impurities from the blood, removes malformed red blood cells, stores the healthy blood cells, and recycles old red blood cells (Newman, 2018).

People may perforate or lacerate their spleens from automobile accidents and, sadly, in the United States from gun violence (Demetriades et al., 2006). Many medical teams assess damage using the American Association for the Surgery of Trauma (AAST) Organ Injury Scale (Tinkoff et al., 2008). The AAST assesses the seriousness of the lesions on a scale that grades them from Grades I through V based on the proportion of the spleen that has been damaged (Kozar et al., 2018).

Surgical interventions following spleen injuries are risky according to Cadeddu and colleagues (2006); therefore, use of nonoperative management (NOM) has increased. Dehli and colleagues (2015) reported that from 2000 to 2007, of patients who hemorrhaged following blunt force trauma, 38.5% received a splenectomy, while from 2007 to 2013, that number decreased to 10.5%. Ruscelli and colleagues (2019) found, in a study of blunt force trauma to the abdomen, 94.7% of patients responded favorably to nonoperative treatment and that failure to respond favorably occurred in only 5.3% of cases. While the spleen is an important organ, its function is also carried out by other components of the lymphatic system, and in the event the spleen has been damaged irrevocably and removed, one can live without it (Newman, 2018).

(T) Mental health clinicians can benefit from understanding technology to understand treatment of AIDS

When AIDS became a problem, the male condom was the most common and effective prophylactic available to prevent infection if used properly. Depending on one's infected partner to use a condom, however, meant negotiating with them either before or during the sex act, making sure the condom was available, and using it correctly. Not all couples were able to manage this process and passed the infection to their partner. A female condom came on the market in 1993; this slipped into the vagina, covered the cervix, provided a reservoir for semen that remained there until the condom was removed (Beksinska et al., 2012), and gave the woman control over her exposure to the virus, other sexually transmitted infections, and pregnancy (Mayo Clinic, 2019). Thus, the female condom (FC) is the only prophylactic barrier that is inserted by the woman and is effective in preventing STDs, including HIV. It is inserted into the vagina before intercourse and prevents the exchange of bodily fluids. As HIV is transmitted through blood that can be present in semen, this type of condom is an important protection from infection.

Unfortunately, male condom use is limited by attitudes that they limit sexual pleasure, are unpleasant to see, touch, or smell, and interfere with the sex act (Ellis et al., 2018). In spite of their efficacy in preventing unwanted pregnancies or sexually transmitted diseases (STDs) in a study of male and female college students in a dating relationship, only half reported using condoms during the first month, and approximately one-third reported that they currently used them (Civic, 2000). In the South African study undergraduate male students who used the FC endorsed the ease of use, curiosity about it, and belief that their partner was more protected from disease and had enhanced pleasure (Masvawure et al., 2014). The male students who did not agree to use the FC explained their refusal as trusting their partner and they were mutually exclusive and that they used another method of birth control. Based on the male's refusal to use FC, the couple has to negotiate use of the male condom which may leave women unprotected from STDs.

These attitudes were also endorsed by urban American men who refused to use the FC (Weeks, 2015). Despite the efficacy in protecting against STDs, FCs are not routinely used, in part because of unfamiliarity, inaccessibility, and expense (Weeks et al., 2015). Weeks reported that men were more likely than women to believe that fate determined whether they became infected, and their partner was responsible for protection against infection. This is counterintuitive because men expressed concern that one of the drawbacks of the FC is that it removed their control of the sexual act. Women who did not endorse use of the FC have reported that they are difficult to insert, and do not feel better than male condoms, or no condoms (Fenwick et al., 2021). These women were less likely to have received training to insert them. However, half the sample of Australian women who used FCs several times as part of a study reported that they would use them for protection from STDs in the future, but only 40% said they would use them for contraception. Thus, it appears that reluctance among women to use the FC was more likely the result of unfamiliarity of the device and among men that they trusted their partner to protect them from infection.

(E) Mental health clinicians can benefit from understanding the engineering of AIDS medications

To date, there is no cure for AIDS, but antiretroviral medication has reduced disease transmission from an infected partner to a seronegative partner (Cohen et al., 2011). The process of bringing medication from bench-side to bedside is difficult and time consuming at any time, but was especially frustrating for HIV[+]

/AIDS patients early its pandemic as they watched their friends die from the disease while the scientific community continued their clinical trials. In response to the lengthy wait, in March 1987 zidovudine, or AZT, an antiretroviral medication, was approved by the Food and Drug Administration (FDA) as the first AIDS drug (FDA, 2019). In 1996, highly active antiretroviral treatment HAART emerged as more powerful as it reduced the disease progression. Overall, the combination of medications effectively lowers the viral load, which is the mechanism that passes along the infection. HAART combined treatment with at least two medications to address the illness and the side effects that emerged, in response to the primary medication, but dosing has been complicated, and simpler medication regimens were needed (National Institute of Allergy & Infectious Diseases [NIAID], 2018). According to NIAID, newer medications are on the market, including non-nucleoside reverse transcriptase inhibitors (NNRTIs), which are cheaper and more accessible for low-income groups.

Women who are HIV$^+$ and aim to become pregnant are counseled to take HAART to reduce their viral load to reduce the chance of infecting their fetus (AIDSinfo, 2020). AIDSinfo (2020) suggested that the woman should take HAART as early in the pregnancy as possible The concept of vertical transmission is based on the logic that because the fetus shares the mother's circulatory system, if the mother's viral load is low, the load of the fetus will also be low (CDC, 2020b). According to the CDC (2020b), the rate of infants born with HIV$^+$ has decreased by 95% since the early 1990s when HAART was introduced (1996) and has declined 54% from 2014 to 2018.

(M) Mental health clinicians can benefit from understanding the mathematics informing epidemiological data

The goal of testing is to identify HIV and AIDS in order to reduce transmission between sexual partners, drug-using partners, and between a pregnant woman and her fetus and to treat individuals who have contracted the illness. In December 2014, the United Nations Program on HIV/AIDS released the 90–90–90 initiative to help end the AIDS pandemic by 2030 (International Association of Providers of AIDS Care [IAPAC], 2021). Specifically, this endeavor set targets for three treatments to have a 90% success rate by 2020: 90% of individuals with HIV would be diagnosed, 90% of those diagnosed would receive treatment, and 90% of those on treatment would succeed in the suppression of their virus. Collaborative efforts across the globe were made to achieve these targets and increase economic, health, and humanitarian benefits. The recent global HIV and AIDS data (UNAIDS, 2021) reported that 84% of all people living with HIV knew their HIV status in 2020; 73% of all people living with HIV had access to antiretroviral treatment and medicines; and almost 59% of people with HIV had suppressed viral loads in 2019. Despite the fact that 90–90–90 global target was not met by 2020, this initiative has generated considerable benefits to reduce the AIDS public health crisis: New HIV infections in 2020 were reduced by 52% compared to the peak in 1997, and AIDS-related deaths were reduced by 64% compared to the peak in 2004.

The World Health Organization (2021) has released HIV data from 2020. By 2020 there were 37.7 million people living with HIV, and 73% of them received antiretroviral therapy. In the midst of the COVID-19 pandemic, there were 1.5 million people who were newly diagnosed with HIV in 2020, and 680,000 died of HIV-related diseases and illnesses in 2020.

Globally, in 2020, of the total number of people living with HIV, 51.19% were women aged 15 years and older (19.3 million), 44.30% were men 15 and older (16.7 million), and 17 million were children younger than 15 (4.51%) (WHO, 2021). In addition, in 2020 there were 660,000 newly diagnosed women (45.52%) among 640,000 men (44.14%) and 150,000 children younger than 15 who were newly diagnosed with HIV (10.34%). It seems that the burden of the HIV epidemic continued to vary considerably across age and gender subgroups (WHO, 2021). According to the CDC (2021), at the end of 2019, there were 1.189 million people living in the United States who were diagnosed with HIV, and 36,801 who were newly infected during 2019. Sexual contact remained the primary source of new HIV infections: 65% of new HIV infections resulted from male-to-male sexual contact; 23% of new HIV diagnoses were from heterosexual contact; 7% of new cases were from intravenous drug use; and 4% of new cases were from a mixture of sexual contact and injection drug use.

Figure 4.3 displays the time-varying trend of new HIV diagnoses in the United States from 2013 to 2018 (CDC, 2021). Although there were more males than females acquiring HIV each year between 2013 and 2018, the total new HIV infections declined during this period, regardless of gender. HIV incidence among males was 31,624 new diagnosed cases during 2013; however, during 2018, the cases were reduced to 30,147 new cases. The female HIV incidence was 7,606 new diagnoses in 2013, which were reduced to 7,139 new cases in 2018.

(H) Mental health clinicians can benefit from understanding how to apply STEM to the health of people with HIV

In addition to unprotected sex, individuals are exposed to HIV[+] when engaged in high-risk drug-using behavior (Batchelder et al., 2016). Piercing the skin with unsterilized needles and exposing the body to antigens by injecting a nonsterile drug solution into one's vein places the illegal drug user at risk of becoming

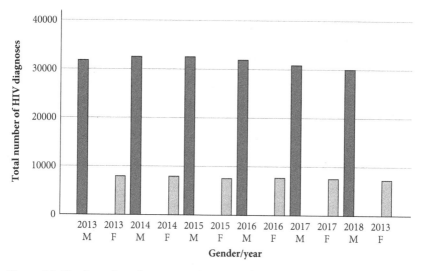

Figure 4.3 Total number of persons with HIV diagnoses, United States, 2013–2018.
Data source: Centers for Disease Control and Prevention. (2021). *HIV diagnoses*. https://www.cdc.
gov/nchs/data/hus/2019/011-508.pdf. Chart created by Dr. Liyun Wu.

infected. Because many persons who use drugs intravenously will resort to using other people's needles and syringes if they do not have clean ones, there was a 7% increase in HIV$^+$ infection rate among IVDU from 2015 to 2019 (CDC, 2020b). Concerns about the high rates of HIV$^+$/AIDS transmitted among IVDUs caused clinicians to promote harm reduction as a way to reduce fatal consequences when addicts continue to use drugs. Public health professionals campaigned to institute a process whereby addicts could trade used needles for sterile ones. Even though the objective was to reduce harm from the HIV$^+$ virus and prevent public health consequences of intravenous drug use, the project faced widespread resistance (Ball, 2007). According to Ball, over time, WHO supported the use of harm reduction methods to curb HIV$^+$ infection among individuals who used intravenous drugs.

Harm reduction has not been as accepted in the United States as it has in other parts of the world because of the focus on criminal justice as a deterrent to drug use rather than viewing it through a public health lens. According to Brocato and Wagner (2003), critics of the harm reduction model argued that providing a means by which to continue drug use safely was unethical as it promoted drug use. Proponents of harm reduction likened it to the carrot-and-stick method of motivation, where the carrot was living drug free, while the stick was fear of contracting HIV$^+$. Public health professionals argued that the carrot-versus-stick method, when applied to punitive drug control measures, had not worked and maintained that it is critical to protect an actively using addict from contracting HIV$^+$ or infecting another addict (Des Jarlais et al., 2014). To support civil liberties, some social workers are encouraged to counsel their patients to stop using, but if they are unable to stop, to at least reduce their usage and incorporate less risky drug-using behaviors into their lives. While trading used needles for sterile ones and cleaning one's drug kit with bleach are two harm reduction techniques, other methods are also important. Clinicians can counsel their clients to use safe sex procedures, including using female and male condoms and enrolling in a methadone program to slowly withdraw from opioids or as a substitute to their addiction to illegal opioids.

HIV$^+$/AIDS is a complicated illness with many consequences to the individual and the family. In addition to access, another factor that predicts improved health is adherence to the treatment regimen and treatment retention. Individuals need ongoing support to continue a complicated treatment regimen and avoid high-risk behaviors. Clinicians can support their clients' success by organizing essential social services, counselling them to discuss safe sex practices with their partner, avoid high-risk behaviors, and remain on a prescribed treatment regimen of HAART.

Conclusion

This chapter has introduced clinicians to the lymphatic system and its structure and function, with special emphasis on WBCs. The chapter compares and contrasts the contribution of innate and acquired immunity and explains how seemingly innocuous WBCs engage in violence to protect the human body. Discussed in detail was HIV$^+$ and AIDS. Each chapter discusses an injury to a bodily system, in this case, the spleen. Discussion surrounding technology included information about the female condom and its use to prevent infection with HIV. The segment on biochemical engineering focused on HAART medication, which has decreased the rates of vertical transmission of maternal HIV$^+$ infection to their fetus significantly. The section on mathematics covered the epidemiology of HIV/AIDs, specifically incidence and prevalence. Finally, this chapter introduced harm reduction as a valid treatment method. A clinician who mastered the material in this chapter will be able to work in a medical setting as a team member or as an individual who treats patients and family members with medical problems.

Glossary

Adaptive immunity   Immunity acquired from earlier experience; has a memory and recognizes a pathogen from past experience and kills it

Antibodies   Released when the lymphatic system recognizes an antigen

Antigen   A pathogen that causes the immune system to release an antibody

Highly active antiretroviral treatment (HAART)   A cocktail of three or more antiviral drugs that are combined to suppress HIV

Innate immunity   Immunity that we are born with; does not have a memory and kills both good and bad cells

Lymph nodes   Groups of cells that capture pathogens

Lymphocytes   White blood cells involved in immune responses to pathogens

Pathogen   A toxin that enters the body and causes an immune response

T cell   Leukocyte made in the thymus gland that kills pathogens

Viral load   Amount of infection in the blood of a person who is HIV⁺

Websites

Centers for Disease Control and Prevention, HIV/AIDS: https://www.cdc.gov/hiv/default.html

Centers for Disease Control and Prevention, HIV testing antigen/antibody versus antibody: https://www.cdc.gov/hiv/basics/hiv-testing/test-types.html

Harm Reduction Coalition: https://harmreduction.org

National Institute of Allergy and Infectious Diseases, HIV/AIDS Research Program: http://www.niaid.nih.gov/topics/hivaids/Pages/Default.aspx

National Institute on Drug Abuse (NIDA) home page: https://nida.gov

5

How Understanding the Sensory System Can Benefit Mental Health Clinicians

Introduction to the Sensory System: The Special Senses

The sensory system comprises two types of senses: the general sense and the special senses. Each is responsible for providing information to the brain from the outside world. We have one general sense, touch, so classified because rather than being limited to one organ (e.g., hearing = ear, sight = eye), it is related to the entire body. In addition to one general sense, we have four special senses. These are responsible for hearing/balance, seeing, tasting, and smelling. This chapter focuses on the special senses. Each is the product of neuroanatomical and biochemical processes that provide the structure of the system. Illnesses and injuries can damage the systems by affecting the organ or nerves that lead to the brain. For example, many persons who have recovered from the coronavirus disease 2019 (COVID-19) state that they lost their sense of taste and smell for a period of time. This phenomenon is studied in detail in this chapter in regard to STEM-H (science, technology, engineering, and mathematics as applied to health).

STEM-H Principles Underlying the Sensory System

(S) Mental health clinicians can benefit from understanding the science that explains the sensory processes

This segment explains the special senses (hearing/balance, seeing, smelling, and tasting) and how they relate to the structures of the brain. The sensory system is examined in terms of its structure and function, illnesses and injuries that are associated with each sense, and the biomedical engineering and technological advances specific to each sense. Prevalence and incidence of each sense are presented, as are the principles that will be applied to clinical work with clients and families that are struggling with deficits in each sensory systems.

STEM-H for Mental Health Clinicians. Marilyn Weaver Lewis, Liyun Wu, and Zachary Allan Hagen, Oxford University Press.
© Oxford University Press 2023. DOI: 10.1093/oso/9780197638514.003.0005

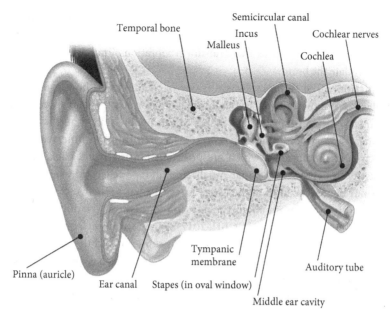

Figure 5.1 The anatomy of the ear.

Auditory System

Structure.   A normal human has two ears: one on either side of the head (bi-lateral). As seen in Figure 5.1, each normal ear has three parts that work in tandem to transform vibrations in the air into sounds. The visible part of the ear, the auricle, is responsible for cupping the airwaves and funneling them into the ear canal. This process concentrates the waves, multiplying their force and amplifying them. The funneled air waves then collide with the eardrum, which separates the outer from the middle ear, causing the membrane to vibrate, much like the skin on top of an actual drum. These vibrations move the three tiny bones (ossicles) in the middle ear (hammer, anvil, and stapes) and cause the stapes to hit the "oval window" in the inner ear, making it vibrate. These vibrations of the oval window cause fluid (perilymph and endolymph) in the inner ear to vibrate. When guitar strings are strummed slowly, the vibrations travel from the oval window to the bottom of the spiral-shaped cochlea. As one plays faster, the vibrations move up the cochlea to the top of the spiral and then back to a "round window." Lower pitched sounds stimulate hair cells at the bottom of the cochlea, but the higher pitched sounds stimulate the hair cells all the way up to the top of the cochlea. When the guitar causes the vibrations to move hair cells, they in turn cause nerve impulses in the auditory cortex to interpret the vibrations as sounds (Campbell, 2011). In addition to the inner ear, hair cells are also found in the outer ear (Thomas, 2019). These hair cells dampen loud sounds and amplify quiet sounds before sending them to the inner hair cells and protect the microphone-like structures that transform vibrations into electrical impulses that stimulate the brain.

Function. The auditory system is one of the doors of the sensory system that leads from the external to the internal environment. When asked to identify the function of the auditory system, most people state that it is to enable hearing. They are only partially correct. Deep within the inner ear lies the semicircular membranes, which are positioned at the front, back, and sides of the cavities. The semicircular canals contain hair cells, and when we tilt or move our heads, the fluid in the canal moves the hairs. Their movement sends information to the brain about the position of the head (National Center for Biotechnology Information [NCBI], 2017). When we are sick or have an inner ear infection, our equilibrium may be compromised, and the room feels like it is spinning. This is called vertigo (American Speech–Language–Hearing Association [ASHA], n.d.).

Hearing begins when the two auricles/pinnae capture sound waves from either side of the head and inform the brain about the direction of the sound. The sound hits the ear that is closer to the sound first. The sounds from each ear are modulated, reducing the louder sound that is closer to one ear and amplifying the softer sound from the farther ear (Thomas, 2019). This sums the two sounds, and you hear one sound.

Illnesses. Sound is perceived differently by individuals, as is deafness. Deafness can occur as the result of trauma or illness, or it could occur during gestation. One illness that causes deafness, or sensorineural hearing loss, is meningitis. There are several types of meningitis (e.g., viral, bacterial). Bacterial meningitis affects 1.2 million people worldwide every year, with 135,000 cases becoming fatal (Gondim, 2021). In 2020, meningitis was responsible for 1,146 estimated deaths in the United States, 89 estimated deaths in Canada, and 265 deaths in the United Kingdom (Meningitis Research Foundation, 2021). For example, hearing loss occurs among 9% of children who have contracted meningitis (Gondim, 2021) due to bacterial-infected fluid in the inner ear killing the cochlear hair cells and damaging the auditory nerve (Singhal et al., 2020).

Meningitis occurs primarily in young children, and identifying the damage quickly is critical so they can receive early intervention services to prevent impaired hearing and speech development (Tuli et al., 2012). Potent vaccines have reduced the occurrence of meningitis because they target four types of bacteria that cause the disease. One vaccine (MenACWY: Menactra® and Menveo®) is recommended for children aged 2 months to 10 years old and older if they have co-occurring illnesses, while the other is a Serogroup B meningococcal vaccine

(MenB: Bexsero® and Trumenba®), which is recommended for people from 16 to 23 years (Centers for Disease Control and Prevention [CDC], 2019). According to the CDC, these vaccines may be given with others. Clinicians should counsel parents who resist allowing their children to receive these high-potency medications to speak to their pediatrician to learn the benefits and risks of the vaccine, as well as the risks of contracting meningitis.

Injuries. Another source of hearing loss is loud noises. According to the National Institute on Aging (NIA, 2018b), hearing can be damaged by exposure to sounds above 70 dB for a long period of time (electronic music), as well as noise over 120 dB on one occasion (an explosion). Sound is measured in decibels, and the level of sound that can be heard depends on the decibels. Damage occurs when the sound-sensitive hair cells are dislodged and are thus unable to convert sound waves to electrical impulses that go to the auditory cortex.

(T) Mental health clinicians can benefit from understanding technological advances to treat hearing loss

According to the NIA, approximately 33% of adults aged 65 to 74 have hearing loss, while almost 50% of adults 75 years and older report hearing loss. Among older adults, hearing loss most often is correlated with exposure to loud sounds or from illnesses that destroyed the hair cells in the cochlea (NIA, 2018a). One technique to replenish hair cells that has been successful with other medical problems has been using embryonic stem cells, but even after years of experimentation, this approach has not been effective. While promising research continues (Waqas et al., 2020), scientists have not been able to translate stem cell research from bench-side to bedside (Senn et al., 2020).

In 2018, the CDC Hearing, Screening, and Follow-up Survey found nationwide that 6,432 newborns demonstrated hearing loss, but that only 46.76% were enrolled in early intervention services before they were 6 months old (CDC, 2020). When evaluated by race, receiving early intervention services was virtually the same among Caucasian, non-Hispanic children who were hard of hearing (64.7%), compared to Caucasian, Hispanic children (68.2%). Substantial differences emerged among African American children. Those who were African American, non-Hispanic (53.2%) were much less likely to receive early intervention services compared to African American, Hispanic children (72.7%) (CDC, 2018).

There are different levels of hearing loss: mild, moderate, severe, and profound. According to Rollop (2019), persons with mild hearing loss are unable to hear whispering or conversations where there is background noise, while persons with moderate hearing loss will have trouble hearing conversations even in quiet environments. Both of these deficits can be corrected with conventional hearing aids. However, persons with severe hearing deficits will be unable to hear people talking or the phone ringing and will need more sophisticated hearing aids. Rollop suggests that lip reading would be helpful at this stage of hearing loss. Persons with profound hearing loss may be able to hear sirens, loud music, and shouting in the ear, but not conversations or a vacuum cleaner, and cochlear implants and sign language may be necessary.

(E) Mental health clinicians can benefit from understanding biomedical engineering to treat hearing loss

Different solutions to hearing loss depend on the location of the damage. Meningitis damages the cochlea, and the most frequently prescribed treatment for severe and profound hearing loss is the use of cochlear implants. Success among patients who have recovered from an episode of meningitis depends on the amount of damage to the cochlea, the length of time the patient has been deaf, and how deep the electrode was inserted (Singhal et al., 2020). Cochlear implant systems have two parts: the microphone that is attached to the top of the ear and the implant that is affixed to the side of the skull next to the auditory nerve. The microphone picks up the movement of the sound waves and converts them into digital signals, which are then directed to the cochlear implant, which sends signals to the auditory nerve that are not heard as sounds, but as sensations that the brain processes as sounds.

(M) Mental health clinicians can benefit from understanding mathematics informing the rate of hearing loss

It has been estimated that there are about 48 million individuals living in America who suffer from some degree of hearing loss (Hearing Loss Association of America, 2021). Hearing loss has become an invisible public health epidemic. The protocol is that all infants are screened, diagnosed, and enrolled in early intervention services for hearing loss. Individuals with hearing loss benefit from hearing aids in various ways, including slowing cognitive decline associated with hearing loss, reducing depressive symptoms, and improving quality of life (Hearing Health Foundation, 2021).

Screening is paramount in order to access treatment. Figure 5.2 presents the proportion of infants that were screened and enrolled in early intervention for hearing loss in the United States from 2000 to 2007. During this

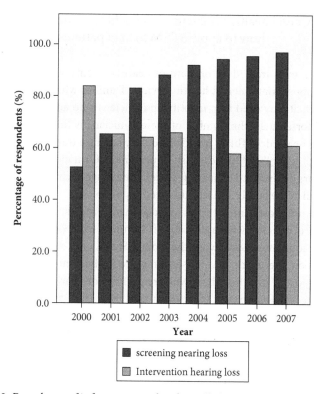

Figure 5.2 Prevalence of infants screened and enrolled in early intervention services for hearing loss, United States, annually, 2000–2007.

interval, the proportion of infants who received screening steadily increased from only 52.1% of them screened in 2000 to 97% of them screened during 2007. However, the proportion of those infants enrolled in early intervention services fluctuated from 2000 to 2007, with the highest rate of infants enrolling in services (83.7%) during 2000 and lowest rate of enrollment (55.4%) during 2006.

Despite the visible benefits, hearing aids are underutilized. The U.S. government, in collaboration with civic organizations, strives to increase the use of hearing aids among adults with hearing loss. The most recent data reported that only 24.4% of adults who were 18 years and older with hearing loss utilized hearing aids (Healthy People 2030, 2021). The adult population aged 70 and older are among those with the highest usage of hearing aids. During the period 2001 to 2012, the usage of hearing aids among adults 70 and older with hearing loss had increase from 25.5% in 2001 to 30.5% in 2012.

(H) Mental health clinicians can benefit from understanding how to apply STEM to help patients

A clinician may treat deaf or hard-of-hearing clients who have problems accessing appropriate mental health services. Families with loved ones with a hearing deficit may need help identifying clinicians who are fluent in sign language. Unfortunately, the number of these clinicians is limited, and an interpreter may be needed. This is not ideal because having a third party in the room may limit the client's willingness to share personal information. Families of loved ones who are deaf or hard of hearing experience a range of challenges throughout the life span of the family and will also need support.

Many, if not most, families enter into a grieving process when they learn that their child is afflicted with a disability (Cherow et al., 1999). This realization can occur soon after delivery. In the United States, each newborn's hearing is assessed soon after birth, and those who score in the abnormal range are formally diagnosed. They, and those who are positive for hearing loss, are referred to early intervention services (Cherow et al., 1999). These services may include referral to mental health clinicians to help the families process their grief due to the loss of their "perfect" child. Cherow and colleagues suggested that the family's coming to terms with this loss is similar to the stages of grief that Kubler-Ross (1969) identified during the dying process. Early intervention services are based on a family-centered model and provide early support during the family's adjustment. These services are considered critical to the well-being of the family and the child. Canadian parents of 10- to 18-year-old children with a hearing loss expressed a sense of loss because they no longer had access to the family-oriented environment found in early intervention services (Jamieson et al., 2011). Jamieson and colleagues reported that the families of deaf and hard-of-hearing children endorsed the need for socioemotional support when working with their children's teachers. They agreed that even though typically these schools are child oriented, they do not have the support they had received from the family-oriented environment of early intervention services. Clinicians may be enlisted to provide emotional support to caregivers when choosing schools to facilitate their child's well-being in addition to their educational needs (Stephens & Duncan, 2020). The participants in Stephens and Duncan's study shared that their children expressed frustration and anxiety that they were unable to follow the class discussion or make friends. Some family focus group participants also shared their need for emotional support while their children struggled to develop relationships at school and become socially involved with their peers. Treatment with parents of hard-of-hearing children is critical because they demonstrate more stress than parents of hearing children and may employ more coercive parenting practices, which are correlated with behavioral problems in their children

(VanOrmer et al., 2019). The maternal and paternal–child relationship should be assessed if there has been hearing loss in very young children. Inability to hear auditory signals can interfere with maternal–child or paternal–child attachment. Early intervention services and clinical interventions can facilitate the attachment relationship, which will increase support and decrease family stress (Mathos & Broussard, 2005).

Visual Processing System

Rather than thinking of sight as the result of seeing something with the eyes, it is more accurate to think of it as the result of a process of the multistructure visual information relay system. There are many components of this relay system, and a variety of things happen during this process of translating objects in the environment to seen objects. The eyes are the beginning: The individual sees an object that is transmitted to the brain, where it is perceived as an image that is flipped upside down. The system and the brain interpret the image as right side up. This chapter's subsection on sight describes the structure and function of the visual information processing system. The illnesses and injuries that are common in the system are discussed, and the technological advances that are used to overcome deficits in the visual system are covered. Biomedical options used to treat blindness (brain implants, nano-diamond lenses, and the bionic eye) are introduced. Mathematical data demonstrating epidemiologic principles pertaining to blindness are covered. Finally, clinically applying STEM-H principles to the visual information processing system is addressed.

Structure.   The normal individual has two eyes; they are bilateral and sit in the bony orbit of the skull on either side of the nose. Their position and the eyelids protect them from damage. The eyelids blink automatically when something touches them or something is coming toward the eyes. The person can close them at will. Eyelashes are attached to the eyelids and trap dust and minute particles to prevent them from entering the eyes. The eye has many parts that work together to send visual information to the brain, where it is perceived as images.

As can be seen in Figure 5.3, the eye is a globe enveloped by several layers: The outer layer, or the sclera ("white of the eye"), is opaque and maintains the round structure of the eyeball. As the sclera comes to the front of the eye, it becomes the cornea, which is transparent and allows light to enter. The second layer of the eye is the choroid, which provides the blood supply to the eye. The choroid layer also contains muscles that allow the iris to constrict or dilate. The third, inner layer is the retinal layer. The retina is the area that is photosensitive, or sensitive to light. Inside these three layers, the eye is hollow and filled with a gel-like substance called humors. These structures form a chamber in the front that is filled with aqueous humor and a chamber in back that contains vitreous humor. They

Eye anatomy

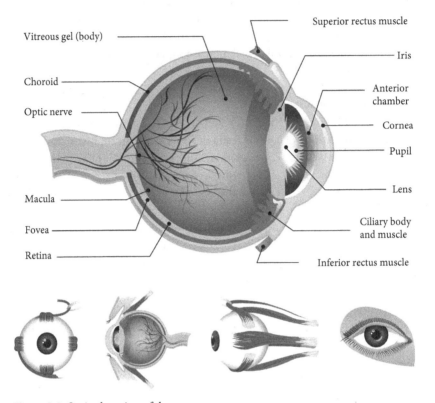

Figure 5.3 Sagittal section of the eye.

leave an opening in the front where the lens sits and lets light go into the eye to reach the photosensitive area. The lens sits behind the iris, the colored part of the eye, which constricts or dilates depending on the amount of light that shines on it. The pupil, the black part of the eye, dilates when the iris lets in more light and constricts when the pupil lets in less light. The retina layer is the innermost layer and sits at the back of the eye. It is populated with cells that are called rods because of their shape and are responsible for recognizing color and seeing in lighted conditions. The cones, also named because of their shape, are responsible for seeing in low light; they do not process color. These cells send electrical signals with visual input to the brain through the optic nerve (Campbell, 2011).

Function. The eyes' function is to detect light and has been integral to the development of most of the species on Earth. They function to ensure our survival, so much so that 96% of all species possess a visual system (Land & Fernald, 1992). The eye transforms light into electrical signals, and the brain processes them as images. These images from the environment pass through the pupil, an opening in the center of the eye that dilates or constricts, depending on the intensity of light. The image is then sent to and through the lens, where it is received by the retina cells of the back of the eye. Specialized cells at the retinal layer respond to dim light (rods), while others respond to bright light and color (cones) (Colbert et al., 2020). Cells that distinguish color are shaped like, and therefore called, cones. Because of cones, individuals are able to discern colors when there is light. Light travels in wavelengths of varying lengths. Cones, but not rods, can transform wavelengths into colors. The human eye cannot perceive wavelengths shorter than 380 (violet) or longer than 700 nanometers (red) (National Aeronautics & Space Administration [NASA], 2010). The cones can discern green and blue and combinations of those colors, reddish-blue and yellow-blue. The cones detect the colors and send that information to the brain. The inability to see color is a recessive gene and is passed to the individual, usually a man, by his mother. According to the National Eye Institute (NEI) (2019a), symptoms of color blindness include inability to see different shades and the brightness of colors. There are individual differences in color deficiencies. They range from mild to severe. Some people cannot perceive color unless they are in bright light, while some people with the most severe deficiency do not see color, but see the world in shades of black, white, and gray (Turbert & Mendoza, 2021).

Illnesses.   Because there are treatments that halt the progression of some illnesses, early intervention is important to achieve this success. But this is not always the case. There are different types of vision dysfunction. Blindness, the most extreme dysfunction, can occur because of several illnesses. This section discusses glaucoma-related blindness.

Glaucoma is associated with older age and is one of the most frequent causes of blindness in adults over 60. It is the leading cause of irreversible blindness in the world (Allison et al., 2020). According to Allison and colleagues, cases of glaucoma are estimated to be 70 million worldwide, which is expected to increase to 111.8 million by 2040 (2020). The worldwide prevalence of glaucoma is 3.54% (Tham et al., 2014). There are two types of glaucoma: open angle and closed angle (acute-angle closure). In the United Kingdom, the most prevalent form of glaucoma is primary open-angle glaucoma (POAG); it afflicts 2% of the population older than 40. POAG is highest in Africa (4.20%), while primary angle closure glaucoma (PACG) is highest in Asia (1.09%). Gender differences are also present, with men more likely to experience POAG than women and persons living in cities more likely to experience glaucoma than those living in the country.

Glaucoma-related blindness is an illness of the retinal layer and is associated with increased fluid in the eye causing pressure, which damages the optic nerve (Mayo Clinic, 2021a). In the normal eye, fluid in the front of the iris (aqueous

humor) drains out of the front of the eye. If the drainage angle is blocked because the angle is too narrow or the iris slips over the angle, fluid builds up
and can damage the optic nerve (Boyd & McKinney, 2020; Panahi et al., 2017).
According to the Mayo Clinic (2021a), symptoms in open-angle glaucoma include blind spots and tunnel vision. Symptoms of acute closed-angle glaucoma
include blurred vision, headaches, nausea and vomiting, eye pain, and auras
around lights. Routine eye exams are necessary to identify this disorder in the
early stages because symptoms may not alert the individual until damage has
already occurred. Vision loss is permanent but early intervention may slow the
progression of the illness.

Some individuals attempt to treat glaucoma by smoking marijuana (Delta-9-
tetrahydrocannabinol, Δ9-THC) because of anecdotal and empirical evidence
that it reduces eye pressure. Relying on anecdotal evidence, some patients use
cannabidiol (CBD), which is a substance that is extracted from the marijuana
plant to isolate the medicinal from the psychoactive properties. Overall, while
some researchers have reported a decrease in intraocular pressure among men
with Δ9-THC but not CBD (Miller et al., 2018), other researchers' reports were
mixed (Flach, 2002; Klumpers & Thacker, 2019; Panahi et al., 2017; Sun et al.,
2015). In extensive reviews on studies testing the effects of Δ9-THC or CBD on
intraocular pressure, Panahi and colleagues (2017) and Passani and colleagues
(2020) reported that while there were positive findings, the benefits were not robust enough to warrant the side effects and recommended that patients continue
to use glaucoma medications that have been approved because using cannabis
to treat glaucoma is impractical, is potentially addictive (Panahi et al., 2017; Sun
et al., 2015; Turbert & Gudgel, 2021), and sensitizes susceptible smokers to the
onset of psychotic disorders (Klumpers & Thacker, 2019). However, Sun and
colleagues (2015) acknowledged that Δ9-THC may be indicated in late-stage,
inoperable glaucoma when other treatments have failed, but that it has been associated with many side effects. Currently, recommended treatment includes
draining the fluid in the eye using drops or surgery. The eye drops have unpleasant
side effects, including changing the color of the iris, lowering blood pressure,
causing burning and stinging, developing corneal deposits, introducing allergic
reactions to the preservatives, incurring financial expense, and causing difficulty
following the treatment regimen (Radhakrishnan & Iwach, 2018). Therefore, it is
not surprising that some patients would choose to use marijuana to treat themselves and avoid having such aggressive treatment (draining fluid from the eye
or surgery). However, a systematic review of studies that examined the effect of
cannabinoids on intraocular pressure (Passani et al., 2020) found that while there
were positive findings, the benefits were not robust enough to warrant the side
effects and recommended that patients continue to use glaucoma medications
that have been approved.

Injuries. Among civilians, most eye injuries occur due to automobile accidents or falls, whereas among military personnel, explosive blasts are responsible for the largest proportion of eye injuries. According to Cockerham and colleagues (2009), there are three types of injuries from blasts: Primary blast injuries to the visual system occur when the force of the blast shakes the brain so forcefully that it collides with the bony skull and the brain tissue is damaged. Secondary blast injuries occur when the eye is struck by shrapnel from explosive devices or debris from flying objects in the environment. Tertiary blast injuries occur when individuals are thrown against stationary objects in the environment. Closed head injuries occur from the brain's rapid back and forth movement inside the skull, which stretches and damages axons. Direct or indirect trauma of the visual system that results in blindness can occur anywhere along the visual pathway from the bony orbit that houses the eyeball to the cornea or lens at the front of the eye, the retinal layer at the back of the eye, the optic nerves that exit the eye and cross over in the optic chiasm, or the fibers that travel from the chiasm to the visual centers in the cerebral cortex (Cockerham et al., 2009).

Damage can result in a range of deficits: partial or total blindness; elimination of central or peripheral vision; inability to entrain both eyes on one image and convert the two images into one; the ability to track a moving object; permanent double vision; and the inability to fixate on an image, causing blurred vision (Cockerham et al., 2009). Some of these deficits occur because the damaged brain is no longer able to distinguish background from an object in the foreground. The ability to see contrasts is reduced, and therefore the patient is unable to recognize outlines and sizes of objects, resulting is poor depth perception and misjudging distances of objects (e.g., steps). These injuries can reduce one's quality of life if they result in the inability to work, read, drive, or even walk without colliding with people or objects or falling down (Powell & Torgerson, 2011, p. 359).

(T) Mental health clinicians can benefit from understanding the technology that treats visual problems

There are a variety of corrections that can be made to overcome problems with the visual processing system. Figure 5.4 depicts three types of vision. Normal vision occurs when the eye is perfectly round and smooth, and the light that passes through the cornea and lens comes in contact with the retinal cells at the back of the eye. However, in cases where the shape of the eye is elongated, the light falls in front of the retina, and the individual's vision is nearsighted (myopic) (NEI, 2021b). Eyeglasses are prescribed, and the corrective lens in the eyeglasses refracts or bends the light so that it falls behind its uncorrected state and falls

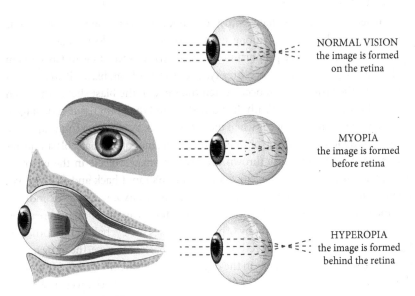

Figure 5.4 Myopia and hyperopia.

on the retina, as it would if the eye were perfectly round. In cases where the eye is shorter than it should be, the light falls on the optic track that is behind the retinal layer, and the person is farsighted (hyperopic) (Mayo Clinic, 2021b). Corrective lenses would bend the light so that it falls in front of its noncorrected state and onto the retina.

Normally, in young people, the eye's lens automatically changes rapidly to accommodate objects that become closer or farther away. The lens' shape is controlled by ciliary muscles that are attached to the outside (sclera) of the eyeball. When the individual looks at something in the distance, these ciliary muscles relax and the curvature of the lens flattens, allowing images in the background to appear clear. In other instances, when the individual looks at an object that is close to the eye, the ciliary muscles contract, causing the lens to thicken, making images in the foreground appear clear (Federov, 2021). With many people who become older, the muscles are no longer able to rapidly accommodate to the changes in distance, and lenses that correct for nearsighted as well as farsighted vision must be prescribed. In other cases, when the cornea's shape is abnormal, astigmatism results, and vision is blurry regardless of its distance. In most cases, a corrective lens can rectify this problem, and the light is bent (refracted) so it falls on the retinal layer.

The first choice of remediation is to determine if the problem can be managed with eyeglasses that correct vision for long and/or near distances. These can generally improve the ability to recognize people at a distance, read printed material, or work on the computer. In cases where the patient has double vision, a prism may be added to the eyeglasses in order to bend light so it falls on the correct area of the retina. The prism in one lens of the eyeglasses will shift the image that the eye is viewing so it falls within the same visual field as the other eye. This allows the brain to process the image as one entity, instead of two.

(E) Mental health clinicians can benefit from understanding the engineering used to treat glaucoma

Diamond nanogel-embedded contact lens. The diamond nanogel-embedded (DNE) contact lens was developed to secrete time-released medications, such as timolol, through the cornea. Timolol is a beta-blocker that has been used to treat high blood pressure and migraines, as well as intraocular pressure. Treatment of intraocular pressure is critical to avoid blindness in cases of glaucoma. Timolol can be used as eye drops or in DNE contact lenses. The soft lenses are made so they are permeable, and their pore size is conducive to dispersion of medication embedded in the contact lenses (Kim et al., 2014), with the medication released when the enzyme comes in contact with tears from the lacrimal gland. The medication is secreted from the lens in a controlled way during a 24-hour period. Fabricating these lenses is very complicated because they have to have not only the right prescription, but also the right shape to fit the eye and the correct drug solution embedded into the lens. They are meant to be replaced every 24 hours, which can be very costly. These difficulties notwithstanding, the benefits include sustained release of the medication rather than receiving a bolus of medication at one time. Benefits also include increased patient adherence to the treatment regimen (Kim et al., 2014).

(M) Mental health clinicians can benefit from understanding the mathematics explaining the epidemiology

Diabetes is widespread. In 2010, it was prevalent in 6.4% of the world's population and was ranked third among people aged 20–79 living in the United States (26.8 million), behind India (first) and China (second). This ranking is projected to hold in 2030, with the prevalence of persons living in the United States increasing to 36.0 million by 2030, when 14.0% of the population is projected to have diabetes. In addition, 13.9% of Canadians are estimated to have contracted the illness and 5.4% of residents of the United Kingdom (Shaw et al., 2009). These numbers are staggering because anyone with Type 1, Type 2, or gestational diabetes is at risk for blindness (NEI, 2019c), and among patients aged 20–74, within

20 years of having been diagnosed, nearly all patients with Type 1 diabetes and over 60% of those with Type 2 diabetes will have developed retinopathy (Fong et al., 2004).

It is clear that the total number of Americans with diabetic retinopathy is projected to double from the year 2010 to 2050, rising from 7.685 million cases in 2010 to 14.559 million in 2050 (NEI, 2020). This growing pattern can be observed for all racial and ethnic groups, as shown in Figure 5.5. Hispanic populations witness the fastest growth rate in cases, rising more than four times from 1.194 million in 2010 to 5.254 million in 2050. Diabetic retinopathy increased in this estimate from 2010 to 2030 but remained at that elevated level in 2050. Other ethnic groups showed an increase during the 20-year interval of 2030 to 2050.

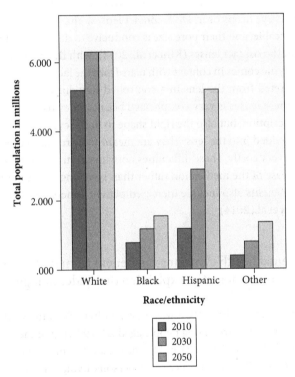

Figure 5.5 Projections for total population diagnosed with diabetic retinopathy, United States, 2010 to 2030 to 2050.

Note: Data are expressed in millions.

Data source: National Eye Institute. (2020). *Diabetic retinopathy tables*. https://www.nei.nih.gov/learn-about-eye-health/outreach-campaigns-and-resources/eye-health-data-and-statistics/diabetic-retinopathy-data-and-statistics/diabetic-retinopathy-tables. Chart created by Dr. Liyun Wu.

(H) Mental health clinicians can benefit from understanding STEM-H principles regarding vision

In a poll conducted by Research!America, McIntosh (2015) reported that participants identified blindness as one of the four top "worst things that could happen." According to the poll, African Americans (59%), Hispanics (60%), Asians (68%), and non-Hispanic Whites (73%) reported that the loss of quality of life was the greatest impact they experienced from vision loss (Research!America, 2014). Some people who struggle with vision loss have expressed suicidal thoughts (Nyman et al., 2012). Overall, persons with visual impairments were over two times more likely to report suicidal ideation during the past year and almost five times more likely to have attempted suicide during the past year (Khurana et al., 2021). This is counterintuitive because Lam and colleagues found that suicide deaths among visually impaired individuals were not higher than among sighted individuals when the level of self-reported health from other medical problems was assessed (Lam et al., 2008). However, completed suicides were higher among males who had greater degree of visual impairment, but not among females (Meyer-Rochow et al., 2015).

One of the defining characteristics associated with suicide attempts is hopelessness (Beck et al., 1979). Patients may be at increased risk when their vision is deteriorating and articulate their hopelessness as: "I am a burden to my family, and they will be better off without me" (Beck et al., 1979). Thus, clinicians should monitor their client's level of suicide risk carefully following eye evaluations. Indeed, Van Orden and colleagues (2010) found that a combination of hopelessness and a perception of burdensomeness is a strong predictor of suicide. Perceiving oneself as a burden was associated with increased dependence on family members secondary to vision loss (Bambara et al., 2009; Khare et al., 2016). According to Marco and colleagues (2016), the client is at extreme risk when he or she has lifelong risk factors (e.g., family history of suicide, past history of suicide attempts) that now were combined with a current risk factor (e.g., hopelessness).

Some family members become depressed and burdened (Khare et al., 2016) from taking on the added responsibilities the impaired loved one can no longer do for him- or herself (e.g., going to the ophthalmologist, obtaining medications). In addition, the family member loses some of his or her access to social support because more time is spent on being responsible for caregiving and having less time for a social life (Bambara et al., 2009). However, friends can provide support as well, and sharing the burden can reduce role strain (Reinhardt, 1996). Identifying persons in the client's environment who will provide at least one type of support is critical. As Sherbourne and Stewart (1991) wrote, people who provide one type of support are more likely to provide another type, as there are several types of social support that are important for one's well-being. Indeed, the Medical Outcome Study Social Support Survey (Sherbourne & Stewart, 1991) identified four types of social support: emotional/informational; tangible; affectionate; and positive social interaction that are conducive to increased well-being.

Increasing social interactions is important when working with depressed families and clients with vision loss. Visual impairment is associated globally with increased social isolation and reduced social roles (Shah et al., 2020), decreased opportunities for social support, and increased loneliness among older Canadians (Mick et al., 2018) and increased depression among Ghanaians (Tetteh et al., 2020). On the one hand, reducing social interactions limits the opportunities to receive support from friends and their families, but on the other hand, it protects the individual from exposing themselves as having a disability (Wang & Boerner, 2008). This was supported by Senra and colleagues' (2011) findings that persons who have become visually impaired struggle with transitioning from (1) their identity as a seeing person to (2) a new, unknown identity as a person with a disability. Some participants cope with vision loss by initiating new strategies to continue or establish social relationships. Some of these strategies included being more transparent and assertive about their abilities and limitations, while in other cases participants reported that relinquishing relationships with sighted people was necessary because maintaining them was too disappointing (Wang & Boerner, 2008).

When working with clients who are adjusting to loss of their visual acuity, it is important for clinicians to support their attempts to become more assertive about their needs and to rely more on their other senses (touch, sound) when interacting with others. This clinical support is critical, as evidenced by a study of emotional well-being among older people with irreversible vision loss (Nyman et al., 2012) that showed that individuals with more severe vision loss were more likely to use clinical services. Therefore clinicians should reach out to those patients with moderate vision loss and support their psychological well-being by working with them to accept their vision loss, as well as increase their social support (Nyman et al., 2012).

The Gustatory and Olfactory Systems

(S) Mental health clinicians can benefit from understanding the science of taste and smell

Smell and taste are part of the chemosensory system and the oldest senses of the human (Sherman, 2019). Taste is primarily due to smell (Spence, 2015), and

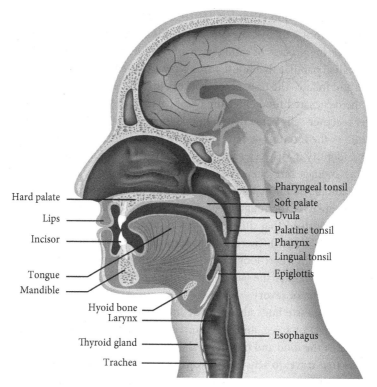

Figure 5.6 Anatomy of the mouth and tongue.

because the gustatory and the olfactory systems work in concert, this section includes information regarding both systems. The function of the gustatory and olfactory systems is to sustain life. When food is eaten, the nerves in the central nervous system transmit the information from the taste buds to the brain, which synthesizes the taste, texture, and smell and decides whether the individual has eaten an apple or a Habanero chili.

Gustatory System

Structure.   Figure 5.6 shows the anatomy of the mouth and tongue. They are housed within the face, behind the lips and teeth; both are necessary for chewing food. Other structures that contribute to gustation include the esophagus and the hard and soft palates. The structure of the gustatory system begins with the taste buds on the tongue and the palate (AlJulaih & Lasrado, 2021). Each taste bud contains gustatory cells and supporting cells and sits in a pocket of the papillae. At birth, the human has approximately 10,000 taste buds, which are replenished on an ongoing basis (National Institute on Deafness and

Other Communication Disorders [NIDCD], 2017). The average life span of a taste bud is from 1 to 2 weeks. Dead taste buds are sloughed off during teeth brushing or the process of eating or drinking. The tongue is covered by small bumps called papillae that house three types of taste buds: fungiform, circumvallate, and foliate. The taste of food occurs in part because gaseous molecules from the desiccated food enter the nasal cavity and stimulate olfactory hairs that let receptor cells know that desirable food is present. When this desirable food enters the mouth, the taste buds give more information about its qualities and identify it as sweet, salty, sour, or savory (umami). Bitter foods, often signaling spoilage, are often rejected (AlJulaih & Lasrado, 2021). In the past, people thought that taste buds that reacted to different tastes were located in particular areas of the tongue, but newer research has refuted this idea and now asserts instead that different types of taste buds are scattered over the tongue (NIDCD, 2017). There are openings, or pores, at the top of the taste bud and at the bottom where long, thin hairs slip through to the surface of the cell. They register whether the gaseous molecules of the food or drink are sweet, sour, salty, bitter, or savory.

Function.   Taste buds also provide information about the food's temperature, the level of spice, and its texture. Taste buds respond to the gaseous molecules of the food and transform that chemical information into electrical impulses that travel to sensory neurons (AlJulaih & Lasrado, 2021). Not everyone tastes the same thing when they eat the same food. Ethnic and gender differences have been found in response to perception of tastes (Williams et al., 2016). African Americans and Hispanics are more likely to perceive salt, sugar, and citrus as intense tastes compared to non-Hispanic Whites (Williams et al., 2016). Bartoshuk and colleagues (1994) found that compared to men, regardless of ethnicity, women were more likely to have more taste buds, were more likely to be classified as "supertasters," and to perceive bitter and sweet tastes as more intense.

Taste buds on the tongue and palate respond to the sweet, salty, sour, bitter, and savory (umami) chemicals in the food (AlJulaih & Lasrado, 2021). Differences in taste perception are also correlated with body mass index (BMI). According to Skrandies and Zschieschang (2015), sensitivity to salty tastes was higher among persons with higher BMI. Elevated BMI is partially a genetic predisposition and partially a socioeconomic problem, although socioeconomic factors play a larger role than the genetic ones in this case.

The Olfactory System

Structure.   As Figure 5.7 shows, the nose is the primary source of smell and contains olfactory and supporting cells and is responsible for directing the air into the lung. A nasal septum, comprising cartilage and bone, supports the

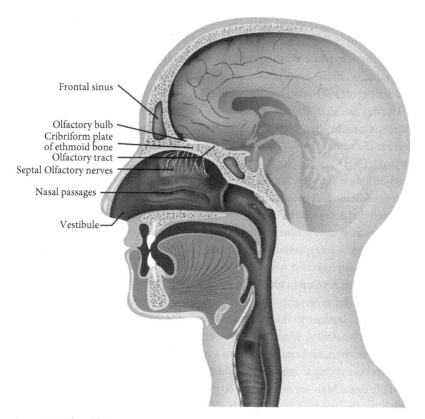

Frontal sinus

Olfactory bulb
Cribriform plate
of ethmoid bone
Olfactory tract
Septal Olfactory nerves

Nasal passages

Vestibule

Figure 5.7 The olfactory system.

bridge of the nose and separates the nasal area into two nostrils. When we examine the nose, we notice slender hairs that protrude down from the top of
the upper epithelial membrane. During gustation, the hairs collect gaseous
molecules from masticated food and send them up to the olfactory epithelial layer at the roof of the nose. At the epithelial layer, nerves extend up into
the tissue and form nerve bundles of approximately 20 nerves that respond
to smells. These smells stimulate the olfactory axons that innervate the olfactory bulb and travel to the front of the cortex, where the smell is identified
(Krusemark et al., 2013).

Function. The olfactory system is one of the oldest sensory systems and
informs individuals about the external environment. The human brain contains
approximately 50 million receptor cells adapted for olfaction (Sarafoleanu et al.,
2009). These cells are intricately bound to the survival of the species because they
facilitate discrimination of odors of potential mates (Savic et al., 2001) and one's
newborn baby (Uebi et al., 2019). The process of olfaction begins when volatile

molecules coming from an odor enter the nasal cavity and stimulate olfactory tissue (Pinto, 2011). As each of these olfactory cells only responds to one odor, each of them must be synthesized into one complex smell (e.g., tomato sauce + pepperoni + cheese + oregano + crust = pizza). This synthesizing occurs in the olfactory center of the brain.

During the sixth month of gestation, the fetal nostrils open, and the fetus inhales amniotic fluid. This process forms the basis of its recognition of its mother (Schaeffer, 1910). By birth, newborns have approximately 10,000 olfactory cells (NIDCD, 2017), which help the fetus recognize the mother's smell. The newborn shows preference for the mother, especially if it received immediate skin-to-skin contact with her (Mizuno et al., 2004). Zhang and colleagues (2018) reported that access to the mother's amniotic fluid reduced scores on a pain scale and shortened crying time during and after collection of blood samples. Zhang and colleagues interpreted these findings to mean that because the baby's response to pain lessened when it smelled the amniotic fluid, the fetus' sense of smell began to develop in utero and provided the newborn with information that is important for survival.

Injuries.   Injuries to the gustatory or olfactory systems can occur because of accidents or assaults. Maxillofacial traumas include any injuries to the face or jaw, are common, and can occur from a variety of sources. These types of trauma can affect the ability to smell or eat and can trouble those individuals throughout their life span. Men are more likely to experience maxillofacial injuries, most of which are the result of traffic accidents. However, assaults account for approximately one fourth (23.45%) of all maxillofacial injuries among either gender, but among women, they account for half (53.61%) of their injuries (Manodh et al., 2016).

Loss of taste or smell may occur following facial trauma. Several areas can be affected: the olfactory bulb, cranial nerves, or olfactory epithelial receptors (Wrobel & Leopold, 2004). Olfactory epithelial cells regenerate every 3 to 6 months; thus, patients may eventually notice a return of the ability to smell and taste. Unfortunately, nasal surgery undertaken to repair damage may result in deficits in the ability to smell and thereby limit the ability to taste. If reduced airflow inhibits molecules from the mixture of saliva and food to enter the nasal cavity, the ability to taste will be impaired. However, when the obstructed airway is repaired, smelling may eventually return. On the other hand, according to Wrobel and Leopold (2004), when the loss of smell results from damage to the olfactory nerves, olfactory bulb, or olfactory center in the brain, the return of the client's ability to smell to its pretrauma level is doubtful. Although one's pretrauma level may not return because there are different levels of dysfunction, the patient may regain some ability to smell.

Illnesses.   Loss of the ability to smell and taste food is of great concern. These deficits were not initially recognized as a symptom of the COVID-19 virus, but this has changed because of overwhelming data to the contrary (Borsetto et al., 2020; Boscolo-Rizzo et al., 2020; Lechien, Chiesa-Estomba, et al., 2020; Lechien, Journe, et al., 2020; Mazzatenta et al., 2020; Spinato et al., 2020). When ill, clients are more likely to lose the ability to smell than to taste. Among severely ill patients with COVID-19 who were hospitalized, 95% had problems smelling, but only 47% had problems tasting (Mazzatenta et al., 2020). When these patients were evaluated for level of sensory dysfunction, most of the patients exhibited symptoms that ranged from moderate (hyposmic) to severe (severe hyposmic), falling under the middle of the curve. Only a few patients had no problem (5%) and were able to smell normally (normosmic). Only a few patients were totally unable to smell (13%) and were considered anosmic, while more had reduced ability to smell (34%) and were diagnosed as hyposmic. Finally, most had severely reduced ability to smell (43%) and were severely hyposmic. The overall data indicated that even among severely ill patients, only a small minority had lost the ability to smell and taste. This reflects findings of a superadditive relationship of smelling and tasting (Escanilla et al., 2015), and that brain activity is stronger when food is paired with an odor rather than in isolation. Because human life depends on recognizing and imbibing nourishment, it stands to reason that neural systems (e.g., smelling and tasting) that are critical for survival would be multimodal systems.

(T) Clinicians can benefit from understanding the technology used to treat gustatory and olfactory deficits

Because most of the perceived problems with taste are actually the result of problems with smell, this section focuses on the olfactory system. Sinus cavities are located in several areas of the face: the forehead, between the eyes, behind the cheekbones, and further back in the center of the head (Medical University of South Carolina [MUSC], n.d.). They are hollow cavities that sit inside bony structures lined with epithelium that is moistened by a thin layer of mucus. Even though the nose filters and humidifies the incoming air, sinus problems are common in societies with air pollution and toxic fumes (Hoffman, 2020). Usually, the sinuses drain into the nose, but when the body is exposed to viruses, bacteria, or fungi, an increased amount of mucus may remain in the sinuses. When this discharge does not drain, it builds up in the sinus cavities. Sinusitis is the result, and the lymphatic system becomes hyperactive and ineffective. There are three kinds of sinusitis: acute (less than 1 month); subacute (1 to 3 months);

and chronic (more than 3 months). When the mucous membranes that line the sinus cavities become inflamed due to infection, sinusitis is diagnosed. Typically, it occurs in over 15% of the American population and is one of the most common chronic illnesses (MUSC, n.d.), but several groups exhibit incidence of the condition more often than other groups.

Many first responders at the World Trade Center (WTC) in New York City following the bombings on 9/11 reported later that they developed breathing problems from searching for survivors through rubble, which contained asbestos, human remains, particles of commercial insulation, dust from pulverized brick and mortar, and gasoline molecules. Active duty and retired firefighters, rescue recovery workers, and first responders worked in these conditions without personal protective clothing and inhaled the particulate matter, some for many weeks. However, when surveyed 9 years postdisaster, approximately 40% (42.3%) of first responders who participated in the WTC clean-up continued to suffer from sinusitis (Wisnivesky et al., 2011), while others (46%) reported inflamed nasal mucosa (Levin et al., 2004) and others (54%) the "World Trade Center cough" (Chen & Thurston, 2002) with nasal symptoms (Prezant et al., 2002).

Empirical evidence of sinusitis from contaminated WTC dust supports clinical findings, regardless of whether the data were self-reported (17.3%) or from a physician's diagnosis (9.7%) (Webber et al., 2011). To identify sinusitis, identify the type and extent of the problem, and determine if it is chronic sinusitis or another physical condition, the least invasive diagnostic procedures are considered first, which include computer tomography (CT) or magnetic resonance imaging (MRI) scans (Hoffmann, 2020). A nasal endoscopy (rhinoscopy) may be used to treat sinusitis to reduce the white blood cells (blood eosinophils) that fight the infection (Honma et al., 2016). During the procedure, the physician threads a flexible tube with a camera attached to it into the nasal cavity. The camera takes pictures to show if there are polyps and the size, number, and location and whether they may be blocking the airway (MUSC, n.d.).

Recurring acute sinusitis is diagnosed when infections return after a medication regimen is completed. The repeated return of these infections can result in chronic sinusitis with nasal polyps, which is the swelling of the membranes, development of nasal polyps, loss of smell (or taste), and difficulty breathing. Some physicians recommend over-the-counter (OTC) nasal irrigation methods with medications to flush irritants out of the nasal canal (Fandino & Douglas, 2021). If OTC medications do not resolve sinusitis, the physician may prescribe antibiotics. The course of action is designed first to kill bacteria that have grown in the sinus cavities and second to reduce inflammation. Oral or nasal steroids, such as prednisone, are used. Medication regimens usually resolve sinusitis within 14 days by reducing swelling that is obstructing the airway.

(E) Mental health clinicians can benefit from understanding how engineering identifies food and liquids

Smells are the result of gaseous molecules, and identifying them using mechanical means is being carried out at several research and development departments worldwide. This is no small feat because the tastes of foods can combine more than 1,000 different chemicals. According to Suslick and colleagues (Lim et al., 2008), this feat is possible because the models are based on olfactory and gustatory systems in nature. Using "mechanical tongues," taste sensors can distinguish liquids by isolating sugar molecules (sweet), pH (sourness), sodium (saltiness), and glutamate (umami). Electronic taste buds have been developed to act as sensors and have distinguished sugar and fructose (Lavigne et al., 1998). They can differentiate 15 different sugars and sugar substitutes (Lim et al., 2008); distinguish bitterness and sweetness of beer, sake (an alcoholic Japanese drink), coffee, and mineral water (Toko, 2000), tomato sauces (Malmendal et al., 2011), and 30 types of fruit juices (Bruker, 2021). Scientists have also used mechanical tongues to differentiate sugars and proteins (Hou et al., 2011) and the presence of umami and L-monosodium glutamate (MSG) in liquid food, such as chicken stock (Lee et al., 2015).

This methodology has practical application because even though the Food and Drug Administration (FDA) has classified MSG as "generally recognized as safe," some susceptible individuals have complained that they have felt nauseous and have had headaches after eating foods with large amounts of MSG. Requiring scientific proof that these compounds are, or are not, present in processed foods is important because in 1906 the Federal Food and Drug Act began to require that all manufacturers list each added ingredient on all food labels to protect the public.

(M) Mental health clinicians can benefit from understanding the mathematics underlying epidemiology

Coronavirus disease (COVID-19) is now an ongoing pandemic and has been transmitted person to person. This infectious disease impacts different people in many different ways, ranging from mild symptoms to severe illnesses and the need for critical intensive care. In addition to fever, cough, fatigue, headache, and shortness of breath, a reduction in the ability to smell and taste was recently recognized as one of the 12 most common symptoms by the CDC (2021). Findings from a telephone survey of 274 symptomatic adults who had tested positive for COVID-19 indicated that loss of smell and taste were symptoms with the longest duration, with a median of 8 days. This ongoing deficit prevents individuals from symptom resolution and returning to their usual health status. Other scholars conducted research related to the dysfunction in smell and taste among COVID-19 patients. Butowt and Von Bartheld (2020) completed a meta-analysis by synthesizing 42 empirical studies reporting data related to smell and taste dysfunction among COVID-19 patients who lived in either East Asia or Western countries. Furthermore, the aggregated data from synthesizing those 42 studies were published in the study by Butowt and Von Bartheld (2020).

The prevalence rate of loss of ability to smell normally was 22.4% among 4,587 COVID-19 patients who lived in four East Asian countries: China, Japan, South Korea, and Singapore. In comparison, the prevalence of olfactory dysfunction was 48.4% among 13,897 COVID-19 patients who resided in Western countries, including the United States, United Kingdom, Canada, France, Germany, and Italy. On average, the prevalence of olfactory dysfunction was 44.1% among 18,484 patients in East Asia and Western countries. There were no olfactory data reported in Africa and South America. The prevalence for loss of taste was 16.2% among 5,747 COVID-19 patients residing in four East Asian countries and 50.3% among 10,168 COVID-19 patients living in Western countries such as the United States, United Kingdom, Canada, France, Germany, and Italy. Overall, the prevalence of loss of ability to smell normally was 43.3% among 15,915 patients living in these two regions. No taste dysfunction data were reported in Africa and South America.

(H) Mental health clinicians can benefit from understanding how to apply STEM to the health of patients with illnesses of the olfactory system

One of the interesting symptoms of COVID-19 is the loss of smell and taste. This phenomenon has also been reported in upper respiratory illnesses, so it should not be surprising that this is a symptom of COVID-19. Furthermore, clinicians now report that loss of smell and taste may be hallmarks of the illness. Treatment of deficits in smell and taste has shown some success. Clinicians who work with clients recovering from COVID-19 can be trained to help them improve their ability to smell. In a review of treatment options, clients can be trained to improve their ability to smell by practicing smelling (1) items as they exist in life, (2) scent strips/tissues dipped into essential oils, or (3) commercially manufactured smell identification tests. There are several online sites with clear directions explaining how to conduct olfactory training. These directions include choosing four strong scents that are recognizable. Many people buy scented oils (lemon, rose, clove, and eucalyptus) from the aromatherapy store (AbScent, 2021), while others use household substances with strong aromas that are similar to flowery, fruity, spicy, and resinous smells (can of coffee) (Fifth Sense, 2020).

The company AbScent (https://www.abscent.org) advises that training should begin with the client creating a sensory log of his or her current ability to smell, which can simply indicate (yes/no) whether the client can smell individual items. That information gives the client and therapist a baseline from which to compare changes. Then, while the client is at home, he or she should saturate a disk of watercolor paper with the scent and place it in its own jar (a dark colored glass jar with a lid, which can be purchased online). The client should write the name of the scent on the jar as well as on the lid, making sure not to place the lid on the wrong jar so the smells do not intermingle. After the client has put several drops of each scent on its corresponding paper disk, he or she should close the jar tightly and place it in the refrigerator (AbScent, 2021). Fifth Sense (2020) added that a patient can obtain scent strips on which drops of the essential oils can be placed or purchase smell identification tests online.

If the AbScent (2021) protocol is used, the client should bring the jars to their session to begin olfactory training. They begin the training by putting on a blindfold so their eyes do not "smell" for them (AbScent, 2021). Then, the client takes a series of short gentle sniffs of the aroma, repeating this two or three more times (approximately 10 seconds for each smell), then resting for 5 minutes (Fifth.Sense, 2020). It's important to keep a log identifying their reaction after testing each aroma. Advise your client to write (a) whether they could smell anything (yes/no); (b) whether the smell was what was written on the jar's label (yes/no); (c) how strong the scent was on a scale of 0 to 3 (0, could not smell anything at all; 1, could smell the scent somewhat; 2, the scent smelled as it normally did prior to losing their sense of smell; and 3 the scent smelled stronger than normal; (d) whether the smell they perceived was distorted (yes/no); and (e) the name of the odor they actually smelled. Then the client moves on to the next smell and answers the questions again. He or she does this twice daily (ideally at the beginning of the day and at the end) (Fifth Sense, 2020). At their next visit, he or she should bring their data to discuss. Clinicians may need to remind clients that it is not unusual for them to be unable to smell during the training period because people regain their sense of smell at different times. Some people notice that their sense of smell has returned after 5 to 14 days (Lechien, Chiesa-Estomba, et al., 2020), while others still have not returned to their pre-COVID-19 sense of smell by 8 weeks (Boscolo-Rizzo et al., 2020).

Conclusion

This chapter on the sensory system special senses discussed the wide variety of special senses that humans use to perceive the world around them. The chapter presented, in detail, information highlighting the structure and function of the auditory, visual, olfactory, and gustatory systems. Illnesses and injuries of each system were examined, and the biomedical engineering and technological advances pertaining to each system were discussed. Finally, techniques that clinicians can apply when they treat clients who suffer from disorders of these special senses were introduced. Mastery of this chapter that combines the special senses will make it possible for students to work with clients and their families in medical settings or as independent clinicians.

Glossary

Auditory System

Chemoreceptors   Nerve endings outside the central nervous that respond to chemicals

Innervated   Provide nerves to an organ, tissue, bone, and other body parts

Nociceptors   A sensory receptor that is sensitive to pain

Ossicles   Three tiny bones in the middle ear that are responsible for transmitting sound by vibrating the tympanic membrane

Photoreceptors   A sensory receptor that is sensitive to light

Thermoreceptors   A sensory receptor that is sensitive to temperature

Visual System

Aqueous humor   Water-like fluid in the anterior and posterior chambers of the eye

Astigmatism   Distortion of vision from abnormal curvature of the eye

Choroid   Layer between the retina and the sclera

Cornea   Curved, clear lens in the front of the eye; allows light to come in

Diabetic retinopathy   Most common cause of blindness in the United States caused by disease (diabetes)

Glaucoma   An illness that is the result of damage to the optic nerve from increased pressure within the eye

Intraocular   Inside the eye, as in intraocular pressure

Iris Colored part of the eye

Myopia Quality of being nearsighted

Pupil Black part of the eye that dilates to let more light in or constricts to reduce the amount of light that enters the eye

Sclera Membrane that covers the eyeball, keeping fluids in the eye in a round ball, giving the eyeball its shape

Vitreous humor Gel-like substance behind the lens and in front of the retinal layer

Gustatory and Olfactory Systems

Chemosensory system A bodily system that senses chemicals through taste or smell

Circumvallate Describes papillae that contain taste buds and are wider at the top and tapered at the bottom and existing at the back of the tongue in the shape of a "V"

Foliate A leaf-shaped papilla that houses taste buds along its sides

Fungiform A mushroom-shaped papilla that houses taste buds on the top and sides of the tongue

Multimodal systems More than one system that work together (e.g., taste and smell)

Nasal septum Cartilage layer that separates the nose into two cavities

Olfactory bulb The sensory area in the front of the brain that responds to odors; passes information to the areas in the cortex that are related to smell

Papillae Protruding bumps on an organ (tongue)

pH A measure of the level of acidity (low pH) or alkalinity/basicity (high pH) of a liquid solution; a body attempts to maintain an acid/base balance between acidity and alkalinity

Receptor cells Cells that recognize stimuli (chemicals, temperature, pressure, light) (e.g., receptor cells that respond to light are cells that exist in the retinal cells)

Rhinitis Inflammation of the mucous membranes of the nose

Websites

Auditory System

American Speech–Language–Hearing Association (ASHA): https://www.asha.org/
Centers for Disease Control and Prevention: https://www.cdc.gov/
Meningitis Research Foundation: https://www.meningitis.org/

National Association of the Deaf (American Sign Language): https://www.nad.org/resour
ces/american-sign-language/
National Institute on Deafness and Other Communication Disorders (NIDCD): https://
www.nidcd.nih.gov/

Visual System

American Academy of Ophthalmology: https://www.aao.org/
American Diabetes Association: https://www.diabetes.org/
Glaucoma Research Foundation: https://www.glaucoma.org/
National Center for Biotechnology Information (NCBI): https://www.ncbi.nlm.nih.gov
National Eye Institute (NEI): https://www.nei.nih.gov
National Health Service (NHS): https://www.nhs.uk/

6

How Understanding the Circulatory System Can Benefit Mental Health Clinicians

Introduction

This chapter in the discussion of STEM-H (science, technology, engineering, and mathematics as applied to health) covers the circulatory system and focuses on its structure and function. Special attention is given to the contribution of smoking to heart disease and the technologies associated with surgical treatments for arrhythmias, a condition whereby the heartbeats become disorganized. Engineering is introduced by explaining medications that treat cardiac problems. A discussion of mathematics related to the field of epidemiology includes the incidence and prevalence of heart disease and the concept of social determinants of health (SDOH). Finally, the section on clinical application to health covers smoking cessation using nicotine replacement therapies and nonmedical interventions, as well as assessing motivation to change using the transtheoretical stages of change model.

STEM-H Principles Underlying the Circulatory System

(S) Mental health clinicians can benefit from understanding the science underlying the circulatory system

Information in this chapter is important when working as a team member treating patients in hospitals, outpatient clinics, private offices, rehabilitation centers, or the patients' homes. Because of the frequency of cardiac diseases, many mental health clinicians will treat family members who suffer because of their loved one's smoking. In order for the clinician to be effective, they must understand concepts and terminology and how it is impacted by nicotine.

STEM-H for Mental Health Clinicians. Marilyn Weaver Lewis, Liyun Wu, and Zachary Allan Hagen, Oxford University Press.
© Oxford University Press 2023. DOI: 10.1093/oso/9780197638514.003.0006

Structure

The circulatory system comprises the heart, blood, and blood vessels traveling to and emanating from the heart. Blood comprises three components: liquid blood plasma, which contains ions, waste, nutrients, and protein; leukocytes, or white blood cells, which are important in the immune response; and (3) erythrocytes, or red blood cells, which carry oxygen and carbon dioxide (Kahn Academy, n.d.-a). There are approximately one-quarter to one-half million blood platelets in one drop of blood, along with 7,500 white blood cells (Colbert et al., 2020). Blood transports oxygen, hormones, and nutrients throughout the body via the circulatory system, which comprises arteries that carry blood away from the heart and veins that return blood to the heart (Ward, 2021). The pulmonary circulatory system provides the exception to the rule, as the oxygenated blood is carried to the heart from the pulmonary veins and the deoxygenated blood is carried away from the heart by the pulmonary arteries (Cleveland Clinic, 2021).

During gestation, the heart is one of the first organs to form and develops rapidly during the first 3 weeks of gestation, when a rudimentary heartbeat can be detected (Curran, 2019). At Week 3, the embryo still needs the mother's circulatory system to survive, and even though the embryonic heart has begun to distribute oxygen and nutrients, it continues to depend partially on the placenta until birth, when the fetus is separated from the mother's circulatory system (Tan & Lewandowski, 2020).

The adult heart is a hollow, three-layer, muscular organ that sits inside the chest cavity and is protected by the breastbone and the backbone (Campbell, 2011). In medicine, the orientation of the heart is opposite of the actual orientation, which can be envisioned by facing forward and imagining the heart facing you. The right side of the heart is on your left side and the left side of the heart is on your right (Pappano & Wier, 2019). Of course, if we line up behind them, facing the same way as they do, the left side of their heart is on our left.

As Figure 6.1 shows, the heart is divided into right and left atria and ventricles by a septum that runs vertically down the middle of the organ and prohibits oxygen-poor blood on the right side of the heart from mixing with oxygenated blood from the left side of the heart (Campbell, 2011). The heart is further "divided" by valves on each side of a septum running horizontally, creating a four-chamber heart (Loukas, 2021).

Blood enters the heart from the superior and inferior vena cavae. After the right atria has filled with blood, the tricuspid valve opens to let the blood go down to the right ventricle (Colbert et al., 2020). Its three flaps then close to prohibit that blood from backing up into the right atrium. Instead, the right ventricle pumps the blood to the pulmonary arteries, which send it to the lungs, where it releases carbon dioxide and becomes oxygenated. This is referred to as the pulmonary circulatory system.

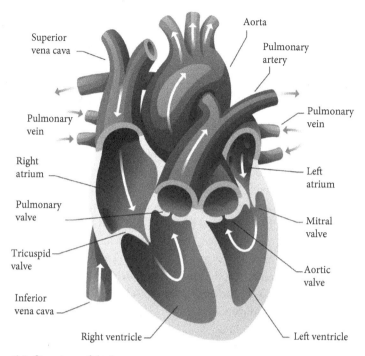

Figure 6.1 Structure of the heart.

On the opposite side of the septum, the oxygen-rich blood enters the left atrium via the pulmonary veins. The mitral valve (also called the bicuspid valve) and the aortic valve allow the blood to enter the left ventricle, which pumps it to the aorta and, from there, the body (Campbell, 2011). This is referred to as the systemic circulatory system. This function requires more effort than just sending the blood to the lungs; thus, the walls of the left ventricle are thicker and more muscular than those of the right ventricle, which only sends the blood to the lungs.

Function

The function of the heart is to pump blood throughout the body to provide nutrients and oxygen to the body. In the healthy heart, the cardiac cycle begins when the cardiac "pacemaker cells" in the upper right atrium are stimulated (Loukas, 2021). When a sympathetic nerve stimulates the pacemaker cells, the circulatory cycle is initiated, and an electrical charge is generated, causing blood to flow into the right atrium from the superior and inferior vena cavae (Loukas, 2021). The pressure builds until the ventricle contracts. When it contracts, it pumps the blood up through the pulmonary artery and into the lungs to receive oxygen to deliver to the body's organs (Colbert et al., 2020). According to Loukas (2021), only milliseconds following the initiation of activity from the pacemaker cells in the right atrium, the pulmonary veins on the left side of the heart receive the blood back from the lungs and force it down into the left ventricle, where it is then pumped up to the aorta. This process sends approximately 5 quarts of the oxygen-rich blood to the body every minute (WebMD, 2021). To accomplish this feat, the healthy heart is beating approximately 100,000 times per day (Mayo Clinic, 2013) or about 70 times per minute.

The oxygen-poor blood on the right side of the heart is kept from mingling with the oxygen-rich blood from the left side by the septum (Colbert et al., 2020). According to Colbert and colleagues, the oxygen-poor blood is sent to the lungs, where it is oxygenated before it is sent to the body. After the blood gives up its oxygen, it returns to the heart (Colbert et al., 2020). When the left atrium receives the incoming blood from the lungs, another heartbeat pushes the blood down into the left ventricle through a valve called the mitral valve. When the heart pumps again, it forces that blood in the left ventricle into the aorta, where it is sent out into the body again before it returns to the right atrium to begin the circulatory cycle again (Mayo Clinic, 2013). This process occurs 100,000 times per day.

The force of the blood depends on the size of the vein. The bigger the surface area, the more force it can withstand. Pressure develops from the blood being pumped through the blood vessels, with the blood pushing against the vessel wall, causing pressure. The pressure can cause ruptures if the wall of the vessel is weak. To check the amount of pressure on the vessel, one's blood pressure is measured. Managing blood pressure, particularly when the heart is at rest, is important in order to avoid a heart attack and damage to the heart (American Heart Association, 2020c).

Illness

Cardiac disease is a major cause of death among adults worldwide. In the United States, it accounted for approximately one fourth of total deaths in 2016 (23.1%) and 2017 (23.0%) (Heron, 2019). Coronary artery disease (CAD) was the most common cause of death in 2019 (WHO, 2020). The longitudinal Global Burden of Disease Study indicated that CAD affected approximately 126 million individuals globally in 2017 (Kahn et al., 2020). The study reported that health disparities have emerged between the more affluent countries and poorer countries, in part because countries with higher socioeconomic indicators have shown reduced CAD prevalence over time. The study attributed the high rates of disease burden to lifestyle factors, including emotional and social factors related to psychological distress and poor social relationships. However, when comparing affluent countries, Kahn and colleagues (2020) reported that in the

United States the prevalence of CAD was 2,929 persons per 100,000, while the prevalence among Canadians was 2,335 per 100,000 residents. Even though the prevalence of CAD in the United States and in Canada are high, they were substantially lower than those in the United Kingdom (3,337 per 100,000) (Kahn et al., 2020). It's clear that CAD prevalence rates were comparable, but the prevalence of disability is not. The United Kingdom and Canada have lower rates of disability compared to the United States, where 2,470 of every 100,000 residents were disabled, compared to 1,837 of 100,000 in Canada and 1,864 of 100,000 in the United Kingdom.

Coronary artery disease is characterized by a buildup of plaque in the arteries. This plaque consists of fat and remnants of bacterial cells, proteins, and calcium that move throughout the bloodstream, clump together, and adhere to the arterial walls (Cleveland Clinic, 2020). According to the Cleveland Clinic, blood platelets are attracted by the plaque and form a clot around it. As the clot enlarges, it takes on additional plaque, which reduces the available surface area of the blood vessel, causing it to constrict. This constriction obstructs the blood's flow and increases pressure on the vessel wall (American Heart Association, 2020c) and, in some cases blocks blood flow to the heart muscle, resulting in a heart attack, which according to the National Heart, Lung, and Blood Institute of the National Institutes of Health (2019) is often the first sign of CAD.

Smoking is a major contributor to heart disease (Alam et al., 2018; Duncan et al., 2019; Tuan et al., 2008; Watanabe, 2018). Its other toxins notwithstanding, a cigarette's main ingredient, nicotine, is a stimulant that increases the action of the sympathetic nerves on the heart. Nicotine also affects the receptors of the neurotransmitter acetylcholine and changes its natural balance in the brain (Advokat et al., 2019). For example, the amine family of neurotransmitters reacts to nicotine. Amines include acetylcholine (Locker et al., 2016), norepinephrine, dopamine, and serotonin (Shearman et al., 2005; Singer et al., 2004). Smoking stimulates the brain's "reward pathway," which reacts by releasing neurotransmitters that are associated with the feeling of euphoria. These neurotransmitters act as if they turn on a "go switch" that tells the brain that it must have more of the substance in order to survive (Inaba & Cohen, 2014). When adding nicotine to the system is stopped, the artificially stimulated neurotransmitters in the reward pathway become depleted, causing withdrawal. Acetylcholine is associated with memory, arousal, attention (Advokat et al., 2019), and rapid eye movement during sleep (Power, 2004). Discontinuing nicotine will result in the reduction of these effects. In addition, the individual may have cravings and thoughts about using the drug again. If they do use again, either through tobacco or a tobacco replacement product, the cravings dissipate. Unfortunately, this relief is time limited, and the brain will need more nicotine to remain satisfied (Advokat et al., 2019; Inaba & Cohen, 2014). The rewarding effects of smoking are from an increase in the neurotransmitter, dopamine, which is made in the substantia nigra region in the brainstem (Advokat et al., 2019). Drugs, including nicotine, that stimulate the reward center trick the brain into believing that it needs to have more of the substance. When smoking is stopped, the person can develop cravings that persist until more nicotine is taken into the body. Nicotine patches and gum supply nicotine and are called agonists because they mimic the effect of smoking. A substance that prevents nicotine from being pleasurable is called an antagonist. A commonly used nicotine antagonist is the antidepressant bupropion.

Acetylcholine's synthesis follows a similar process as other neurotransmitters. Figure 6.2 demonstrates that it is synthesized by the joining of two substances that are by-products of food, choline (Ch) and acetyl coenzyme (AcCoA) (Advokat et al., 2019). If nicotine enters the body, acetylcholine is released artificially, which excites the receptors of the postsynaptic membrane unnecessarily. Thus, the receptors receive more stimulation than they normally would. However, if the individual stops taking nicotine, the postsynaptic membrane of the reward pathway will not be stimulated and the person will feel dysphoric until withdrawal passes.

Injury

There is an epidemic of firearm violence in the United States. According to the Educational Fund to Stop Gun Violence (EFSGV, 2021), during 2019 there were 39,707 mortalities in the United States from gun violence. The data showed that 7.69/100,000 homicides and 12.27/100,000 suicides were of men, while 1.42/100,000 homicides and 1.85/100,000 suicides were of women (EFSGV, 2021). According to the World Population Review (2021), during 2021 in the United States alone, 12.21/100,000 deaths were gun related: 4.46/100,000 were homicides, and 7.32/100,000 were suicides. This is compared to the United Kingdom, where there were only 0.23/100,000 gun-related deaths, and among those, 0.06/100,000 (64%) were homicides and 0.15/100,000 (27%) were suicides (World Population Review, 2021).

When someone fires a gun with intent to kill, their target is often the heart. In addition to the number of bullets, the amount of damage depends on the caliber of the bullet; how many objects, including shrapnel, enter the heart; the location of the wounds; the trajectory of the wounds; whether there is an exit wound; and the distance of the gun from the heart (Shrestha et al., 2021). According to Shrestha and colleagues, death may result from infection or hemorrhage as well as organ damage from the bullets or fragments of bone, clothes, and other objects that enter the body.

Gunshot wounds to the heart are typically fatal (80%) because the victim often bleeds to death. But in cases when the shooting victim is alive when a medic

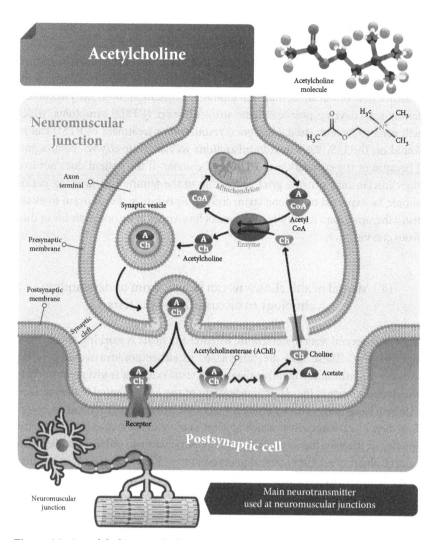

Figure 6.2 Acetylcholine metabolism.

or physician attends to them, the first objective, according to Willacy (2021), is to begin standard A, B, C trauma procedures: airway, breathing, circulation, and resuscitation. According to Kawall and colleagues (2020), the goal is to stop the bleeding; stabilize the vital signs; assess the extent of the injury; locate and remove the bullet and shrapnel; and repair the wound (Kawall et al., 2020). According to Kawall and colleagues, a firearm injury is classified as a "(1) myocardial contusion; (2) chamber laceration or perforation; (3) valve injury; (4) injury to the septum; and (5) injury to the coronary vessel" (Wani et al., 2012).

Based on what we have learned about the structure of the heart from this chapter, we can visualize where the injuries take place.

Patients who survive may suffer from long-term disabilities because of their wounds, and clinicians will be called on to help their families adjust to the patient's new physical, mental, and emotional condition. Both the patient and family may develop post-traumatic stress disorder (PTSD) symptoms, which will need to be addressed. Very good resources for treatment of PTSD can be found on the U.S. Veteran Administration's website (https://www.ptsd.va.gov/) because of the correlation of PTSD and combat. If the patient does not live, the clinician may provide grief counseling to the family. This grieving period should be expected to be long term, and it may behoove the clinician to establish a therapy group for family members of loved ones who took their life or died from gun violence.

(T) Mental health clinicians can benefit from understanding technology to discuss diagnostic tests

There are several tests to determine whether the heart is working at less-than-optimal level. These tests are categorized as either noninvasive or invasive. Among the minimally invasive diagnostic tests, one that is given routinely in the doctor's office is the electrocardiogram or the EKG (United States) or ECG (United Kingdom). The technician places electrodes on the chest to record heartbeat electric activity s, which appears as waveforms. If the shape or the frequency of the waveforms is abnormal, the physician will order more definitive tests (Colbert et al., 2019). An adjunct test to the EKG is the stress test; a patient walks on a treadmill at an increasingly difficult pace, and incline, to stress the heart. Data from the electrodes indicate whether the blood supply to the heart is normal. Another minimally invasive test is the echocardiogram. During the procedure, an ultrasound transducer is moved over the chest and emits a high-frequency sound that bounces back from the heart to the computer to create images (Johns Hopkins Medicine, 2020).

If after these noninvasive tests the doctor observes abnormalities, the doctor may order an invasive procedure, a catheterization. During the catheterization, a long, thin, hollow tube is inserted into an artery, often through the groin or wrist, and is guided to the heart (Mayo Clinic, 2019). The doctor views the image of the heart on a monitor in real time to determine whether an artery is blocked. If so, the surgeon may then perform an angiogram (Mayo Clinic, 2019), during which time a radioactive dye is infused into the blood vessels to increase the visibility of the x-ray images. If the surgeon identifies a blocked artery, they may perform angioplasty through the inserted catheter. The angioplasty is performed to open the size of the vessel by inflating a balloon at the tip of the catheter. This pushes the clump of platelets against the walls of the artery, which increases its diameter and allows blood to flow past the clump. A stent, which is a metal coil that provides scaffolding, may also be inserted through the catheter to keep the artery open (American Association of Neurological Surgeons, 2020). After the angioplasty, the doctor prescribes a treatment regimen to keep other blockages from forming in the vessels, as well as on the stent. The regimen usually consists of anticoagulation medications and changes to the person's behaviors. The changes include smoking cessation, increased exercise to strengthen the heart muscle, reduction of food high in cholesterol, controlling diabetes, lowering blood pressure, and controlling weight to reduce the amount of work the heart has to expend to pump blood throughout the body (Fogoros, 2020).

(E) Mental health clinicians can benefit from understanding the engineering of medical treatments

Chemical engineering develops medications for heart disease, while mechanical engineering develops surgical apparatuses to correct the problem if medication alone does not suffice. One type of heart disease that often requires products developed using chemical and mechanical engineering is atrial fibrillation (Afib). Atrial fibrillation occurs when the atrium beats erratically and is unable to force blood into the ventricle efficiently. This results in the atrium fibrillating in a disorganized way and blood collecting in the atrium, where a blood clot may form. When blood does finally flow from the atrium to the ventricle, the blood clots are released into the bloodstream along with the blood. These blood clots enter the arteries, which can cause strokes. This is why patients with atrial fibrillation are often on long-term blood thinners. This causes disorganized heart contractions that reduce the heart's pumping efficacy (Mayo Clinic, 2020). Because the heartbeats are irregular and weak, blood can collect in the atrium and coagulate. When the heart organizes itself and produces a strong beat, it may push a blood clot through the atrium and into circulation (Mayo Clinic, n.d.). Therefore, when someone is in Afib, the first objective is to restore the rhythm of the heart either pharmaceutically or mechanically so clots do not form and cause a stroke.

Often the first treatment for Afib is a medication regimen that may include medications to prevent blood clots from forming (anticoagulants/blood thinners or antiplatelets/aspirin) or slow the rate of the heart (beta-blockers or calcium channel blockers) (American Heart Association, 2020a). Other medications that may be prescribed change the heart rhythm (sodium channel blocker or potassium channel blocker.

If medication (chemical cardioversion) does not return the heart to its normal rhythm, the doctor may reset the rhythm with a process termed mechanical cardioconversion (American Heart Association, 2020b). Two paddles are placed on the patient's chest, or their chest and back, to deliver a mild shock to stop and restart the heart and restore it to its normal rhythm (American Heart Association, 2020b). If a mechanical cardioversion does not resolve the issue, a cardiac ablation may be performed (Mayo Clinic, 2020) to destroy the cardiac cells that are beating irregularly. When the physician orders a cardiac ablation, the physician guides a catheter, using a thin wire, up through the groin or wrist to the right ventricle of the heart (Loukas, 2021). When the wire reaches the heart, it emits radio frequencies that are either very cold or very hot to kill the heart tissue causing the irregular heartbeats.

(M) Mental health clinicians can benefit from understanding the mathematics underlying the epidemiology

Understanding the SDOH has increasingly become one of the major research areas in public health and epidemiology and is one of the key focuses of *Healthy People* initiatives, led by Office of Disease Prevention and Health Promotion (ODPHP), part of the U.S. Department of Health and Human Services. Since 1980, this initiative has gone through *Healthy People* 1980, *Healthy People* 1990, *Healthy People* 2000, *Healthy People* 2010, and *Healthy People* 2020, and the fifth iteration, *Healthy People* 2030, which was launched on August 18, 2020, sets the ten-year objectives to improve American's health. As a key focus of *Healthy People*, SDOH is defined as "conditions in the environments where people are born, live, learn, work, play, worship, and age that affect a wide range of health, functioning, and quality-of-life outcomes and risks" (Healthy People 2030).

The World Health Organization Commission on Social Determinants of Health published its report in 2008 to highlight health equity. SDOH refers to a wide array of conditions that affect people's health risks and outcomes, including socioeconomic and environmental factors. Although numerous factors can impact population health outcomes, the Healthy People 2020 (Healthy People 2020, 2021) document outlined five key areas of determinants, including economic stability, education, social and community context, health and healthcare, and neighborhood and built environments. Each area contained a number of influential factors, ranging from individual levels to societal levels.

Since 1957, the U.S. Census Bureau has collected National Health Interview Survey (NHIS) data annually to monitor the health status, healthcare access, and progress toward achieving national health objectives (U.S. Census Bureau,

2020). Empirical results from the 2019 NHIS data set (U.S. Census Bureau, 2020) indicated several disparities in the prevalence of cigarette smoking among adults in the United States. Of the total number of 31,916 adults aged 18 or more years, 13.8% identified themselves as current smokers, a combination of "everyday smokers" and "some cigarettes/day smokers," and 25.6% were known as "former smokers" and 60.7% as "never smokers." Current smoking status significantly differed by SDOH, including gender, age, race, and ethnicity. The prevalence of cigarette smoking in 2019 varied by gender: 15.3% of men were smokers versus 12.5% of women, which was statistically significant ($p < .001$). In terms of age groups, smoking prevalence was highest among adults aged 45–64 years (17.6%), the second highest among those aged 25–44 (15.9%), the third highest among young adults aged 18–24 (9.0%), and the lowest among the elderly (8.3%). These age differences were significant ($p < .001$). Racial and ethnic differences in smoking also existed. Prevalence was highest among African Americans (15.3%), then Caucasians (14.0%), and lowest among other racial/ethnic groups (11.8%). These findings were significant in terms of racial and ethnic differences in smoking ($p < .001$).

Current smoking status also differed by SDOH indicators, including education, total earnings, and region of the country. Prevalence differed among educational attainment ($p < .001$): less than high school (21.4%); high school diploma or general equivalency degree (GED) certificate (19.8%); some college (15.4%); baccalaureate degrees (7.2%); and graduate degrees (4.3%). Prevalence also differed among total annual earnings ($p < .001$): less than $19,999 (24.6%); $20,000–$49,999 (17.7%); $50,000–$100,000 (11.5%); $100,000 and above (5.9%). Regional area of residence showed disparities, with the highest prevalence of smoking found in the Midwest (16.0%), followed by the South (15.3%), Northeast (12.3%), and West (10.5%) ($p < .001$).

Based on the 2020 National Health Interview Survey data, researchers estimated that there were 47.1 million adult smokers aged 18 years old in the United States who consumed any commercial tobacco product (Cornelius et al., 2022). Tobacco use imposed a heavy burden at the societal level, with 480,000 deaths each year (CDC & National Center for Health Statistics, 2019). As indicated by Figure 6.3, there were 124,800 adults who died from heart disease each year during the period 2005–2009. The mortality rate was higher among male smokers than among female smokers: 75,200 male smokers (60.26%) versus 49,600 female smokers (39.74%).

When evaluating the incidence of smoking by age and gender among smokers who either smoked every day, some days, or had smoked at least 100 cigarettes during their lifetime when evaluated in 2019, middle-aged adults 45 to 64 years old had the highest incidence (17.0%), followed by young adults 25 to 44 years old (16.7%), people 65 and older (8.2%), and emerging adults

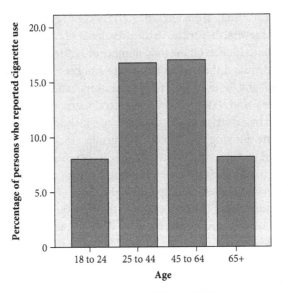

Figure 6.3 Smoking incidence by age, United States, 2019.

Note: Data are expressed as percentage of persons with reported cigarette use.

Data source: Center for Disease Control & Prevention. (2021). *Burden of cigarette use in the U.S.* https://www.cdc.gov/tobacco/campaign/tips/resources/data/cigarette-smoking-in-united-states. html. Chart created by Dr. Liyun Wu.

18 to 24 years old (8.0%). When evaluated by gender of adult among current cigarette smokers in 2019, there were more male smokers (15.3%) than female smokers (12.7%).

(H) Mental health clinicians can benefit from understanding STEM and the health of the circulatory system

Smoking tobacco products can initiate or exacerbate cardiac problems, including cardiovascular disease and stroke, as well as contribute to intermediate and chronic illnesses. Cigarette smoke contains 7,000 chemicals (CDC, 2011), but its teratogenic effects depend, in part, on the number of cigarettes smoked per day and the number of years the individual has smoked. These are significant risk factors for short- and long-term health problems but can be ameliorated if the individual decreases or ceases smoking as smoking is the cause of most preventable deaths in the United States and is responsible for 480,000 deaths each year (CDC & National Center for Health Statistics, 2019). In the United States alone, 23.0% (*n* = 647,457) of all adult deaths were cardiac related during 2017 (Heron, 2019). Fourteen percent of all adults (34.1 million) were current smokers in 2019

(CDC & National Center for Health Statistics, 2019). These included 15.3% of all men and 12.7% of women.

Because of the association of the toxic effects of smoking cigarettes and cardiac problems, many people have stopped, or tried to stop, using nicotine products. According to the NHIS of 2017 (Healthy People, 2021), during the period 1965 to 2017, in large part due to a U.S. Surgeon General's report and public health campaigns, prevalence of smoking decreased among men living in the United States, from 52% to 15.8%, and among women from 34.1% to 12.2%. Those findings notwithstanding, there are still large numbers of people living in the United States that put their health at risk by smoking, including those who substituted cigarettes for vaping electronic cigarettes (American Health Association, 2021).

Because of the deleterious effects of smoking on cardiac function, stopping or at least reducing smoking is critical. The benefits of stopping are substantial. Former smokers, depending on the length of time since their last cigarette, may significantly reduce their risk factors for cardiac disease even though they continue to have higher risk factors than their counterparts who have never smoked (U.S. Department of Health & Human Services, 2020). In cases where total smoking cessation has not been possible, a harm reduction model focusing on decreasing the number of cigarettes has resulted in ameliorating some of the adverse health effects (Hughes, 1995). The transtheoretical stages of change model was developed by Prochaska and DiClemente to identify the client's level of commitment to the recovery process so the clinician could tailor treatment recommendations to that stage (LaMorte, 2019). Clinicians who use the stages of change techniques work with their client regardless of their level of readiness to change and regardless of their commitment to total abstinence or reducing their use to moderation.

The stages of change, as developed by Prochaska and DiClemente (DiClemente & Velasquez, 2002), include the following: the precontemplation stage, which is characterized by a total lack of awareness that smoking is a problem. In this case, treatment may be focused on increasing motivation by probing if the client may have any concerns about their smoking. During the next stage, the contemplation stage, the client begins to acknowledge that there may be a problem (e.g., shortness of breath) as the result of smoking but is not yet motivated to take steps to stop or decrease use. Treatment for this level of motivation may be to provide medical data and other information about the harm smoking is causing this individual (National Institute of Alcohol Abuse and Alcoholism, 2005). In the action stage, clients may make appointments (and break them and make them again) with a clinician or seek services (e.g., go to Nicotine Anonymous). Treatment during this stage is to increase motivation by addressing barriers and "seemingly irrelevant decisions" that put the individual in danger of continued use.

An example may be that the individual decides to go into the drugstore to buy a non-nicotine product for themselves (fingernail polish, shampoo) that could be purchased elsewhere where nicotine is not for sale. However, because they are in a setting where cigarettes are available, they impulsively buy a pack of cigarettes. The treatment objective at this time is to help the client look at the concept of cravings and how their emerging motivation to resist smoking may be jeopardized by decisions that place them within easy access to the substance. During this stage, the clinician will work with the client to identify the triggers that precede their cravings. The fourth level of change is maintenance. During this time the clinician works with the client using relapse prevention techniques, such as refusal skills, and assertiveness training. This stage can, and hopefully does, last indefinitely.

Conclusion

After learning the material in this chapter, clinicians know the terminology associated with the structure and function of the circulatory system and are familiar with common illnesses, injuries as the result of gun violence, the epidemiology of smoking's contribution to the public's health problem, as well as SDOH. The transtheoretical stages of change model was introduced. Clinicians who successfully learn this material will be in the position to participate as an effective team member or independent clinician with cardiac patients and their families. Treatments for cardiac ailments, including Afib were discussed. Some illnesses related to smoking can be ameliorated by the individual, and clinicians may have occasion to work with patients who are motivated to cease or decrease their smoking.

Glossary

Acetylcholine   Neurotransmitter involved in transmission of nerve cells
Angioplasty   Medical procedure using a small balloon to open a blocked artery
Arrhythmias   Conditions where the heart's rhythm is abnormal
Fibrillation   Abnormal rhythm of the heart where atria of the heart flutter
Norepinephrine   Neurotransmitter that increases heart rate and blood pressure
Serotonin Neurotransmitter that stimulates smooth muscles to contract

Websites

American Heart Association: https://www.heart.org/
Centers for Disease Control and Prevention: https://www.cdc.gov/heartdisease/index.htm
National Heart, Lung, and Blood Institute: https://www.nhlbi.nih.gov/

7

How Understanding the Respiratory System Can Benefit Mental Health Clinicians

Introduction

Even though we are examining the bodily systems individually, they work in tandem. This chapter explains the structure and function of the respiratory system and how it is affected by illness, specifically the severe acute respiratory syndrome coronavirus 2 (SARS-CoV-2; causes the disease COVID-19), as well as injuries that result in a collapsed lung. Examples of medical technologies that include noninvasive and invasive breathing treatments are presented, as well as examples of pharmaceutical engineering. Transmission and prevalence and incidence of COVID-19 are discussed using epidemiologic models. STEM-H (science, technology, engineering, and mathematics as applied to health) is presented concerning treatment of individuals and families suffering from COVID-19.

STEM-H Principles Underlying the Respiratory System

(S) Mental health clinicians can benefit from understanding science related to the respiratory system

Unlike many other bodily functions, breathing through our mouth and nasal passages can be voluntary and involuntary. Even though most breathing is involuntary and is controlled by the medulla oblongata in the brainstem (Ikeda et al., 2017), individuals also can consciously cause themselves to breathe. This is important as Li and colleagues (2018) found that consciously slowing one's breathing decreases the heart rate and blood pressure. While breathing through our nasal passages and/or mouth is what we typically think of as respiration, it is actually ventilation and refers to inspiration and exhalation of air through our mouth and nose (National Cancer Institute, Seer Training Modules, n.d.). On the other hand, there are three types of respiration: external, internal, and cellular.

STEM-H for Mental Health Clinicians. Marilyn Weaver Lewis, Liyun Wu, and Zachary Allan Hagen, Oxford University Press.

External respiration occurs when air is inhaled and travels to the millions of tiny alveoli that are in sacs in the lungs. Carbon dioxide in the air is then exchanged for new oxygen in a process of gas exchange (Powers & Dhamoon, 2021). Internal respiration occurs when cells within our body tissues exchange carbon dioxide for oxygen through blood vessels. The third type of respiration is cellular, where oxygen is used in the creation of energy molecules by breaking down glucose molecules from food (Kahn Academy, n.d.). The use of oxygen in cellular respiration is referred to as aerobic respiration. However, this chapter refers only to the biologic structure that facilitates external respiration.

You may think that the abdomen and the chest are in a closed system because increasing the volume of one component decreases the volume of the other. However, on taking a breath, the rib cage moves up and out and the diaphragm pushes down in the thoracic cavity (Campbell, 2011a). This movement causes the lungs to inflate with air to bring in oxygen. On the other hand, when the diaphragm moves up, the space inside the lungs is reduced, and air is expelled. Thus, the expansion or contraction of the lungs causes inspiration and expiration, allowing our body to inhale new oxygen and exhale carbon dioxide.

Structure

The development of the respiratory system occurs in stages. Even though it begins when lung buds begin to emerge around 7 weeks of gestation, the lungs have not begun to develop until 17 weeks, and a "normal airway template" is not found until the 24th week (Bush & Collins, 2021). According to Bush and Collins, fetal breathing must begin in utero to develop lung volume. By the third trimester, the fetus is breathing one-third of the time. However, the placenta is responsible for fetal respiration until birth. Premature babies have immature lungs at birth, and more than half of them develop respiratory distress (Bush & Collins, 2021).

Figure 7.1 depicts the structure of the adult respiratory system, which consists of the nasal cavity and mouth as part of the upper respiratory tract, including the windpipe, or trachea. The air travels down the trachea, which is a tube that comprises a column of rings of cartilage and connective tissue (Campbell, 2011a). The rings of the trachea are similar to those of a vacuum hose and provides structure to the tube, causing a firm, open airway. The trachea resembles an upside-down tree that branches into two bronchial tubes, each one ending in a lung. The trachea receives the air from the environment and distributes it to one of two bronchial tubes (Fogg, 2021). These branches further divide approximately 15 to 20 times to resemble a plant's root system of small "roots" or bronchioles. The ends of these bronchioles are alveoli, or air sacs mentioned above, which are small grape-like structures that are responsible for exchange of carbon dioxide for oxygen (Weinberger et al., 2019).

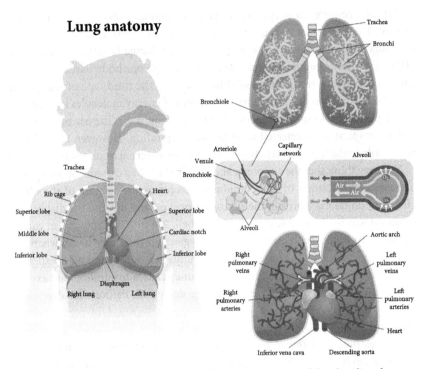

Figure 7.1 The respiratory system, including magnification of the alveoli and bronchiole.

There are two lungs that lie on either side of the heart. Although there are two, they are not identical. The lung that sits in the right side of the body has three lobes (superior, medial, and inferior) and is wider than the left because of the liver's position in the abdominal cavity. The left lung has only two lobes (superior and inferior), possibly because because its space in the chest cavity is constricted as it shares the left chest cavity with the heart (Chaudhry & Bordoni, 2019). According to Fogg (2021), when the lungs are examined postmortem, the impressions of the neighboring organs that had been next to the lung in the thoracic cavity are visible. On average the right lung in the male weighs 15.7 oz compared to 12.0 oz for the female. The left lung of the male weighs 13.9 oz compared to 10.5 oz for the female.

Within the chest, the lungs are between the thorax and the abdomen and lie above the diaphragm, which is a relatively flat sheet of muscles and tendons. The adult lungs can move, as they are only attached at the central compartment of the chest (Fogg, 2021). Each is encased by a two-layer membrane called the pleura and the pleural cavity, which is a fluid-filled space between the two membranes that reduces the friction of the lungs moving during inspiration and expiration (Colbert et al., 2020b).

Lungs are the main organs for breathing and supply a large surface area to house the alveolar sacs. According to Ochs and colleagues (2004), in a study of adult human lungs, the number of alveoli sacs formed at the end of the bronchioles ranged from 274 to 790 million. These grape-like structures that form sacs at the end of the bronchioles provide a large surface area for gas exchange to take place (Weinberger et al., 2019). A thin membrane around the alveoli allows for diffusion of oxygen and carbon dioxide during gas exchange (Colbert et al., 2020a).

Function

The main function of external respiration is to take in air through the nose and the mouth, extract oxygen from it, and distribute the oxygen throughout the body via the blood. During each exhalation, external respiration also releases the carbon dioxide that was formed during cellular respiration. On the other hand, the goal of internal respiration is to transport the blood to the body's organs and tissues and distribute oxygen while collecting carbon dioxide. This process occurs through gas exchange in the alveoli, which allows the blood to take on more oxygen before sending it back to the heart (Colbert et al., 2020a).

This process has several components: ventilation, circulation, and diffusion (Weinberger et al., 2019). The process begins with ventilation; thus, the function of the nose is critical because its membranes are coated with micro cilia that protect the nasal passages and lungs from dust and pathogens from the environment. It also warms and humidifies the air before it enters the lungs (Naclerio et al., 2007) in order to protect the bronchioles from becoming dried (Campbell, 2011a). The circulatory system is intimately involved with pulmonary circulation as the heart sends blood to the lungs to be oxygenated, which is then returned to the heart.

Movements of the lungs during inspiration and expiration cause friction as the external surface of the lung and the internal surface of the chest wall slide against one another (Weinberger et al., 2019). However, because the lungs are encased by the pleural membrane, they are protected. One inner membrane of the pleura is attached to the surface of the lung, while the outer pleura is fixed to the chest wall. Because a liquid layer of pleural fluid exists between the two pleural membranes, they are suctioned together and cushion the lungs (Colbert et al., 2020b). If the two membranes become unattached, negative pressure of the lung causes it to collapse, and the inner pleural membrane will become separated from the outer pleura (Campbell, 2011a) and the space between them will fill with air. This is called pneumothorax and is a common injury cause by chest trauma.

The trachea dilate when they are stimulated by the sympathetic nervous system, which allows air to rush into the lungs. Conversely, the trachea constricts when stimulated by the parasympathetic system, and air is limited from reaching the lungs. While it's important to have access to increased air during an experience that causes a fight-or-flight reaction, according to Campbell (2011b) if the bronchi remained dilated, they would be at risk for infection, which would cause them to become inflamed and swollen. On the other hand, the layer of epithelial cells that line the wall of the trachea fights infection. These cells have cilia, or microscopic hairs, emanating from the top of the cells and brush debris, pollen, dust particles, and excessive mucous out of the trachea so it can be expelled (Fogg, 2021). According to Fogg, even though lungs are protected within the body, because they are attached to the trachea they are in contact with the environment and subjected to drying out, freezing, and coming in contact with microbial particles. To protect the lungs, the body can engage its cough reflex, which is an important defense mechanism that, in a healthy person, dislodges and clears the trachea from thick mucosal secretions that trap foreign bodies (Bustamante-Marin & Ostrowski, 2017).

Illness

There are four types of pathogens that can cause diseases and attack the respiratory system: bacteria, fungus, parasites, and viruses (Mayo Foundation, 2020). COVID-19 is an infectious viral disease and has an affinity for the respiratory system (Hatipoglu, 2020). COVID-19 may cause an immune response that breaks down the alveoli and capillaries, causing them to slough off debris that attaches to the walls of the alveoli like plaque, or splattered paint (Cleveland Clinic, 2020). This debris thickens and damages the walls of the alveoli, inhibiting gas exchange. Even though COVID-19 is microscopic, within 5 months from the time it was identified, it infected 4 million people around the world and killed more than 280,000 (Bernstein & Cha, 2020).

The incubation period for COVID-19 is estimated to be from 2 to 7 days (Attia et al., 2021), or approximately 5 (Wong & Saier, 2021) days, while the incubation period for the Delta variant is approximately 4 days (WebMD, 2021). In some cases, the symptoms (COVID-19) may be so mild that the infected individual remains asymptomatic and does not know they are contagious. In a study of 4,841 asymptomatic individuals, 2.2% were positive for COVID-19 antibodies (Dinerstein, 2021). The variety of symptoms is part of the reason that the virus has been able to spread so effectively. Person A may be young and healthy and only experience mild cold symptoms (e.g., cough, loss of their sense of smell) or be asymptomatic. Regardless, they can still produce and disseminate viral particles into the environment for up to 14 days (WebMD, 2021). For instance, if they went shopping while asymptomatic, they could come in close contact and spread the virus to 10 people.

It was not until COVID-19 patients developed severe symptoms that infectious disease doctors and epidemiologists became aware that it was something other than an upper respiratory tract illness (Hatipoglu, 2020). It is highly contagious because it is transported through moisture droplets expelled during everyday activities, such as speaking, laughing, sneezing, coughing, and kissing (Centers for Disease Control and Prevention [CDC], 2021a). These droplets are much smaller than the droplets of other common viruses like the flu and may remain suspended in the air for a much longer time after they have been expelled. A typical distance between individuals that is considered safe for "social distancing" is 6 feet because it is unlikely that moisture molecules travel farther during social interactions that are not intimate (CDC, 2020).

Those with underlying medical conditions are more likely to develop life-threatening complications because their body is already compensating for their underlying disease, and a relatively small insult to the organ system may cause complete failure (World Health Organization [WHO], 2020a). For example, a healthy individual may be able to survive a severe respiratory illness, but if a smoker who is already living with less effective gas exchange at baseline contracts COVID-19, they may develop severe respiratory symptoms (Shastri et al., 2021). Thus, some individuals who contract COVID-19 are more at risk for poor medical outcomes, including death, than others. Persons who have chronic preexisting illnesses such as heart disease, kidney disease, or obesity are not more at risk for contracting the disease, but more at risk medically after they contract it (Galiatsatos, 2020). According to Galiatsatos, other factors that determine whether one recovers are disease severity, the kind of treatment one receives, and how quickly treatment is obtained.

Parsons (2020) advised that people should eliminate behaviors that put their lungs at risk, including smoking nicotine, marijuana, and vaping and practice deep breathing, manage their allergies, and avoid pollution. Maintaining good hygiene, as well as effective handwashing, disinfecting surfaces, and social distancing, are suggested (CDC, 2021a). Social distancing can include the choice to self-quarantine. Quarantine is defined as "separating exposed versus non-exposed persons, whereas isolation is separating sick individuals from those who are well" (CDC, 2020). Self-quarantine removes oneself from the risk of becoming infected and is suggested by public health officials as the best way to "flatten the curve," or slow transmission of the infection. When the growth rate of new cases is halted, the curve flattens. A decrease in the incidence of new cases ultimately decreases mortality rates and protects the medical system from being overwhelmed.

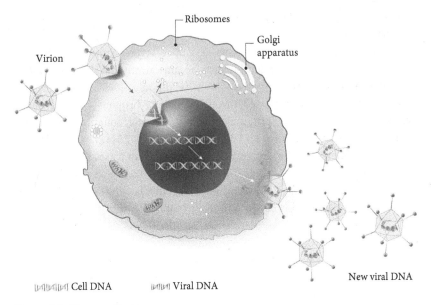

Figure 7.2 Virus replication.

There are several caveats in the treatment of the virus. First, because COVID-19 is a virus, antibiotics do not have an effect, and the body is left to fight it un-aided. Second, we do not know what the long-term trajectory of COVID-19 will be. It may resemble other viruses that have an asymptomatic stage when the host is not aware that they are infectious, followed by an acute stage when the infected person is symptomatic (CDC, 2021c). As shown in Figure 7.2, viruses have ge-netic material, but they need a living host in order to replicate (Steckelberg, 2017). First the virus attaches to the receptors of the living cell and penetrates it by fusing its membrane with the host cell's membrane (Grove & Marsh, 2011). Once inside the cell, the enzymes in the normal cell cause the coating of the viral cell to dissolve and use the host cells own enzymes to produce more viral DNA. This DNA can then be converted to viral proteins using the host cell, with the viral proteins then assembled into infectious viral particles. These particles are then either released by crossing the host cell membrane or when the host cell dies and its membrane breaks down. After the newly infected cells are released, they can infect other cells (Grove & Marsh, 2011).

Injury

Pneumothorax, or collapsed lung, can occur from several types of trauma: blunt force, penetrating trauma, medical procedures, or fractured ribs (Cleveland Clinic, 2021), but the most common cause that is not war related is road traffic accidents among adults (Anisuzzaman et al., 2019). Collapsed lungs can even appear spontaneously, most typically in tall, thin individuals. Trauma to the thoracic cavity is the cause of approximately 10%–15% of traumas globally and is more prevalent in high-income countries (Hajjar et al., 2021), ostensibly due to traffic accidents. In a study of 434 patients diagnosed with pulmonary contusion, the most common injury contributing to the 15.2% mortality rate was blunt force trauma (Mardani et al., 2021).

Blunt force injuries that result in collapsed lungs can cause air to leak out of the lungs and enter the pleural space between the lung and the thoracic cavity causing symptoms that include pain in the chest area, shortness of breath, coughing, and skin that appears blue. Diagnosis typically entails taking images of the lungs and judging the levels of oxygen and carbon dioxide in the blood. While this condition is infrequent, it can cause severe problems and must be treated as soon as possible by extracting the air occupying the space where the lung should be so it can refill with air.

(T) Mental health clinicians can benefit from understanding technology to treat respiratory illness

There are several technological advances that support the main function of the respiratory system, delivering oxygen to the brain. The level of oxygen in the blood is a measure of how well the lungs are working. Too little oxygen and too much carbon dioxide cause the system to work harder to deliver enough oxygenated blood to the brain (National Heart, Lung, and Blood Institute, n.d.). Correcting the imbalance of oxygen and carbon dioxide is critical for treating diseases of the respiratory system. There are several types of support when there is too little oxygen in the blood. The most basic and least invasive type of respiratory support is "oxygen therapy" using a two-prong nasal cannula or face mask (K. Wang et al., 2020). If the blood still has too little oxygen and too much carbon dioxide after oxygen therapy, more support is warranted, and a "continuous positive airway pressure (CPAP)" machine may be prescribed (Shelly & Nightingale, 1999). According to Shelly and Nightingale, the CPAP forces air into the lungs in a continuous way, without the trauma of intubation. Its function is to inflate the thoracic cavity and fill the alveolar sacs with oxygen. An airtight mask is fitted around the patient's nose and mouth, allowing a ventilator to provide constant pressure and increase the amount of air movement through the lungs.

If noninvasive oxygen therapy does not resolve the problem of hypoxemia or the individual is still struggling to breathe, a more severe pathology such as acute respiratory distress syndrome (ARDS) may have developed, in which case the physician may recommend more invasive methods. ARDS is characterized by trouble breathing, catching one's breath, taking deep breaths, rapid breathing, increased heart rate, and dizziness (Cleveland Clinic, 2020). ARDS is a syndrome, not a disease, and is diagnosed if symptoms occur or worsen within 1 week of the infection; opaque images are identified in the lungs in an imaging examination; and problems identified in the respiratory system are not because of cardiac problems. The severity of the diagnosis depends on the level of oxygen depletion in the lungs (Weinberger et al., 2019). Prompt action needs to be taken as ARDS is associated with death among persons with COVID-19 infection, especially if they are elderly or have chronic cardiac or kidney problems (D. Wang et al., 2020; Zhou et al., 2020).

There are several types of intubation, the most common is endotracheal intubation, where the tube is inserted through the mouth, through the vocal cords, and into the trachea. While this is extremely invasive, it is the preferred method of airway control (Shelly & Nightingale, 1999). If nonintubated treatments have not increased the individual's ability to breathe, ventilation may be the next step. This is the treatment of choice to reduce the work it takes to breathe by using a machine to assist the patient to breathe or to completely take over breathing for the patient. It is important to determine if the patient decides they don't want to be "on a machine the rest of their life" (Weinberger et al., 2019). The patient's preference on whether or not they would like to be intubated and placed on a ventilator is often found within their Medical Order for Life-Sustaining Treatment (MOLST). If the patient does not already have a MOLST, the clinician will have to work with the patient and the family to discuss treatment options and potential end-of-life decisions.

(E) Mental health clinicians can benefit from understanding the engineering of medications for COVID-19

It is important for clinicians to support clients who are hesitant to be inoculated against illnesses, including COVID-19. There are currently several types of corona viruses, four of which are minimally contagious and produce mild symptoms, while the other three are virulent highly contagious and can be lethal. They are: the severe acute respiratory syndrome coronavirus (SARS-CoV), the Middle East respiratory syndrome coronavirus (MERS-CoV), and the virus that is responsible for the current pandemic, SARS-CoV-2 and its variants. In December 2019, the coronavirus was isolated in Wuhan city in the province of Hubei, China. Ten weeks later, at the end of February 2020, WHO declared that the virus had caused a global emergency, and 2 weeks after that, in mid-March, COVID-19 was designated as a pandemic. Many cities went on "lockdown" to attempt to control the spread of the disease, with stores and schools closing, international travel restricted, and individuals warned to remain in their homes (Zhao et al., 2020).

Scientifically, the virus that causes COVID-19 is a pathogen that causes an infection, most severely in the respiratory system. Because COVID-19 is caused by a pathogen, it has antigens on its surface that the immune system can detect as foreign (Campbell, 2011b). When the body recognizes the antigens as something foreign, it attempts to kill them (George & Kishore, 2021). In the case of COVID-19, people whose immune systems are compromised are often unable to kill the virus, and it takes over their body.

Unfortunately, there is not yet a cure for COVID-19, and the public health community's best advice is to avoid contracting the illness. In addition to methods that provide personal protection, such as social distancing, wearing masks, and sanitizing hands and hard surfaces, in order to protect the public during this pandemic the medical community recommends that individuals be inoculated with a vaccine. The body reacts to the vaccine as if it were the pathogen and jump-starts the body's immune reaction by mobilizing its lymphatic system. In the process, acquired immunity is established, and if the individual comes in contact with the virus in the future, the body will recognize it as an invader that it has destroyed in the past and try to destroy it. As can be seen in Figure 7.3, the first vaccinations required the individual to be injected with the messenger ribonucleic acid (mRNA) molecule of COVID-19. The mRNA molecule is not a live virus like that of the flu vaccine (CDC, 2021b). When it enters the healthy host cell, it tells it to make spike proteins that tell other cells that the host has become viral. This causes the white blood cells to recognize them

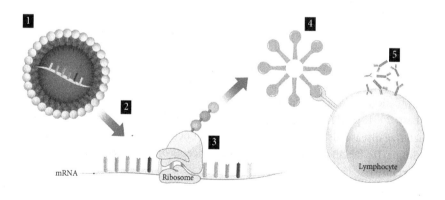

1. The encapsulation of mRNA into a lipid nanoparticle

2. Messenger RNA (mRNA) delivery into target cells

3. Ribosomes read the mRNA and produce antigens

4. Antigens presented to T cells and B cells

5. Antigens stimulate cellular immunity, and humoral immunity

Figure 7.3 The mRNA vaccine.

as invaders. Because they think the spike proteins are invaders, the cell makes antibodies that attach themselves to the spike proteins of the virus and inhibit them from infecting other cells.

Figure 7.3 shows the way the mRNA vaccine works to provide immunity. Vaccines are designed in several ways. One way is to develop an inoculation with live strains of the virus that have been made less severe, while the second way is to develop the vaccine from inactivated viruses that have been developed in the laboratory. After the vaccines are developed, they are tested on animals and then put through clinical trials with humans to determine their efficacy and safety. Several companies developed vaccines for COVID-19 that were made available to individuals who were most at risk of poor medical outcomes if they contracted the disease, as well as front-line workers and those with preexisting medical conditions. These individuals were encouraged to receive their vaccines first, followed by persons by age, beginning with older individuals (Singh et al., 2021). After individuals received the initial round of doses, booster doses were developed to fight new variants of the virus.

According to Zhao and colleagues (2020), the coronavirus has several variants, and many new variants will likely emerge as the pandemic progresses. Two of the three initial companies that had available vaccines early in the pandemic strongly encouraged the public to receive two inoculations. The variant that the public was infected with in 2019 and 2020 was the beta variant. All companies then encouraged the public to receive a booster shot to protect against a new highly virulent variant of COVID-19, the Delta variant. Because more variants developed, a second booster was recommended.

(M) Mental health clinicians can benefit from understanding the mathematics underlying epidemiology

According to the *Dictionary of Epidemiology*, epidemiology is "the study of the distribution and determinants of health-related states or events in specified populations, and the application of this study to the control of health problems" (Last, 2001, p. 61). The epidemiologists therefore need to collect data to characterize disease distribution and health event occurrence. Several key measures summarize health events, including the concepts of incidence, prevalence, and mortality.

Incidence measures the total number of newly diagnosed cases of a disease in a population during a certain period. WHO (2021) began releasing the Coronavirus Disease (COVID-19) Situation Report January 21, 2020. The situation reports summarize surveillance data such as total confirmed new COVID-19 cases, total confirmed cumulative cases, total deaths, and transmission classification. The COVID-19 data in this chapter were obtained from the WHO situation reports.

As the pandemic continued to spread like wildfire and become a regular part of the global landscape, the president of the United States declared a nationwide emergency March 13, 2020, and the country began to shut down to prevent the spread of COVID-19. Nationwide, the school districts and colleges and universities responded to the outbreak quickly, and states began widespread school closures to fight this infectious disease. Other organizations and businesses also switched their daily operations from in-person to virtual mode.

Starting May 1, 2020, the WHO situation report provided aggregated total confirmed new cases in six WHO regions: Africa, Americas, Eastern Mediterranean, Europe, Southeast Asia, and Western Pacific. The distribution of COVID-19 new cases varied across the regions: 45,727 new cases in Americas; 26,764 in Europe; 6,168 in Eastern Mediterranean countries; 3,067 new cases in Southeast Asia; 1,950 in Africa; and 1,095 new cases in the Western Pacific.

The first confirmed COVID-19 case in the United States was reported on January 21, 2020, in the state of Washington (CDC, 2020). Since then, the total number of cases grew exponentially over time. As of November 19, 2021, the cumulative confirmed cases of COVID-19 in the United States reached 47 million (47,030,792 cases), as reported by WHO (2021). The incidence of COVID-19 new cases in the United States is shown in Figure 7.4, which displays the total new COVID-19 cases in the United States using the weekly data based on the last week of each month from March 2020 to March 2021. During the last week of March 2020, there were 175,981 new confirmed cases of COVID-19. Between March and October 2020, there were some fluctuations in terms of total new cases. However, the total new cases dramatically increased during the holiday travel season from November 2020 to January 2021, and there was a surge in the chart. Then the total new cases decreased starting February 2021.

Prevalence is another measure of the occurrence of a disease. Prevalent cases are the total number of cases of a disease that exists in a population over a specified time of period. By the end of January 2020, there were only 9,826 confirmed cases in the world. However, the total cases grew continuously during the year. By the end of December 2020, the total number of confirmed COVID-19 cases in the world reached 79,231,893. With that said, 1% of the total world population was estimated to be diagnosed with this infectious disease.

Mortality is a measure for number of deaths associated with a disease. According to National Cancer Institute (2021), mortality is the total number of deaths in a certain group of people in a certain period of time. By the end of January 2020, the confirmed deaths from COVID-19 globally was 213. However, by the end of December 2020, the number of confirmed COVID-19 deaths in the world was 1,754,574, which had devastating effects on families and communities.

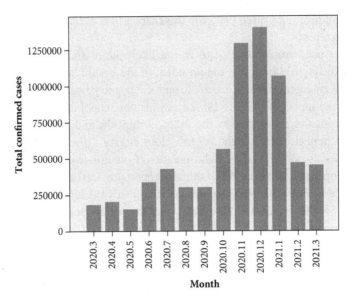

Figure 7.4 Total confirmed new cases of COVID-19, United States, March 2020 to March 2021.

Data source: WHO (2021). https://covid19.who.int/region/amro/country/us. Chart created by Dr. Liyun Wu.

Clearly, protection from exposure to the COVID-19 virus is vital for the health and security of the community.

As of November 19, 2021, total deaths from COVID-19 in the United States were 759,388 cases (WHO, 2021). Total deaths from COVID-19 in the United States from March 2020 to March 2021 are displayed in Figure 7.5. In the last week of March 2020, when the country was locked down, there were 6,658 deaths from COVID-19. The death toll doubled in the last week of April 2020, reaching 13,623 cases. However, the total deaths surged during the holiday travel season from November 2020 to January 2021, with the peak of 22,196 deaths in the last week of January 2021.

(H) Mental health clinicians can benefit from understanding how to apply STEM to health

Clinical work with patients who are making the decision to become inoculated against COVID-19 will necessitate some knowledge of viruses and vaccines. This chapter reports findings from WHO (2020b) that indicated that the COVID-19 pandemic infected many persons on each continent. Some of the

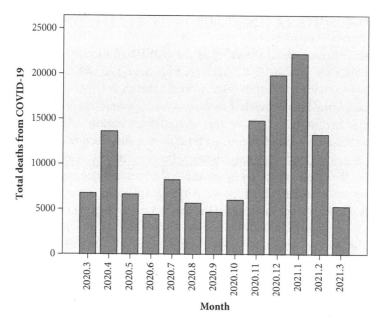

Figure 7.5 Total deaths from COVID-19, United States, March 2020 to March 2021.
Data source: WHO (2021). https://covid19.who.int/region/amro/country/us. Chart created by Dr. Liyun Wu.

people who have been infected were more at risk than others because of preexisting health problems or advanced age. While it is important to triage patients, WHO cautioned that older patients with COVID-19 are entitled to medical care equal to younger patients, even though the older patients are at higher risk for mortality. It is important for mental health clinicians who treat older clients with COVID-19 to involve the family and the individual, if possible, in decision-making and to impress on them the importance of practicing preventive measures to avoid exposure. In spite of public health officials strongly urging citizens to become inoculated against the virus, many people refused. The SAGE Working Group on Vaccine Hesitancy (2014) found three factors impeded compliance with medical advice to become vaccinated: complacency, confidence, and convenience. Confidence refers to having trust in the vaccine, while complacency refers to believing that the danger of contracting the illness is low. Convenience, the third component of the model has been addressed by public health officials, who have provided free vaccines to all citizens and made a concerted effort to provide them to low-income neighborhoods without easy access to medical facilities. The SAGE group makes a distinction between individuals who completely agree that there is a need for vaccines compared to those who completely reject the message that there is a need to be vaccinated.

They focus on the group of people in the middle group who are willing to accept some vaccines but not others.

Misinformation about the safety of the COVID-19 vaccine interfered with the compliance with the CDC's message to become vaccinated because many people were concerned that the vaccine would alter their DNA and feared losing their autonomy by biochemical manipulation. A second concern the authors presented is concern of a governmental conspiracy against citizens. This concern was also mentioned by SAGE (2014) as they discussed the contributions of the individual's cultural group's history. The concerns discussed by SAGE underscore the historical abuses by the medical community during the Tuskegee experiments, during which poor, African American sharecroppers were recruited to participate in a study of the natural course of syphilis even after penicillin, the cure for syphilis, was discovered. More recently, the case of Henrietta Lacks, an African American woman whose cancer cells were used without her or her family's knowledge or recompense, became the foundation for the cancer cell line used in clinical research. These historical abuses still are in the collective consciousness of persons of color and contribute to medical distrust.

As mental health clinicians understand, the working alliance between the client and the provider can predict adherence to a treatment regimen. As shown in a large study of adults receiving treatment for substance misuse (Connors et al., 1997), the working alliance of the clinician and client predicted treatment participation. Thus, empirical evidence suggests that the relationship of the clinician and the client may support the client's decision to accept the vaccine.

Conclusion

In conclusion, students who learn the information in this chapter will understand the science that underlies the respiratory system and the illnesses that attack the system, such as COVID-19. Mastering this material will make it possible for mental health clinicians to contribute as a medical team member or independent clinician who works with patients with illnesses of the respiratory system. Evaluating the effect of blunt force trauma to the lungs that results in a collapsed lung was discussed as well. Development of vaccines for protection against COVID-19 was discussed in the engineering section. Understanding the technology of a breathing apparatus allows the social worker to know how to discuss the patient's and family's concerns about tests and treatments that may be prescribed. While a mental health clinician is not a physician, they can help the family identify questions for the physician and work with them to problem-solve how they can carry out the physician's instructions. Finally, mathematics underlying incidence and prevalence is important to understand morbidity and mortality associated with infection. Clinicians can benefit from understanding basic scientific concepts underlying the respiratory system because their job may require them to provide clinical treatment to patients with respiratory problems. While compassion is a necessary component of clinical practice, it is not sufficient. Clinicians must rely on practice-informed research and research-informed practice.

Glossary

Disease distribution   An epidemiologic term denoting the who, what, when, and where aspects of disease profiles

Flatten the curve   When the number of new cases of an illness decreases, the slope of the line on the corresponding graph decreases

Hypoxemia   Condition that occurs when there is too little oxygen in the body

Pandemic   An epidemic that affects the entire world rather than one country

Pathogen   A microorganism that causes a disease

pH   The relationship between the acidity and alkalinity (base) of a substance; a measure of the acidity and alkalinity of a solution

Social distancing   Distancing oneself from people to stop infection from disease; current rule of thumb for respiratory illnesses is 6 feet

Websites

American Lung Association: https://www.lung.org/
American Public Health Association: https://apha.org/
Centers for Disease Control and Prevention: https://www.cdc.gov
General Provider Telehealth and Telemedicine Tool Kit: https://www.aafp.org/dam/AAFP/documents/advocacy/prevention/crisis/CMSGeneralTelemedicineToolkit.pdf
National Heart, Lung, and Blood Institute, National Institutes of Health: https://www.nhlbi.nih.gov/health-topics/how-lungs-work

8

How Understanding the Integumentary System Can Benefit Mental Health Clinicians

Introduction

There is a lot of interest in skin, particularly the color of one's skin. Pigmentation has been politicized for hundreds of years in many countries. This chapter does not address the politics involved with skin color, but instead considers STEM-H (science, technology, engineering, and mathematics as applied to health) and focuses on the scientific facts, technology, and engineering used in treating diseases and injuries to the skin and the mathematics underlying the epidemiology of diseases and injuries of the integumentary system.

STEM-H Principles Underlying the Integumentary System

(S) Mental health clinicians can benefit from understanding the science of the integumental system

Structure

The skin is the largest organ and weighs approximately 15% of total adult body weight (McGrath & Lai-Cheong, 2021). It has the property of elasticity, expanding when the individual grows in height or width and if the individual gains weight. Skin covers the entire surface area of the body as well as parts of the gustatory (nasal cavities, mouth); respiratory (throat); reproductive (genitalia); auditory (auricle, ear canal); and visual (eyelid) systems (Campbell, 2011a).

According to Singh and Archana (2008) by the 11th week of gestation, skin comprises three layers: the epidermis, the dermis, and the hypodermis. The top layer or epidermis includes the hair, nails, and sweat and sebaceous glands. It is responsible for protecting the body from environmental toxins and is the body's first layer of defense. The layer directly below the epidermis is the dermis and is responsible for housing the immune cells, lymphocytes, mast cells, and macrophages (Slominski et al., 2012). The bottom layer of the skin is the

STEM-H for Mental Health Clinicians. Marilyn Weaver Lewis, Liyun Wu, and Zachary Allan Hagen, Oxford University Press.
© Oxford University Press 2023. DOI: 10.1093/oso/9780197638514.003.0008

hypodermis and is characterized by connective and fatty tissue, which protects tissues deep within the body and provides insulation and temperature regulation (Colbert et al., 2020).

The hypodermis is also responsible for housing skin cells that divide and re-plenish dead cells. Those skin cells are renewed on a continuous basis by pushing up to the surface, where they are sloughed off daily. Approximately 500 million dead cells are replaced by new skin cells each day from the deeper regions of the epidermis (Colbert et al., 2020).

As Figure 8.1 demonstrates, the epidermis does not have a blood supply and receives its nourishment from oxygen in the environment. On the other hand, the dermis contains a blood supply and can feed nutrients up to the epidermis (Campbell, 2011a). The cells at the hypodermis are nourished by the blood supply, while the cells above them, in the epidermis, lose their moisture because,

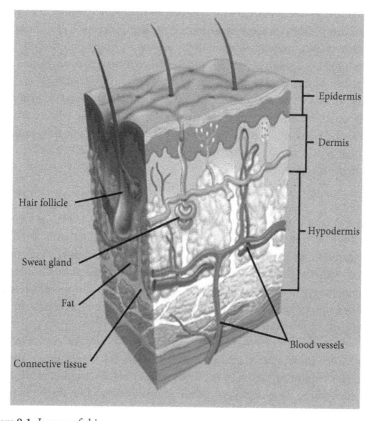

Figure 8.1 Layers of skin.

https://www.istockphoto.com/vector/human-skin-layered-epidermis-with-hair-follicle-sweat-and-sebaceous-glands-healthy-gm1262260786-369328776

as they are pushed up from the basement layer, they dry out and are sloughed off and replaced by the newer cells (Colbert et al., 2020). The corrugated-like juncture between the epidermis and the dermis keeps the cell layers from sliding off each other. In cases where there is friction between the epidermis and dermis, a blister may develop that provides a fluid-filled space between the layers (Campbell, 2011a). The hypodermis lies below the dermis and is the bottom layer of the skin. It is primarily connective tissue, adipose or fat cells, and elastin and provides insulation and energy storage (Colbert et al., 2020).

When skin ages, it loses its structural integrity, and wrinkles occur. Each layer contains collagen fibers, which lose their strength and flexibility (MedlinePlus, 2022) and become tangled, which contributes to wrinkles (Campbell, 2011a). Biochemical remedies to counteract wrinkles can alleviate the visual results somewhat, but only temporarily. Injections of fat deposits in the wrinkles are needed to hide them. Regardless, skin ages, partly because it becomes dry and partly because the juncture of the epidermis and dermis flattens, and the epidermis no longer receives hydration from the dermis (Campbell, 2011a). The individual can slow the process by hydrating the skin, perhaps by relocating to a more humid environment, or drinking more water. Aging, thinning skin that loses its moisture does so in part due to loss of activity to sebaceous glands and is easier to bruise and tear (MedlinePlus, 2020). According to MedlinePlus (2020), wounds are slower to heal and can take up to four times longer to heal in the aging population. Another consequence of aging skin that can be dangerous for patients who remain in bed or a chair for extended periods of time is the development of ulcerated sores on pressure points, often called bedsores (Mayo Clinic, n.d.).

Function

One of skin's most fascinating functions is that it contributes to neurotransmitter production (Slominski et al., 2012), accomplishing this function by producing neurohormones in response to stress, via the nerves of the spinal cord. In conjunction with the internal and external environment, the skin manufactures serotonin, acetylcholine, endorphins, opioids, cannabinoids, thyroid-releasing hormones, and corticosteroids, all of which are used in the nervous system for neurologic transmission.

In addition to protection, the skin's function is to prevent excessive water loss in order to support thermoregulation (Kolarsick et al., n.d.). The epidermis can send information to the brain about the temperature, to which the body responds by developing gooseflesh and shivering when the body is cold (McGrath & Lai-Cheong, 2021) and sweating when the temperature is hot. There are approximately 2 to 4 million sweat glands in the average person, although they differ among people depending on the climate where they reside

(Campbell, 2011a). As their function is to cool the body, they are more plentiful in people who evolved in hotter climates. The eccrine sweat gland begins in the lower part of the dermis layer and extends up to the surface of the skin, where it releases an odorless sweat from a duct at the surface of the skin (Kolarsick et al., 2011). According to Kolarsick and colleagues, the other type of sweat gland is the apocrine sweat gland, which is found at the scalp, armpits, groin, and anus areas. It has an odor that is thought to have sociosexual components and develops at puberty.

The dermis houses the immune cells: the lymphocytes, mast cells, and macrophages (McGrath & Lai-Cheong, 2021). The number and activity of these cells depend on internal and environmental homeostasis and thermoregulation (Slominski et al., 2012). Below the dermis, the hypodermis protects tissues deep within the body, nourishes the epidermis with nutrients, and provides insulation and temperature regulation to the body (Colbert et al., 2020). The layer below the epidermis, the dermis, comprises the bulk of the skin and provides the give and take the skin needs to maintain its shape and remain intact with the individual's movement (Kolarsick et al., 2011).

Illness

There are two types of skin cancer: nonmelanoma and melanoma. Nonmelanoma skin cancer (NMSC) is the most common type of cancer and begins in the epidermal layer of the skin. It is estimated that 5.4 million Americans will develop NMSC during their lifetime (American Cancer Society, 2020). The death rate from skin cancer in the United States is 2,000 per year (cancer.net, 2020) These types of cancer are typically more common in older people but are becoming more prevalent among young people, perhaps because of exposure to more ultraviolet (UV) light from suntanning beds and because exposure to natural light that is more dangerous because of loss of the protection from the ozone layer (Christensen et al., 2005). Skin cancer is the most common type of cancer; however, because of its superficial location, it is often treated before spreading to other parts of the body.

Basal cell cancers (BCCs) and squamous cell cancers (SCCs) are the most common type of nonmelanoma skin cancers and occur most often as the result of overexposure to sunlight (American Cancer Society, 2020). People with light skin are more at risk for these types of cancer than persons with darker skin because dark skin is protected by melanin. Persons with dark skin, however, can acquire squamous cell cancer of the skin that is damaged by burns and scars.

Squamous cell cancers comprise approximately 20% of the skin cancers and occur in the upper layer of the epidermis. They grow rapidly and are more likely to invade adjacent areas than basal cell cancers (McDaniel et al., 2022). SCCs are related to sun exposure and mainly occur on the face, neck, and hands, but occasionally in scars (Xiang et al., 2019). They appear as discrete, solitary, demarcated growths that are scaly, pink-to-red pustules or thin plaques.

Basal cell cancers are more common and less deadly. BCCs are responsible for 25% of all cancers and for 75% of all skin cancers. They occur in the deeper layer of the epidermis and rarely metastasize. BCCs grow slowly, but if not treated they can grow down into deeper layers of the skin and ultimately to the bone (cancer. net, 2020). They can be removed by surgical methods but can grow back, often in the same area. Although this type of cancer rarely metastasizes, if it does, the average survival time ranges from 8 to 10 months.

Melanoma skin cancer (MSC) is the rarest (comprising 1% of skin malignancies) and the deadliest (cancer.net, 2020). It is responsible for 60% of skin cancer deaths, an estimated 6,850 deaths per year in the United States. It is more common among Caucasians, persons who use tanning beds regularly before age 30, those who have a family history of melanoma, and those who have sensitivity and burn in the sun (Strayer & Reynolds, 2003). The clinical identification of melanoma skin cancer can be thought of as meeting the ABCDE criteria: asymmetry; border (irregularity is more likely cancerous); color (multiple colors in one lesion); diameter (>6 mm); and evolution (change over time) (Strayer & Reynolds, 2003).

Marjolin's ulcers have been termed "burn scar carcinomas." Although they are rare, occurring in 0.7% of patients seeking medical treatment, they are potentially lethal (Yu et al., 2013). In an extensive literature review of 412 cases, 95% of those with burn scar carcinoma had not had their injuries excised or grafted (Kowal-Vern & Criswell, 2005). With the practice of modern medicine in developed countries, burn scar carcinomas are rare. The authors found that presence of burn scar carcinomas were more common than cancers from squamous cells (71%), while basal cell cancers (12%), melanoma (6%), sarcoma (5%), and other types of cancers (6%) were evident in the study sample. Persons who were burned while they were young had a longer latency before cancer was evident, whereas patients who were burned later in life had a shorter latency period. The patient's average age of tumor diagnosis was 50 years, with latency since the burn 31 years. The mortality rate was 12%.

Injuries

Burns can be caused by several sources, including fire, electricity, radioactivity, and chemicals. They are the fifth most common cause of accidental death in the United States and the sixth most common cause of deaths among persons aged 5 to 14 years (Mock et al., 2008). Burn-related deaths are common in countries with primitive cooking and heating methods, causing 70% of burn injuries (World Health Organization, 2018). Persons in less developed countries who use oil fires for heat and cooking are susceptible to experiencing accidental burns, with persons living in Southeast Asia most at risk for burn-related deaths (Mock et al., 2008). Among military personnel, burns are a common result of explosions of improvised explosive devises (IEDs). According to the U.S. Department of Homeland Security, IEDs are homemade explosives made with a fuel source comprising combustible material (e.g., fertilizer, gunpowder), an oxidizer to ignite the fuel (ammonium nitrate), and usually an enhancer (e.g., shrapnel, metal fragments, nails) to inflict damage from flying debris. IEDs are designed to kill, maim, and incite terror and may be in the form of a pipe bomb (explosive capacity = 5 pounds), a delivered package (explosive capacity = 1–10 pounds), or a delivery truck (explosive capacity = 10,000 pounds) (Department of Homeland Security, 2020). In addition to burns, they can cause damage from extreme pressure to the bodily organs, flying fragments, and the impact from being thrown or hit by flying objects, which are uncommon in noncombat situations (Centers for Disease Control and Prevention, 2020).

One way to assess the severity of burns is by the Wallace "rule of nines" (A. B. Wallace, 1951), which depicts the amount of the affected area of the body. The body is visualized as divided into smaller areas that are approximately 9% of the full-body area. The head and neck of the adult represent 9% of the body, each upper limb 9%, and each side of the lower limbs is 9% (18% total for each leg), the front of the torso represents 18%, as does the back of the torso and the buttocks, 18%. The peritoneum and the anal and urogenital areas are represented by 1% (Colbert et al., 2020). Generally the size of an adult palm represents approximately 1% of the total body surface area, and this estimation may be used to determine the size of smaller burns. The child's measurements differ. The head and neck constitute 18%, each side of the torso is counted as 18%, the upper extremities are 9% each, the lower extremities are 13% each, and the anus. The prognosis depends in large part on the total body surface area that is affected.

Jeschke and colleagues (2015) reported that among adults, TBSA greater than 42% was correlated with infection and 44% or more with mortality. Among pediatric patients, a total surface area greater than 50% was associated with infections, while total body surface area greater than 60% was correlated with mortality. Elderly patients were most at risk from burns, and mortality was associated with total body surface area greater than 30%. Jeschke and colleagues suggested that these differences in morbidity and mortality were related to the difference in the immune systems of these groups.

In addition to the total body surface area that is affected, burn severity may be correlated by location of the burns. Burns that involve joints, the face, hands, or genitals are considered more severe. Burns that completely surround a part of the body are considered "circumferential," and their healing process can constrict the affected body part. In some cases, the burn is so severe in the chest wall that the charred skin must be surgically split to prevent the burned skin from restricting the patient's breathing (Campbell, 2011b). Because of complications that occur with these extensive burns, individuals who have suffered burns with the above risk factors are required to receive specialized burn care to minimize complications.

Burns are also categorized based on the depth of the burn, as shown in Figure 8.2. There are two types of burns: partial thickness and full thickness (Colbert et al., 2020). According to Colbert and colleagues, first-degree burns damage the first layer of the epidermis, which becomes painful and turns red, but doesn't blister. The burned skin sloughs off, or peels, but doesn't result in scarring. First-degree burns often occur from too much exposure to the sun and are more common in persons with very light skin, as they produce less melanin to protect from sun exposure. Second-degree burns damage the first and second layers of epidermis and typically cause a blister, the size of which also depends on the depth of the burn. The length of time it takes for the skin to recover depends

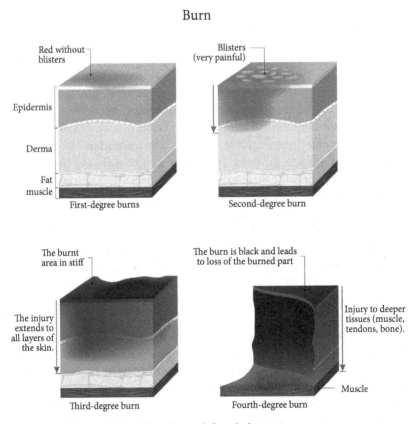

Figure 8.2 Degrees of burn: First through fourth degree.

on the depth of the burn. Second-degree burns that involve only the epidermis can take up to 14 days to heal, while second-degree burns that extend deep into the dermis can take up to 14 weeks to heal and typically involve scarring and the potential for infection (Warby & Maani, 2021). Full-thickness burns include third- and fourth-degree burns and extend down into the entire layer of the skin, often to the bone. The wound is healed in part from regeneration of the viable skin that is around the wound (Campbell, 2011b). Third-degree burns are so deep that the pain receptors are destroyed. The skin can turn waxy and white, dark brown, or black and result in scarring. Third-degree burns are susceptible to infection, thereby threatening recovery, which can result in death. Fourth-degree burns are also considered full-thickness burns because they damage all layers of the skin. The skin becomes charred and changes colors as it does with third-degree burns. Fourth-degree burns damage the structure of the skin by killing the pain receptors, hair follicles, and sweat glands. They can extend down to the muscle, tendons, and bone. Fourth-degree burns are life threatening, and while victims of fourth-degree burns do not feel pain, the risk of infection is very high, often resulting in amputations and death (Colbert et al., 2020).

Consequences of burns include the possibility of introduction of bacteria into the body. Burns disrupt the function of skin and can result in dehydration and inability to regulate temperature. Burns destroy the composition of the skin and can place the wound at risk for invasion of toxins, including those from accelerants and charred particulates circulating in the air. Treatment involves avoiding infections (Souto et al., 2020), which can range from those caused by bacteria (e.g., *Escherichia coli, Staphylococcus*, and methicillin-resistant *Staphylococcus aureus*); to viruses (e.g., herpes simplex, varicella-zoster) to fungi (*Candida, Aspergillus*).

Burns that kill cells disrupt the body's natural immunity, and the body becomes unable to make antibody-secreting cells that normally fight off the infection. The body loses plasma after third- and fourth-degree burns, and the person is susceptible to shock (Bruslind, 2020). When bacteria or fungi enter the wound, they adhere to it and cause changes that allow them to avoid immune system responses that would ordinarily kill them. According to Bruslind, the changes in the immune response cause more bacteria to migrate to the site of the wound. The bacteria are coated in a slime layer that protects them from being destroyed by antibiotics and white blood cells responsible for devouring bacteria (phagocytes) and helps the bacteria adhere to and infect other cells. Burn patients also require large volumes of intravenous fluids as their burned skin can no longer insulate the area of the burn.

Skin repair occurs in four stages: Stage 1 is a critical stage because burns cause leakage of blood to the interstitial fluid outside of the blood vessels; the first reaction of the body is to initiate hemostasis to stop the bleeding. During that first stage the blood vessels vasoconstrict to stop the bleeding. Vasoconstriction causes platelets to stick together and form a clot to prevent microorganisms from entering the body (Koh & DiPietro, 2013). In electrical burns, this vasoconstriction will often hide damage to underlying blood vessels, and significant bleeding can occur hours to days later once these vessels are no longer constricted. The second stage of wound healing is the inflammation stage, during which swelling occurs that protects the wound. Inflammation allows blood clots to secrete enzymes that cause the white blood cells (lymphocytes) to migrate to the wound to kill the invading microorganisms that inhibit healing (Koh & DiPietro, 2013). During the third stage of proliferation, new cells are created that are involved with nerve regeneration and secretion of proteins (cytokines) that initiate the immune response (Zhang & An, 2007). They fill the wound with new tissue and blood vessels, which results in drawing the edges of the wound together, thus creating a scaffold of cells to cover the wound. The cytokines initiate the formation of a temporary extracellular matrix (ECM), which maintains homeostasis and water retention and provides structure to the wound (Frantz et al., 2010). During the fourth stage, the ECM remains until a scar forms during the remodeling stage (Souto et al., 2020). During remodeling, the wound becomes firmer because elastin fibers attach themselves to the wound bed. The phase can last up to 12 months. Depending on whether the wound is kept dry and not traumatized or infected, the length of time it takes for the wound to recover depends on the depth of the wound. The tissue never reaches its pretrauma strength and only recovers approximately 80% of its strength (H. A. Wallace et al., 2020). Often, skin grafts from nonburned areas are required to speed up skin regeneration. Common donor sites include the thighs and buttocks.

(T) Mental health clinicians can benefit from understanding the technology used to treat injuries from improvised explosive device

Improvised explosive devices (IEDs) caused 5% of all casualties from Operation Iraqi Freedom and Operation Enduring Freedom (Kauvar et al., 2006). According to Kauvar and colleagues, over half of burn injuries were the result of explosive devices. While most of the troops were injured while driving and received injuries to multiple body parts, their hands and their face sustained most of the burns (hands 80%; face and head 75%). Combat burns often injure multiple body systems from inhalation of toxic chemicals and trauma (Driscoll et al., 2018). The military developed an array of burn care advances during wartime that have benefited the general public, including stabilization of burn injuries during war zone evacuation (Driscoll et al., 2018); autofluorescent imaging for identifying underlying bacteria and evaluating debridement (Blumenthal & Jeffery, 2018); hemofiltration for treatment of burn-related renal failure during in-flight evacuation (Driscoll et al., 2018); and wound care using ketamine and immersive virtual reality procedures for pain (Maani et al., 2011).

Because burn injuries can be extensive and difficult to manage, a variety of technological devices are needed to respond to each symptom. Treatment of burns includes repairing the integrity of the skin. Several techniques have been used, including application of grafts to the affected areas. There are several common sources of material for grafts. Grafting human fetal cells or cadaver or animal skin is the primary technological technique used to treat burns (Shpichka et al., 2019). An autograft is made from tissue from the burn victim's own body and is preferred because it avoids immune rejection. A drawback is that the number of healthy cells needed may be more that the patient (host) has that are available for transfer to the wound site. An allograft is tissue from another person or species. The source is potentially unlimited but is associated with a high rejection rate. Human fetal cells, especially the epidermal layer, provide another type of tissue for an allograft. It is effective because the cells release growth-facilitating substances. They show plasticity and can divide into new cells and differentiate into different cell types. They also inhibit growth of natural killer (NK) cells and T cells, which decrease the immune response to a graft, but ethical dilemmas limit its acceptance (Shpichka et al., 2019). While the human fetal cell is the preferred material for skin grafts following burn injuries, it is not the treatment of choice on the battlefield because human fetal cells require extensive chemical processing to prepare them for application (Magnusson et al., 2017). Fish skin, on the other hand, doesn't require the harsh processing that is needed for fetal cell grafts and protects the structure from breaking down and eliminating helpful antiviral and antibacterial components. Fish skin grafts have been shown to act as a barrier against bacteria while remaining porous and initiate cell growth at the graft. The authors maintained that because fish skin is effective and more practical on the battlefield, it is preferable to stem cells (Magnusson et al., 2017).

(E) Mental health clinicians can benefit from understanding engineering in burn treatment

Preventing infection is paramount in burn care. Topical and systemic antibiotics as well as newer use of oral probiotics have been used to prevent resistance of the body to antibiotics (Fijan et al., 2019) and stimulate the immune reaction. There are several classes of medications that are common treatments for burns. For first-degree burns, people are advised to use aloe vera gel, an antibiotic cream, and over-the-counter analgesic. Victims of second-degree burns are advised to use an antibiotic cream containing silver (silver sulfadiazine) and over-the-counter pain medications (Cleveland Clinic, 2020). For more serious and life-threatening burns, however, there is a range of medication that is typically used that includes medication to combat dehydration (intravenous fluids of Ringer's lactate); infections (burn creams/antibiotic and antibacterial/antimicrobial/silver sulfadiazine or silver-impregnated dressings); tetanus (tetanus shot); anxiety (benzodiazepines); and pain (opioids/morphine, fentanyl) (Mayo Clinic, 2020b).

According to Patterson and colleagues (2004), burns that require hospitalization often cause severe pain and are the most difficult to treat compared to other sources of acute pain. There are several origins of severe pain: background pain from the burn (although very deep burns kill many nerve endings associated with pain); pain from tissue damage; pain from procedures, including cleaning the wound, debridement (excising necrotic tissue and making a clean wound bed), surgical processes of harvesting and applying grafts, applying and removing gauze and staples; breakthrough pain when the analgesics are inadequate (Patterson et al., 2004) and postsurgical procedures to repair wounds and scars (Griggs et al., 2017).

There are several medications that are often prescribed for analgesia. The gold standard includes opioid derivatives, primarily morphine, but also including fentanyl, clonidine, oxycodone, and rarely even methadone. Some patients develop anxiety and even post-traumatic stress disorder from painful medical procedures during treatment and are prescribed anxiolytics (benzodiazepines) before the procedures (Patterson et al., 2004). Because the patient often needs extended medical care, chronic administration of opioids results in physiological tolerance, and the physician must increase the dose to achieve the results that were previously met with a lower dose. A balance between titrating the amount of the opioid needed to alleviate pain while still protecting the patient from overdosing may be difficult. There are patient differences that need to be addressed in the treatment of pain. They include the site of administration, the medication, and the route of administration (oral, intravenous, transdermal patch). Clinical decisions depend on the location, the severity, and the extent of the burn, as well as the health of the patient and potential for infection (Patterson et al., 2004). Early in burn treatment, intravenous pain medication is often required, and patients are preferably switched to oral pain medication before discharge home.

Patterson and colleagues (2004) stated that patient-controlled analgesia (PCA) may be effective in reducing the patient's anxiety from inability to manage their treatment. The patient may activate the pump whenever they perceive pain until they have reached their limit medication they have been prescribed. The machine is programmed to administer a predetermined dose of the narcotic within a prescribed window of time. The patient cannot self-administer more doses per hour or more drug per dose than prescribed by the physician. The patient self-administers the medication by using a handheld device that when activated causes a machine to dispense a measured dose of the medication through an intravenous line that is inserted into the patient. When the patient has received the prescribed number of doses, the patient is "locked out," and the machine stops infusing the medication.

While there have been examples of tragic overdoses from runaway pumps or apparatuses that were incorrectly installed, PCA has been used successfully since 1975 to treat pain by putting pain control into the patient's own hands. PCA pumps may also partially protect a patient from overdose, as the patient will often be sedated and no longer able to press the button. However, this protection also requires the prescribed dosages to be appropriate. Perception of pain is subjective and is difficult to quantify. The PCA provides the patient the opportunity to alleviate their pain rather than rely on nurses, who may perceive their pain to be less than the patient or the family reports, thereby undertreating it (Hla et al., 2014).

The subjective perception of pain can be exacerbated by anxiety, making it difficult to control the pain. The patient's anxiety is related to an increase in their perception of pain and the increased need for medication. According to Griggs and colleagues (2017), anxiolytics are used for anxiety about upcoming painful procedures and have been shown to be effective. Antipsychotic medications have been successful in reducing procedural pain, especially in the case of anxiety. Ketamine, originally used to sedate animals, has been used as an alternative to anxiolytics and as an adjunct to morphine (Maani et al., 2011). The euphoric dosages of ketamine used recreationally are far above the amount of medication needed for pain control, making psychoactive side effects of appropriately dosed ketamine rare.

(M) Mental health clinicians can benefit from understanding the mathematics of the incidence of burns

Data reporting burn injuries from the National Hospital Ambulatory Medical Care Survey (NHAMCS) were collected by the National Center for Health Statistics (NCHS, 2021) to provide nationally representative sample surveys on ambulatory care visits to hospital emergency departments in the United States. All the burn injury data from 2011 to 2018 were collected that were accessible at the NCHS websites (NCHS, 2021). According to the 2011 NHAMCS emergency departments, there were 460,000 patients with burn injuries receiving medical treatment. The American Burn Association (2016) estimates were 406,000

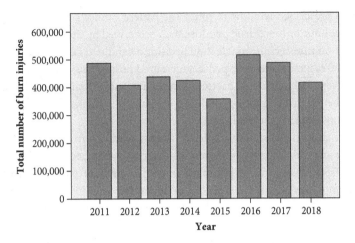

Figure 8.3 Number of burn injuries receiving medical treatment at emergency department visits, United States, 2011–2018.

Note: Data are expressed as total number of injuries.

Data source: National Hospital Ambulatory Medical Care Survey—Emergency department summary tables 2011 to 2018. https://www.cdc.gov/nchs/ahcd/web_tables.htm#2011. Chart created by Dr. Liyun Wu.

burns occurred during 2012; 436,000 in 2013; 424,000 in 2014; 356,000 in 2015; 516,000 in 2016; 489,000 in 2017; and 416,000 in 2018. Figure 8.3 summarizes the total number of patients with burn injuries who received treatment in an emergency department in the United States from 2011 to 2018. The total number of burns was elevated in some years and lower in other years. Thus, there was no clear increase or decrease in burn incidence during the previous decade.

Skin cancer has been recognized by the American Academy of Dermatology (AAD) as the most common cancer in the United States, and one in five Americans will develop skin cancer by the age of 70 (AAD, 2021). These alarming numbers raise the awareness needed to bring about necessary improvements. As stated previously, there are two main types of skin cancer: melanoma and nonmelanoma. This section presents the latest data about melanoma skin cancer. As indicated by Figure 8.4, at the beginning of the millennium, the rate of new skin cancer cases increased from 16.1 per 100,000 in 2000 to 23.1 new cases per 100,000 people during 2017. In addition to the increase in annual rates of new cancers, annual number of new melanoma cases rose rapidly over the past two decades.

As indicated by Figure 8.5, there were only 44,171 new cases of melanoma skin cancers in 2000. However, the total new cases were nearly doubled in 2017, with an alarming number of 87,211. Despite the fact that there was a small decrease of

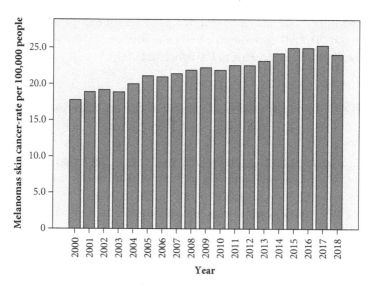

Figure 8.4 New cases of skin cancer melanomas, United States, 2000–2018.

Note: Data are expressed as rate per 100,000 persons.

Data source: Centers for Disease Control and Prevention. United States Cancer Statistics home. https://gis.cdc.gov/Cancer/USCS/#/Trends. Chart created by Dr. Liyun Wu.

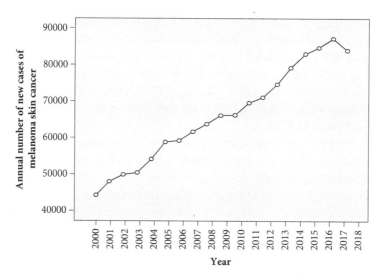

Figure 8.5 New cases of skin cancer melanomas, United States, annually from 2000 to 2018.

Data source: Centers for Disease Control and Prevention. United States Cancer Statistics home. https://gis.cdc.gov/Cancer/USCS/#/Trends. Chart created by Dr. Liyun Wu.

new cases in 2018, the melanoma incidence rate remained high in the previous decade, and the AAD encouraged everyone to perform regular skin self-exams and protect skin from exposure to UV light (2021).

(H) Mental health clinicians can benefit from applying STEM to the health of burn victims

Patients who are recovering from burn injuries are often cared for by family members. According to Kauvar et al. (2006), 91% of the servicemen and servicewomen who were being treated in a U.S. military burn unit returned home to their family's care. Caregiving can be burdensome for the family and tax their economic, emotional, and physical resources. The degree of caregiver burden experienced by those family members depends, in part, on caregiver demographic characteristics. Hughes and colleagues (1999) reported that lower levels of burden were experienced among caregivers who were older than 65 years old, African American, not living in poverty, residing with the patient, or when less care needed by the patient. As caregiver burden is higher when the patient suffers from a mental illness, mental health problems that develop among patients in response to facial disfigurement, loss of social and economic status, and lack of function can increase caregiver burden (Hughes et al., 1999). Bonsu et al. (2019) reported that higher levels of quality of life among caregivers was correlated with increased social support, which decreases the caregiver's burden, regardless of whether it is actually received or simply perceived to be available. This is critical because providing support is essential as it is associated with the caregiver's objective and subjective quality of life (Hughes et al., 1999) and ultimately the quality of care they provide and their decision to maintain the patient at home (Shah et al, 2010).

Clinicians provide tangible support to patients and families of burn victims by instructing caregivers about the medical consequences of their loved one's condition and recovery process, which improves their ability to communicate with the medical team (Walton, 2011). Clinicians identify sources of financial support for patients who have lost income when they are unable to work, providing linkages and often arranging for services to restore the patient's residential space that was damaged by the fire (Christiaens et al., 2015). Clinicians often provide assistance in coordinating posthospital care with the medical team (Walton, 2011) or with in-home burn care professionals, who provide instruction regarding application of lotions, salves, pressurized garments (Christiaens et al., 2015), and wound care, which Schultz and colleagues (2018) found were 24.2% of caregivers in a study of severely ill patients. Clinicians can also provide emotional support to caregivers, which lessens their burden and improves their quality of life (Hughes et al., 1999). As patients and caregivers often experience isolation and need support to engage in social relationships, providing emotional support may be required, often using telemedicine. Clinicians who interact with caregivers or patients who have experienced serious burns provide important aspects of tangible, instructional, and emotional support. They are valuable members of medical teams that interface with physicians, nurses, physical therapists, plastic surgeons, and psychiatrists in their role as providers of care.

Conclusion

Students who have mastered the information in this chapter will be prepared to work in hospitals or at home with patients who have experienced burns or developed cancer. Mental health clinicians will be able to work as team members on medical units or in private practice if licensed. Having an understanding of the structure and function of the integumentary system will give clinicians the vocabulary needed to understand clients' conditions and to communicate with medical team members. Knowing the different types of cancer is important because it is a common problem that clients and families may have. Clients may have been burned because of military action, house fires, or fires as the result of car accidents. Understanding the suffering inherent in treatment of burns will help the mental health clinician develop empathy for the patient and understand the difficulty with pain management. Information about skin grafts has been presented as well as incidence and prevalence of treatment at emergency departments for burn-related injuries. Overall, this chapter provided the clinician with information needed to understand basic concepts and terminology used when treating persons with problems related to the integumentary system.

Glossary

Allograft   Skin graft made from skin other than the patient's skin
Autograft   Skin moved from one place on a patient and moved to another place
Dermis   Layer of skin below the epidermis; contains blood vessels, lymph vesicles, nerves
Ectoderm   Outside layer of embryo that gives rise to the nervous system and some body parts

Epidermis   Superficial layer of skin containing nerves but no blood vessels
Hemostasis   Stopping flow of blood
Hypodermis   Bottom layer of skin

Websites

American Cancer Society: https://www.cancer.org/
World Health Organization: https://www.who.int/

9

How Understanding the Musculoskeletal System Can Benefit Mental Health Clinicians

Introduction

There are three types of muscles in the human body: skeletal, cardiac, and smooth. Skeletal muscles are the focus of this chapter because they are intricately dependent on the muscular system and vice versa. The skeletal muscular system encases the skeleton from the head to the feet. If the body did not have bones, we would not have a three-dimensional form. On the other hand, muscles are critical for voluntary movements, which support the ability to carry out intentional behaviors. Muscles work in tandem with the skeleton to allow movement and to effect change in the environment (Clemente, 1985). While many researchers have devoted their careers to finding a cure for catastrophic diseases that afflict motor neurons, they have not been altogether successful. Clinicians need to become familiar with the concepts and terminology of the musculoskeletal system because it is impacted by serious diseases and injuries their clients may face. As Figure 9.1 shows, these two systems are intertwined. Thus, this chapter focuses on the structure and function of each system and their application to STEM-H (science, technology, engineering, and mathematics as applied to health).

STEM-H Principles Underlying the Musculoskeletal System

(S) Mental health clinicians can benefit from understanding the science underlying musculoskeletal systems

Structure

Structure of the muscular system. The muscular system is a collections of muscle cells that form cables in the body (Adams, 2021). Their main property is that the fibers are able to contract and relax. Skeletal muscles are under a healthy person's voluntary control. Figure 9.2 depicts the anatomy of muscle fiber, which consists of a group of rod-like structures that are encased by a layer of connective

STEM-H for Mental Health Clinicians. Marilyn Weaver Lewis, Liyun Wu, and Zachary Allan Hagen, Oxford University Press.
© Oxford University Press 2023. DOI: 10.1093/oso/9780197638514.003.0009

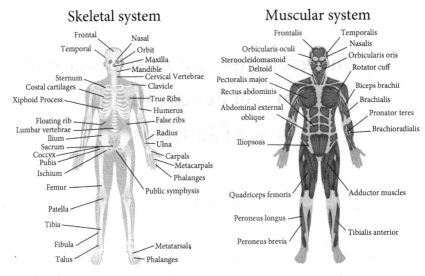

Skeletal system

Frontal
Nasal
Temporal
Orbit
Maxilla
Mandible
Cervical Vertebrae
Sternum
Clavicle
Costal cartilages
Xiphoid Process
True Ribs
Humerus
False ribs
Floating rib
Lumbar vertebrae
Radius
Ilium
Ulna
Sacrum
Coccyx
Carpals
Pubis
Metacarpals
Ischium
Phalanges
Femur
Public symphysis
Patella
Tibia
Fibula
Metatarsals
Talus
Phalanges

Muscular system

Frontalis
Temporalis
Nasalis
Orbicularis oculi
Orbicularis oris
Sternocleidomastoid
Rotator cuff
Deltoid
Pectoralis major
Biceps brachii
Rectus abdominis
Brachialis
Abdominal external
oblique
Pronator teres
Brachioradialis
Iliopsoas
Quadriceps femoris
Adductor muscles
Peroneus longus
Peroneus brevis
Tibialis anterior

Figure 9.1 Muscular and skeletal systems.

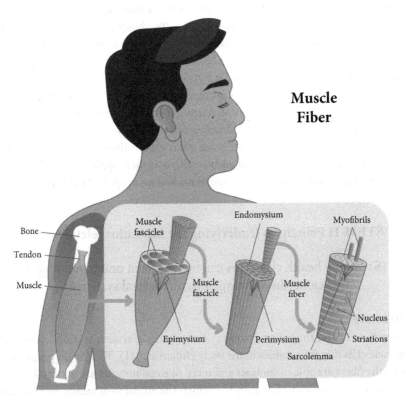

Muscle Fiber

Bone
Tendon
Muscle
Muscle
fascicles
Endomysium
Myofibrils
Muscle
fascicle
Muscle
fiber
Epimysium
Perimysium
Nucleus
Striations
Sarcolemma

Figure 9.2 Anatomy of the muscle fiber.

tissue. Smaller cable-like structures comprise the fiber. The word *myo-* means muscle, and myofibrils denote muscle fibers, which are smaller groups of rods that run parallel. If you have ever seen a metal cable that tows a car or a boat, you can see that even though the cable looks as if it is one entity, on closer examination you will see that the cable consists of smaller cables that are grouped together. If those smaller cables are inspected, you would be able to see that they comprise smaller cables. The small muscle fibers run parallel and are encased by a sarcolemma, or sheath, providing even more strength.

Ligaments are connected to bones to create levers and pulleys to move the skeleton. For example, each tapered end of the bicep muscle becomes a tendon. The tendon is attached to the bones of the upper and lower arm to create a joint that allows the individual to move their arm up and down. Muscles are arranged in pairs that work opposite of each other (Campbell, 2011): The bicep can contract to pull the arm, while the tricep relaxes to allow the arm to be pulled. The arm cannot move sideways at the elbow. If the tendons were not attached, the elbow would not move. When the muscle fibers contract, they pull the tendons closer together, which in turn pulls two bones together. This movement takes place as the muscles shorten and lengthen when they slide back and forth (Davis et al., 2020). Bones are only pulled together, never normally pulled apart (Britton, 2018), and are unable to do so without muscles.

According to Westbrook and colleagues (2020), there are 650 skeletal muscles in the human body. Those muscles can be broken down into 11 major muscle groups, with each of these groups made up of many muscles: four in each arm (forearm, bicep, triceps, and shoulder); three in each leg (quadricep, hamstring, and calf); and four in the body's core (abdomen, chest, upper back, and lower back) (Kahn Academy, 2012). Muscles are further named based on their location (e.g., pectoralis major, gluteus maximus); shape (e.g., deltoids, trapezius); action (flexors, extensors); number of divisions (biceps, triceps, quadriceps); direction (e.g., obliques, transversus abdominis); and where they are attached (omohyoid) (Clemente, 1985; Colbert et al., 2020). There are 42 muscles in the face! They are responsible for expressions and the ability to move the eyes and the mouth and tongue for chewing and talking.

The muscle size and shape can change in response to voluntary use, or they can atrophy, or waste away, from lack of use. When muscles are stimulated by muscle neurons, they secrete the neurochemical acetylcholine, which changes the membranes that cover the muscle neurons and cause the muscles to extend or contract (Colbert et al., 2020). When the muscles extend and contract, they stretch and then recoil much like an elastic band. Because of elasticity, the muscle is able to stretch easily but retain its ability to resume its original form after stretching (Clemente, 1985). If the neurochemical conduction between the nervous system and the musculoskeletal system is impaired and the muscles no longer receive input from the nervous system, they can atrophy, or waste away. In cases where individuals have diseases that affect the muscles, the person may not be able to contract or relax their muscles and lose their range of motion.

The muscles are connected by tendons that are malleable and allow the muscles to move. Several muscles extend from the pelvis to meet at the same place (patella). Their strength is further reinforced by wrapping around the bones and providing stability and strength. Without the muscular system, the bones would not be able to move, and without the skeletal system, the muscles would not be attached to the body.

Structure of the skeletal system . The cartilaginous bones develop on the outside and in the inside simultaneously. At the inside center of the bone, a cavity is formed by calcium, which creates crystal-like forms that act like a scaffold, holding up the spongy bone around the vacant space, while the outside of the bone is sheathed by a hard calcium substance that creates a compact bone that provides structure (Clemente, 1985). The compact bone contains yellow marrow of fat and stem cells that can become fat, cartilage, or bone. The ends of the bones contain red marrow that houses the stem cells that can become red or white blood cells or platelets (National Cancer Institute, n.d.).

The structure of the skeletal component of the musculoskeletal system comprises a total of 206 bones that make up the axial skeleton (vertebra [26 bones], skull [28 bones], hyoid bone [1], ribs, and sternum [25]) and the appendicular skeleton (upper [64] and lower [62] extremities) (Clemente, 1985). Bones are classified based on their shape: long bones, which are found in the arms (e.g., humerus, radius, ulna) and legs (e.g., femur, tibia, fibula); short bones, which are found in the wrists (e.g., carpals, metacarpals, phalanges) and ankles (e.g., tarsals, metatarsals); flat bones (e.g., ribs, scapula, breastbone); and irregular bones (coxal hip bones, mandible, cervical vertebrae, inner ear bones) (Colbert et al., 2020).

There are 22 bones in the skull; 8 are cranial bones that protect the brain, and 14 are facial bones that give the face its form (Anderson et al., 2021). There is only one bone that can move, and that is the jawbone, or mandible. At birth, the cranial bones have not joined together, and the baby has a "fontanelle" or soft spot on top of their head until the bones grow together. In the adult, all the other bones fit tightly together with sutures. The skull has two holes: One, the external auditory meatus, is in the lower temporal area and is the opening for the inner ear (Anderson et al., 2021). The other hole is at the base of the brain for the spinal cord.

There are three sections of the bone, as you can see in Figure 9.3. The distal area that is at each end of the bone is the epiphysis and is the part of the bone that grows and lengthens in children. The epiphyseal plate is the area below the epiphysis and above the shaft of the bone, or the diaphysis. The area between the

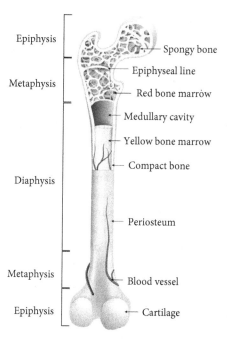

Epiphysis

Metaphysis

Diaphysis

Metaphysis

Epiphysis

Spongy bone

Epiphyseal line

Red bone marrow

Medullary cavity

Yellow bone marrow

Compact bone

Periosteum

Blood vessel

Cartilage

Figure 9.3 Bone anatomy.

epiphysis and diaphysis is known as the metaphysis. The shaft contains the nutrient canal where marrow is made (Clarke, 2008). Bones are living things that are made of minerals, specifically calcium. They begin to develop as cartilage during gestation and do not become calcified until the child is several years old. A normal human's bone growth is rapid, begins during gestation, and continues during early childhood and into adolescence. Bone constantly undergoes "remodeling" through actions of osteoblasts and osteoclasts. Osteoblasts lay down new bone and mineralize it (Wolf, 2008). Later, vitamin D and certain hormones signal osteoclasts to resorb the old bone by removing its minerals, thus breaking it down. This cycle repeats itself unless it is disrupted, as is the case with osteoporosis, when the actions of the osteoclasts outpace the actions of the osteoblasts (Wick, 2009).

Function

Function of the muscular system . A healthy individual does have control over the movements of the musculoskeletal system because of the skeletal muscles, which make it possible to engage in purposeful acts. While most skeletal muscles are classified as either under or outside of voluntary control, muscles that cause movement of the lungs and the diaphragm in the respiratory system have qualities of both (Colbert et al., 2020). The diaphragm normally contracts or relaxes automatically, causing the lungs to expand and deflate without our awareness. But the person can "will" the lungs to expand or deflate. An example is how people respond to an anxiety attack. When a person becomes anxious, he or she may begin to automatically breathe rapidly or hyperventilate. However, if the individual becomes aware that they are breathing rapidly, they can purposely inhale a large amount of air and hold their breath, which can result in the brain receiving more oxygen and relaying messages to the lungs to slow down.

There are four main functions of skeletal muscles: (1) providing locomotion, (2) maintaining posture, (3) stabilizing joints, and (4) generating heat (Clemente, 1985). In fact, according to the National Cancer Institute (n.d.), nearly 85% of the body's heat comes from muscles. Increasing bulk or developing a lean physique are the goals of many athletes. So much so, that worldwide, the fitness center market share was $87.23 billion in 2019 (Policy Advice, 2021). This interest is not all cosmetic, however. If not used, skeletal muscles atrophy, become weakened, and waste away when their movements are limited, perhaps when a bone was broken and needed to be immobilized for a long period of time in order to mend.

Function of the skeletal system . There are several functions of the skeletal system; the most obvious ones are to provide structure, stability, and form to the human body, without which the person could not hold up their head, sit, stand, or move. But the skeletal system contributes so much more than structure that its value cannot be overstated. In addition to posture, bones are necessary to protect the organs (e.g., lungs, brain matter) from damage: The ribs form a fence to protect the lungs and the heart, the pelvis provides a barricade that protects the ovaries and female reproductive system, and the skull encases and protects the brain (Clarke, 2008).

The third function of the skeletal system is to make bone marrow. As Longaker stated, the skeletal stem cells provide a nurturing environment for development of red and white blood cells, as well as bone, cartilage, and marrow (Conger, 2018). There are two types of marrow, red and yellow. At birth, the human has primarily red marrow throughout their body, but with age, the yellow marrow predominates, and red is primarily found in the hip, pelvis, scapula, ribs, and skull (Saladi-Schulman, 2018). The red marrow is extremely critical for health. It makes all the blood cells, red and white, that are in the peripheral bloodstream. Its red blood cells carry oxygen throughout the bloodstream to the cells of the body (Myelodysplastic Syndromes Foundation [MDS], 2014). Without red marrow, the person would be anemic. According to MDS, red marrow also makes white blood cells that are critical for immunity and fighting infections, and without red marrow, the person would have no defense against viruses, bacteria, or fungi. The red marrow also makes blood platelets, which are critical for resolving blood clots. Without them, the person would bleed excessively if injured. The red as well as the yellow marrow make pluripotent stem cells, so named because they can become any kind of cell in the blood system. They are critical for health because without them bones would not regenerate after trauma (MDS, 2014).

Illnesses

Illnesses of the muscular system. Motor neuron diseases (MNDs) are the result of dysfunctional nerves in the nervous system that fail to tell the brainstem and spinal cord to move voluntary muscles (Motor Neurone Disease Association [MNDA], 2018). According to MNDA, there are approximately 5,000 people who suffer from MND in Great Britain, although the disease differs among patients and is difficult to diagnose. Ultimately, it results in loss of movement, wasting of muscles, weakness, and death. Because failure to move the muscles weakens them, causing them to atrophy (National Institute of Neurological Disorders and Stroke [NINDS], 2021], patients may lose the ability to walk, speak, swallow, or even breathe.

Motor neuron diseases are not reversible, and there is no cure. Symptoms become progressively worse over time. MND can progress quickly, and ultimately the person's life is shortened, with most people dying within 3 to 5 years after onset of symptoms (Foster & Salajegheh, 2019). However, Dr. Steven Hawking, perhaps the most famous contemporary victim of ALS, lived 50 years with the disease. One theory why he lived so long is because he could afford state-of-the-art medical care as well as 24-hour, 7-days-a-week private nursing and exemplary personal care that most other people cannot afford (Fox, 2018).

Amyotrophic Lateral Sclerosis (ALS). The prototypical MND is ALS, or Lou Gehrig's disease in the United States, or is referred to as MND in Great Britain. It is a fatal MND that is thought to be inherited. It can result from at least one parent passing on a dominant gene, both parents passing on recessive genes, or the mother who is a carrier of the defective gene on her X chromosome passing on a defective gene (NINDS, 2019). While the formal name for the disease is amyotrophic lateral sclerosis, people in the United States began calling it Lou Gehrig's disease after a much beloved baseball player for the New York Yankees was diagnosed with ALS in 1939.

Caucasians are more likely to contract the disease compared to non-Hispanic persons of African descent, Hispanics, and non-Hispanics of other races when socioeconomic status is not a factor (Roberts et al., 2016). Some researchers have found that men are more likely to develop ALS/MND than women (ALS Association, 2022; McCombe & Henderson, 2010), while other researchers have not (Roberts et al., 2016). According to McCombe and Henderson (2010), on the one hand, compared to females, males tend to contract ALS/MND when they are younger even though those who do contract the disease are typically in their late middle age (40–60 years). On the other hand, cases of juvenile onset motor neurone disease, such as Spinal Muscle Atrophy II (SMA type II), have been found to affect children as early as 6 months old, making them unable to reach developmental milestones (NINDS, 2022).

Treatment options for ALS/MND are scant, and at this time pharmaceutical interventions are limited to two medications: riluzole, which has a neuroprotective function and potential antidepressant and antianxiety effects (Gourley et al., 2012); and edaravone, an antioxidant that slows the decline of disease progression (NINDS, 2021).

According to NINDS, the symptoms of ALS reflect that the affected cells are upper and lower motor neurons that direct muscles responsible for voluntary as well as involuntary movements. Symptoms are the result of the myelin sheaths of nerve cells becoming damaged and unable to transmit signals to contract the muscles. The progression of the illness culminates with death, primarily because the muscles are unable to facilitate breathing, usually within 2 to 4 years after onset (Foster & Salajegheh, 2019). Turner and colleagues found that in a sample of 769 patients with an MND, the mean survival rate was 3.6 years ($SD = 2.8$) with a median of 3.3 years and ranged from 3 months to 24.9 years, with only 3.9% surviving more than 10 years (Turner et al., 2003).

Because of ALS's involvement with muscles that support the respiratory system, and that most deaths are the result of respiratory failure, treatment that supports breathing is critical. ALS is a progressive illness, and breathing is affected in the early, middle, and late stages. According to Beukelman and colleagues (2011), in the early stage the amount of air needed to produce normal speech may occur intermittently but may be difficult to understand because of the effort needed to produce it. According to Beukelman et al., during the middle stage, muscles may be weakened substantially, and patients may have difficulty breathing without ventilation. During the final stage, breathing may fail, and death occurs. Scala and Pisani (2018) suggested that noninvasive positive pressure ventilation (NPPV) should be started early in the disease course because it slows respiratory deterioration and helps the patient avoid invasive procedures such as inserting an endotracheal tube to provide an artificial airway.

The choice of treatment for ALS/MND depends in large part on the stage of illness. In the early stage, lower limb muscles become weak, and reducing the number of falls is paramount. Strengthening the lower limbs by mild-to-moderate exercise has been shown to strengthen the legs, but vigorous aerobic exercises has been detrimental (Paganoni et al., 2015). According to Paganoni and colleagues, braces to stabilize the lower extremities may be fitted during the early stage, but during the middle stage, weakening of the muscles has usually progressed to the point where walking is difficult, and wheelchairs are beneficial. Obtaining medical benefits for a wheelchair can be time consuming, and Majmudar and colleagues (2014) recommended renting a manual wheelchair while the patient is waiting to acquire an electric one. Obtaining an electric wheelchair is critical because over time the patient will not have the body strength to maneuver one that is nonelectric (Majmudar et al., 2014). Cramping in the legs, because of spasticity, can result in muscular pain and require medication, including benzodiazepines, to relax the muscles (Majmudar et al., 2014; Paganoni et al. 2015). Because MND attacks the muscles, physical therapy, massage, stretching, and yoga can help improve balance, slow muscle atrophy in the early stage of the illness, and reduce shoulder and hip pain (Paganoni et al., 2015).

Paganoni and colleagues (2015) reported that the most distressing symptom endorsed by patients during the middle stage of the illness was loss of the ability to communicate. The ability to speak becomes limited as time progresses, and if patients cannot rely on caregivers to facilitate communicative devices they operate by noncomputerized boards, they may need to use computerized speech synthesizers that translate eye movements to a keyboard projected onto a computer screen. Use of an electronic eye-tracking communicative device has been shown to improve the patient's quality of life, reduce depression in the patient, and reduce caregiver burden (Hwang et al., 2014). During the late stage, caregivers are needed to satisfy all basic needs, including feeding, bathroom functions, and bathing. During the end stage, muscles have generally deteriorated to the point that unassisted breathing is impossible, and if the patient has not written a living will, the caregiver must decide whether the patient will be placed on invasive mechanical ventilation or entered into palliative care that is focused on increasing the patient's comfort. However, with the eye-tracking communicative device, the patient can retain control of their medical care as long as the eye muscles are functional.

Illnesses of the skeletal system. Osteoporosis literally means porous bones. It is a debilitating disease of the skeletal system that attacks the structure of the bones and is defined by the Association of Professors of Medicine Consensus Development Conference (1991) as "microarchitectural deterioration of bone tissue" (Kanis et al., 1994). Osteoporosis primarily occurs among postmenopausal women, although it also occurs among men (Burge et al., 2007; Chen et al., 2019) and persons who have received chemotherapy (cancer. net, n.d.). Osteoporosis is, in part, due to genetic factors that are responsible for several conditions: low bone mass related to low bone mineral density (BMD; Koromila et al., 2013); the balance between bone formation and resorption (Wolf, 2008; Yang et al., 2019); and estrogen deficiency (Sharma et al., 2018; Yang et al. 2019). Some contributors to these factors can be addressed medically, and if the client heeds medical advice this deterioration can be mitigated. If care is not taken to ameliorate the condition, the skeletal tissue can break down further, increasing the probability that the person fractures a bone during everyday activities like standing and walking.

According to the World Health Organization (WHO), osteoporosis is responsible for more than 4.5 million fractures occurring in the Americas and Europe (WHO, 2007). The WHO Scientific Group on the Assessment of Osteoporosis at Primary Health Care Level (WHO, 2007) found in 2000 that the estimated number of hip fractures in the Americas and Europe among men and women aged 50 years or older was 931,000 annually. These findings are greatly concerning because of the profound effect hip fractures have on quality and length of life. Up to 30% of patients with hip fractures will die in the year following the injury (Brauer et al., 2009), and this number continues to rise as the population of the United States ages.

Injuries

Injuries to the muscular system.   One way to categorize muscle injuries is by their onset. Acute injuries happen quickly, often from traumatic events, whereas chronic injuries occur from extended overuse. There are three types of muscle injuries: lacerations, contusions, and strains. Lacerations can occur when the muscle is cut after coming in contact with a sharp object like shrapnel from an improvised explosive device (IED) or shards of metal or glass from an automobile accident. Contusions, the second type of muscle injury, can occur when violent force is applied to the muscle, for example, during trauma from domestic violence or vigorous contact during sports (e.g., hockey, football). According to Campagne (2021), the third type of muscle injury is a strain, which is the result of excessive tension that breaks muscle fibers, often from overstretching. There are three levels of strains. Grade I strains occur when only one or two muscle fibers snap, but the overall muscle remains intact and strong. Grade II strains occur when many muscle fibers snap and the entire muscle loses some of its strength. Whiplash to the neck is an example of a Grade II strain that can occur when the head is moved forward and backward rapidly as in an automobile accident or if a baby is shaken too vigorously by their caretaker. In a Grade III strain, the entire muscle snaps and no longer functions. A Grade III strain can occur from sports injuries from overextending or work injuries from carrying heavy equipment or furniture (Haver, 2021). This notion is supported by findings that the most frequent injuries among disabled male veterans were back and neck problems (Wu & Lewis, 2015), potentially from carrying heavy equipment and weapons for long periods of time.

Injuries to the skeletal system.   The prototypical injuries to the skeletal system are fractures, and among the elderly with compromised bone density, the most common injury is the hip fracture, often from falling. The National Osteoporosis Guideline Group (NOGG) (2020) reported that in the United Kingdom approximately 550,000 new fractures occur annually, including 105,00 hip fractures and 86,000 vertebral fractures. These data reflect an increase from

2013, when 536,000 new fractures were found to occur annually, including 79,000 hip fractures and 66,000 fractures to the vertebrae (Svedbom et al., 2013). More than one third of all adult women in the United Kingdom will incur a "fragility fracture" during their lifetime. A fragility fracture is a fracture that occurs without trauma and can be precipitated from everyday behaviors that include coughing or getting out of a car. Fragility fractures have also been called "spontaneous fractures" (Wick, 2009), which is a term used interchangeably with compression fracture, insufficiency fracture, as well as fragility fracture, which Wick defined as "falling from a less-than-standing height." Fragility fractures indicate extensive deterioration of the bone, and more than half (53%) the women who experience them will no longer be able to live independently. Because the costs of institutionalization are exorbitant, long-term assisted living is virtually unaffordable with private funds. While the average cost for a shared room in a nursing home facility in the United States was $93,075 annually, after government subsidies, out-of-pocket expenses for individuals in America are, on average, $11,000/year.

Several researchers have noted that patients who experienced a hip fracture were more likely to die within a year, compared to their counterparts who did not fracture their hip (Association of Professors of Medicine [Washington, D.C.] Consensus Development Panel, 1991; Hernlund et al., 2013; Ong et al., 2018; Svedbom et al., 2013; Tajeu et al., 2014). There were similar findings among Svedbom and colleagues (2013), who reported that the incidence of death within a year was 28.7%, while the Consensus Development Panel (1991) reported the incidence as 12% to 20%, and Ong and colleagues (2018) reported that the mortality rate was 20.0% to 26.9% within 1 year. In a study of 27 countries in the European Union, Hernlund and colleagues (2013) found that 142,687 people died within 1 year following a fracture, with 26,389 life-years lost. The drastic and permanent lifestyle changes that often occur due to the hip fracture may contribute to the deaths, as most patients are no longer able to perform activities of daily living without assistance or to live independently (Ong et al., 2018).

(T) Mental health clinicians can benefit from understanding technology associated with the care of musculoskeletal system

Technological Advances to Treat the Muscular System

Computerized aids have been found to improve communication and the quality of life of the patient (Bongioanni, 2012; Hwang et al., 2014) and to reduce caregiver burden (Hwang et al., 2014; Pagnini et al., 2010). These devices are so important that in England, the National Health Service funds "augmentative" and "alternative" devices (National Health Service, 2016). In 2001, the

U.S. government adapted the Medicare and Medicaid benefit systems to include alternative and augmented communication devices or, as Medicare refers to them, speech generative devices. Augmentative systems are appropriate for persons who can still produce some speech even though it is often difficult to understand or hear, while alternative communication systems are for people who have lost the ability to speak entirely. As stated previously, the average length of life following a diagnosis of ALS is 3 to 5 years. During that time, case managers and counselors must facilitate access to communicative devices soon after the diagnosis. Because a patient with ALS/MND can deteriorate during the time social workers organize services, the caregiver will need to anticipate the patient's needs until they are able to communicate again.

Technological Advances to Treat the Skeletal System.

Bone marrow transplants . Osteoblasts are responsible for creating new bone, while osteoclasts are responsible for breaking it down. Normally, this process keeps bone growth in balance while the two groups of cells work together to "remodel" the bone. The disease of osteoporosis occurs when this balance is disrupted. The osteoclasts dominate the process and continue to break down the bone while the osteoblasts are unable to lay down new bone fast enough to build it back up. Implanting stem cells from bone marrow has been an effective treatment because of their ability to generate new bone and reverse the demineralization process (Paspaliaris & Kolios, 2019). Current medications that treat osteoporosis aim to decrease the activity of osteoclasts to rebalance the relationship between osteoclasts and osteoblasts.

The study of bone marrow transplantation introduces a new technical vocabulary and concepts that a clinician in the medical field will need to understand in order to support their client's treatment. The probability that a clinician will have the occasion to work with a client, or the client's child, who undergoes a bone marrow transplant will depend on their patient population, but it is not outside the realm of possibilities. The transplantation procedure is carried out routinely. For example, Passweg and colleagues (2016) reported that in a study of 47 European countries in 2014, more than 40,000 stem cell transplants were carried out each year. During 2018, in the United States alone, 9,275 bone marrow and cord blood stem cell implants were performed (Health Resources & Services Administration [HRSA], 2021a). When the total number of bone marrow transplants was analyzed by donor, the data showed that 21% (1,048) of the total number of stem cells were harvested from bone marrow donors who were not related to the recipient (allogenous), and 26% (1,112) were from donors who were related (autologous) (HRSA, 2021b). From 2014 to 2018, bone marrow donors were far more likely to be unrelated persons (9,987 from 2014 to 2018) than autologous ones (133 from 2014 to 2018).

(E) Mental health clinicians can benefit from understanding biomedical engineering

Engineering Advances to Treat the Muscular System

COVID-19 (coronavirus 2019) is not the only pandemic that has affected us in the past. Poliomyelitis is also caused by a virus and was responsible for the polio pandemic during the mid-20th century. It is transmitted through feces and primarily affects children under 5 years old. It typically enters the organism through the mouth, travels down the alimentary canal, and is defecated (Oshinsky, 2005). Although the first six cases of polio were diagnosed during June 1916 in Brooklyn, New York, by that October the virus was responsible for 8,900 cases and 2,400 deaths (Oshinsky, 2005). Ultimately, it was responsible for 6,000 deaths and 27,000 cases of paralysis in the United States alone (Oshinsky, 2005). Notwithstanding the eradication of the disease in North America and Great Britain currently, it continues to be a pandemic in Pakistan, with 11,915 cases, and in Afghanistan, with 3.969 cases (WHO, 2020). Because polio has not been eradicated yet, persons who have not been immunized with the polio vaccine are at risk for contracting and spreading the disease.

The poliovirus enters the central nervous system (brain, brainstem, and spinal column) and attacks the motor neurons (Hogle, 2002). Symptoms include not only the inability to move muscles of the limbs, but also, in some cases, the inability of the muscles in the diaphragm to move. Most deaths that were attributed to polio were caused by an inability to inflate and deflate the lungs. In the mid-20th century, before a reliable vaccine was discovered, individuals with severe cases that affected breathing were confined to an "iron lung." The apparatus forcibly expanded and contracted the lungs and was so effective that the U.S. government provided benefits to cover their expense (Center for Medicare & Medicaid Services [CMS] (2021). Many children survived the polio pandemic because of the iron lung, and although modern ventilators are not as cumbersome, a handful of polio survivors still use their iron lung today.

Today, people can be protected from polio with a vaccine, but there is no cure. The vaccine halts the illness by recognizing the virus as an invader and creating an immune response. The white blood cells within the lymphatic system release antibodies that attach to the virus and destroy it. Similar to other viruses, the poliovirus attaches itself to the host's cells, where it injects the virus into the genetic component (RNA) of the cell, which is then replicated.

Engineering Advances to Treat the Skeletal System

Biomedical technology is also used to treat osteoporosis. Antiresorptive agents halt the resorption process that breaks down the bone. These medications include bisphosphonates, isoflavones, and hormone replacement therapies (i.e., estrogen, estrogen/progesterone) (Chen et al., 2019). They have been used to reduce loss of bone mineral density (BMD) among postmenopausal women.

In a meta-analysis of nine studies, Zhao and colleagues (2015) reported that, compared to exercise alone: (1) Antiresorptive medication plus exercise increased BMD at the spine, but not the femoral neck; (2) hormone replacement therapy (HRT) plus exercise increased the BMD of the spine as well as the femoral neck; but (3) isoflavones plus exercise failed to show a difference in BMD at the spine and hip. When the effects of antiresorptive treatment plus exercise were compared, Zhao and colleagues reported that impact exercises (e.g., walking, running, skipping, jumping) had greater benefits than resistance exercises (e.g., strength training). On the other hand, Daly (2017) found that progressive resistance training with weight-bearing exercises was the most effective regimen in preventing bone or muscle loss among older adults and frail elderly, especially when paired with protein and multinutrient supplements. Muir and colleagues showed that antiresorptive therapy was also effective in increasing BMD at the spine and femoral neck, and that exercise and medication delayed bone loss (and potentially prevented fractures) among elderly women. They suggested that moderately strenuous exercise improves BMD at the hip region, which is helpful because that is the area of the body that commonly absorbs most of a fall. These effects can be long lasting. Although Mugnier and colleagues (2019) failed to find group differences in refracture rate at 12 months, among participants who received antiosteoporosis medication (68%, bisphosphonate) for 1 year, at 31 ± 7 months follow-up, those who were receiving antiosteoporosis medication had fewer refractures compared to those who did not receive the medication. Thus it appears that the combination of antiresorptive medications and exercise is effective in preventing fractures.

(M) Mental health clinicians can benefit from understanding the mathematics of the prevalence of illness

In 1988, a coalition of public and private partnerships was founded, and the World Health Assembly launched the Global Polio Eradication Initiative (GPEI), spearheaded by governments; WHO; the Centers for Disease Control and Prevention (CDC); United Nations International Children's Emergency Fund (UNICEF), now known as United Nations Children's Fund; Rotary International; and recently joined by the Global Alliance for Vaccines and Immunization (GAVI) and the Bill & Melinda Gates Foundation. Data have indicated remarkable success since GPEI's foundation: Global incidence of polio was reduced by 99.9%; 16 million people were prevented from becoming paralyzed

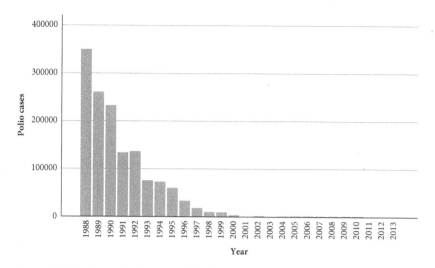

Figure 9.4 Number of polio cases, globally, 1988–2013.

Data source: Centers for Disease Control and Prevention. (2014). *Infographic: The time to eradicate polio is now.* Retrieved November 10, 2021 from https://www.cdc.gov/globalhealth/immunization/infographic/eradicate_polio.htm. Chart created by Dr. Liyun Wu.

(CDC, 2021a). Globally, Afghanistan and Pakistan are the only two countries experiencing wide poliovirus type 1 transmission (CDC, 2021b). Figure 9.4 displays the total cases of polio in the world from 1988 to 2013. In 1988, there were 350,000 polio cases among 125 endemic countries. The prevalence of polio was reduced to 233,000 cases in 1990. By the end of the 20th century, the total number of cases of polio was lowered to 10,000 cases. The 21st century witnessed massive improvements in polio eradication, and there were only 403 polio cases worldwide in 2013.

As presented by Figure 9.5, more women than men have osteoporosis, regardless of their age. For adults aged 50–64, 13.1% of women were diagnosed with osteoporosis and only 3.3% of men. For adults aged 65 and over, the proportion of women with osteoporosis increased to 27.1%, four times higher than among men (5.7%). Overall, for adults 50 years and over, the prevalence of osteoporosis is 12.6%, with 19.6% among women and 4.4% among men.

The prevalence of low bone mass is also higher among women than men. As displayed by Figure 9.6, the overall prevalence of low bone mass among adults aged 50–64 years old is 39.3%. Among women, it is 50.3% and among men 27.5%. In addition, the overall prevalence of low bone mass among the adults 65 and over is 47.5%. Among women, it is 52.9% and 40.7% among men. Thus, for adults 50 years and over, the prevalence of low bone mass is 43.1%. Among women, the prevalence is 51.5% and is 33.5% among men. Because low bone

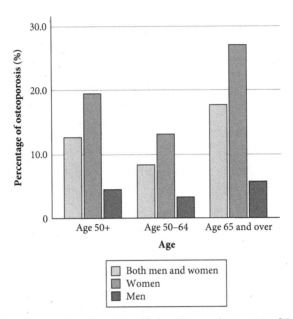

Figure 9.5 Prevalence of osteoporosis among adults aged 50+, United States, 2017–2018.

Data source: Centers for Disease Control and Prevention. (2021c). *Osteoporosis or low bone mass in older adults: United States, 2017–2018.* Retrieved November 10, 2021, from https://www.cdc.gov/nchs/data/databriefs/db405-H.pdf. Chart created by Dr. Liyun Wu.

mass increases the risk of developing osteoporosis, it is important to take actions to keep bone strong.

(H) Mental health clinicians can benefit from understanding the application to health

The Muscular System

Amyotrophic lateral sclerosis is irreversible and always fatal. Because of this, it is important that mental health clinicians become comfortable discussing preferences regarding advanced medical directives and options for palliative care with the patient and family members. There may be a limited window of opportunity to discuss the patient's wishes because if and when they lose the ability to communicate, the medical team will have to rely on the family member to make decisions based on their understanding of the patient's wishes. Decisions may include whether the patient will receive long-term mechanical ventilation (LTMV) (Blackhall, 2012). Long-term mechanical ventilation

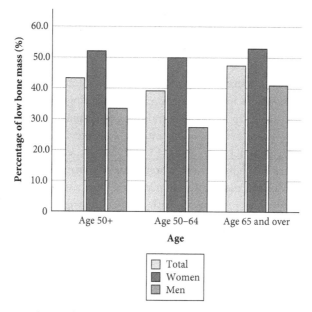

Figure 9.6 Prevalence of low bone mass among adults aged 50+, United States, 2017–2018.

Data source: Centers for Disease Control and Prevention. (2021c). *Osteoporosis or low bone mass in older adults: United States, 2017–2018.* Retrieved November 10, 2021, from https://www.cdc.gov/nchs/data/databriefs/db405-H.pdf. Chart created by Dr. Liyun Wu.

requires intubation and is used when noninvasive positive-pressure ventilation (NPPV) that had been used during an earlier stage of the disease is no longer effective. According to Blackhall, long-term mechanical ventilation is typically permanent, but it may be desirable because it can extend life for 10 years or more. However, the question becomes whether the patient will enjoy an acceptable quality of life. When the patient's illness has progressed to the point that they are suffering, clinicians need to initiate discussions exploring palliative, or end-of-life, care. Blackhall (2012) urged family members to begin the discussion of advanced directives early in the disease process because its progression is unpredictable. The patient's decline can be rapid. If a patient does lose the ability to communicate their wishes, and no advanced directive is set, family members become surrogate decision-makers in a very specific order. The first contact is the spouse, followed by the children, then the parents, then siblings. This order may be remembered by the pneumonic "Spouse ChiPS in" (spouse, children, parents, siblings). If no direct family members are alive to become the surrogate, the best effort must be made to identify a friend, or even a neighbor, that may know the patient's final wishes. It is especially important for a clinician to know this order of medical surrogates as they are often the lead in coordinating end-of-life care for a patient.

Lillo and colleagues (2012) found that most caregivers of ALS/MND patients are family members (97%) and demonstrate elevated levels of caregiver burden, which is positively associated with anxiety and depression (Pagnini et al., 2010). In the United States, because of the parameters regarding the patient's expected length of life, hospice care is often contraindicated for patients with ALS/MND. Hospice is reserved for persons whose anticipated longevity is 6 months, but the course of ALS is often not predictable (CMS, 2021). If the patient is not a candidate for hospice care, palliative care at home can be managed, but as the patient's condition deteriorates, the family will need help from a mental health clinician who can support their relationship with a physician willing to prescribe pain medications or other symptomatic treatments.

The Skeletal System

Interpersonal violence (IPV) is the major cause of injuries to women. Lifetime prevalence of IPV in Canada (25%) (WHO, 2021a) and Western Europe (21%) were similar to worldwide rates of 23.7% for women aged 50 and older (WHO, 2021b). But, when 12-month IPV rates among 15- to 49-year-old women from the least developed countries (22%) were compared to global averages (13%), differences emerged. Bhandari and colleagues (2006) found that for 43% of women who reported physical abuse at a clinic, 40% of the injuries were to the head and neck, 28% were musculoskeletal injuries, and 36% required medical care. Santos and colleagues (2019) discovered that physical aggression was the primary abuse reported by 84.7% of the participants in the victim survey, but only 14.8% of the population sample. Santos and colleagues added that 29% of participants in the victim survey reported physical abuse by children or grandchildren, 26% reported physical aggression by a spouse or partner, and 18% reported physical and psychological abuse by children/grandchildren. Only 50% stated that they had "plenty/enough" perceived social support, and 23.6% reported that they had "few/no one" to go to for support (Santos et al., 2019).

Gosangi and colleagues (2021) found that while there were half as many patients who reported any IPV during the COVID-19 pandemic, victims were more likely seen in the emergency department (38% vs. 18%) than other medical settings, were 1.8 times more likely to experience physical versus nonphysical abuse, to have experienced "severe" abuse (19% vs. 8.7%), and "very severe" abuse (19% vs. 13.7%). They concluded that because of "shelter-in-place" orders, only victims who experienced extreme physical abuse sought treatment; therefore, even though fewer victims sought healthcare for their injuries, their cases were more severe.

During the COVID-19 pandemic, public health and government officials ordered citizens to shelter in place, which has been found to be related to increased abuse among older adults (Makaroun et al., 2020). The lack of support is concerning because being sequestered with the abuser is associated with increased abuse, especially among vulnerable older adults (Han & Mosqueda, 2020). Because of the health consequences of IPV, clinicians working in the medical field may be able to engage with victims with suspicious injuries. Each clinician, whether they treat clients in a hospital, outpatient clinic, or long-term rehabilitation facility or provide in-home care, must be alerted to the pattern of injuries sustained by victims of IPV so they can investigate injuries in a sensitive manner and provide protection while meeting with the client. The clinician can provide up-to-date contacts for online addresses, telephone and text numbers, as well as engage in face-to-face interactions with patients and advocate for their safety. Most cities will have a designated hospital or emergency department with staff trained to care for victims of IPV or sexual assault. These locations are also trained to take confidential evidence for use in criminal investigations if so desired by the victim. When clients cannot attend face-to-face meetings because of social distancing or the limitations due to their illness, Han and Mosqueda (2020) urged clinicians to reach out and contact their clients on a frequent basis. Makaroun and colleagues (2020) recommended frequent telehealth appointments so the medical care provider can monitor the patient for evidence of abuse. Clinicians are mandated reporters of suspected abuse and must report evidence of suspected abuse by alerting an adult protection service to make an in-depth assessment. Clinicians are in a unique, and powerful, position to help victims of abuse because they are the first line of defense (Gosangi et al., 2021).

Conclusion

In conclusion, while the musculoskeletal system comprises two bodily systems, each is a system in its own right. This chapter introduced both the muscular and the skeletal systems in depth, discussing their structures and functions and how they are interdependent on each other. ALS, a devastating motor neuron disease was presented as the signature illness of the muscular system, while osteoporosis was presented as the prototypical illness of the skeletal system. Injuries to the skeletal system as the result of fractures related to intimate partner violence or falls and fractures were discussed. The section on mathematics discussed the prevalence of polio, a muscular disease, and osteoporosis, an illness that attacks the skeletal system. Finally, this chapter discussed how discussion of end-of-life care needs to be addressed by families that are struggling with ALS and how clinicians should be alerted to potential increase in IPV as the result of isolation.

Glossary

Atrophy   Decrease in size from wasting away

Autologous   From one's own body (root = "auto," which means "self")

Cartilaginous   Made from cartilage

Pluripotent cells   Can develop into many different cells

Resorption process   Process by which old bone is destroyed and new bone is made

Websites

FRAX® Fracture Risk Assessment Tool: https://www.sheffield.ac.uk/FRAX/tool.aspx?country=1

National Osteoporosis Guideline Group (NOGG): https://www.nogg.org.uk/ (sheffield.ac.uk)

10

How Understanding the Gastrointestinal System Can Benefit Mental Health Clinicians

Introduction

People are hardwired to receive pleasure from eating and drinking, but among some people this straightforward function is overshadowed by eating for emotional reasons and vain attempts to satisfy psychological needs. Some researchers maintain that eating can become compulsive because it engages the same neurochemicals as addictive drugs. Professionals in the medical field may attribute obesity to genetic effects (Farooqi & O'Rahilly, 2006; Stunkard et al., 1990), while psychologists may attribute it to childhood sexual, physical, or emotional abuse or physical neglect (Danese & Tan, 2014). Public health professionals may attribute it to the density of, and distance from, fast-food restaurants (Cobb et al., 2015; Galvez et al., 2010), and social workers may attribute it to poverty-like conditions that provoke intermittent access to sugary and fatty foods (Corwin, 2011). Some nutritionists blame obesity on fried fast foods, junk foods, and processed foods that quickly metabolize to sugar, as well as sugary desserts and drinks (Fuhrman, 2018). In reality, it is most likely a combination of all of these factors that drives today's obesity epidemic, including the brain's response to substances that are high in sugar and fat.

Using STEM-H (science, technology, engineering, and mathematics as applied to health), this chapter gives clinicians a basic understanding of the science of the gastrointestinal (GI) system: injuries and illnesses associated with the system, technology used to treat obesity, engineering of medications prescribed for obesity, the mathematical data showing empirical evidence of the prevalence of obesity, social determinants of health, Type 2 diabetes, and how clinicians can intervene to impact an individual's illness.

STEM-H for Mental Health Clinicians. Marilyn Weaver Lewis, Liyun Wu, and Zachary Allan Hagen, Oxford University Press.
© Oxford University Press 2023. DOI: 10.1093/oso/9780197638514.003.0010

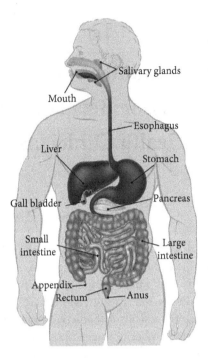

Figure 10.1 The gastrointestinal tract.

STEM-H Principles Underlying the Gastrointestinal System

(S) Mental health clinicians can benefit from understanding the science explaining the GI system

Many clients suffer from eating disorders and obesity-related medical problems. In order to separate the emotional component of eating from its mechanics, becoming familiar with the concepts and vocabulary of the structure and function of the GI system is important.

Structure

According to Colbert and colleagues (2020), in conjunction with the stomach, the GI system includes three organs (liver, gallbladder, pancreas) that work with the GI tract and facilitate eating and drinking and elimination of waste. As can be seen by Figure 10.1, the stomach is the largest organ of the GI system and is able to be distinguished from the esophagus as early as 4 weeks' gestation (Collins, 2021). The small intestine itself is divided into three segments (in descending order): the duodenum, the jejunum, and the ileum. Each segment has a specific role in digestion, as do the stomach and large intestine.

According to Berkovitz (2021), the adult GI system begins with the mouth and comprises the lips; teeth; tongue, which primarily provides the floor of the mouth; the soft and hard palate, which form the upper area of the mouth; and walls of the oral cavity of the mouth and the cheeks. There are three pairs of major salivary glands and many minor glands that aid in digestion and are located in front of and under the ears, under the tongue, and under the jaw (Berkovitz, 2021). The salivary glands aid in moistening the mouth, help to chew and swallow the food, and provide antibodies to kill bacteria in the mouth (National Institute of Dental and Craniofacial Research [NIDCR], n.d.). In addition to the mouth, the nose and nasal cavity are considered part of the GI system because of their important role in smelling and tasting food (Hopkins, 2021). According to Hopkins (2021), swallowing occurs from 600 to 1,000 times per day. There are classically four phases of swallowing: the oral preparatory, oral transit/transfer, pharyngeal, and esophageal phases.

When food and drink are swallowed, they travel down the esophagus, a long tube that extends in the upper GI tract and ends when it meets the stomach. The "gastroesophageal sphincter" prohibits food and digestive juices to be regurgitated back into the esophagus, as is the case with acid reflux reactions (Going et al., 2021). In the adult, the stomach lies between the esophagus and the juncture of the small intestines. The small intestines, which are convoluted and lie within the abdominal cavity, connect to the large intestines, which terminate in the rectum and end in the anus.

In addition to the GI tract, three organs aid in digestion. The liver, the largest organ in the abdominal cavity, is divided into two lobes. The right lobe is larger and comprises two smaller lobes. According to Colbert and colleagues (2020), the liver is essential in digestion and serves a variety of important functions, including metabolizing alcohol and drugs, as well as impurities in food substances; manufacturing bile, which is essential in metabolism of fats; and storing sugars, vitamins, as well as producing cholesterol. The second ancillary organ that is a component of the larger digestive system is the gallbladder. The gallbladder is a pear-shaped organ that lies next to the liver. Its main function is the release of bile, which is important in the absorption of fats. The third ancillary digestive gland is the pancreas, which secretes enzymes to help digest carbohydrates, lipids, and proteins (Conrad, 2021). The pancreas has a head, neck, body, and tail. It is oriented with its head lower than the body and curving up and toward the left side of the body with its neck, body, and tail pointed to the left. It is tucked between the stomach and the large intestines and is shaped like a shepherd's crook that is laid on its side, which may make it difficult to see on examination. The healthy pancreas has a yellow hue with small lobules that give it a bumpy appearance. According to Conrad, it is an exocrine tissue that drains into the GI tract and secretes enzymes that aid in digestion of lipids, carbohydrates, and proteins. The pancreas is also an endocrine gland that participates in glucose–insulin balance.

The walls of the organs of the GI tract, from the esophagus to the stomach, intestines, and rectum, consist of membranes (Campbell, 2011). For example, the inside of the stomach wall is the mucosa, or mucous, layer, which is the outermost layer of the membrane. This layer is lined with mucus to aid the contents in passing through the stomach without damaging the organ. Interior to, or under, the outer mucosal layer is the submucosal layer, which houses a network, or plexus, of nerves and produces digestive enzymes. The next innermost layer is the muscle layer, with three segments: the oblique, circular, and longitudinal layers. These layers of muscles contract and relax, which make it possible for contents to pass along the structure while they are being mixed and digested further. The final layer is the serosa layer, or layer that includes serum/plasma, which further lubricates the bowel (Campbell, 2011). Figure 10.2, which shows the structure of the mucosal layers of the stomach wall, gives an indication of the undulations of the tissue of the membrane. There are deep grooves in the mucosa that provide a large surface area for absorption in a small space. The linings of the organs provide layers of mucous cells, nerves, and muscle cells. The folds are lined with villi, which are structures that absorb water and nutrients (National Institute of Diabetes and Digestive & Kidney Disorders [NIDDKD], 2017). The epithelial cell include stem cells, which replenish the dead and damaged cells. The gut has one of the highest cell turnover rates in the body.

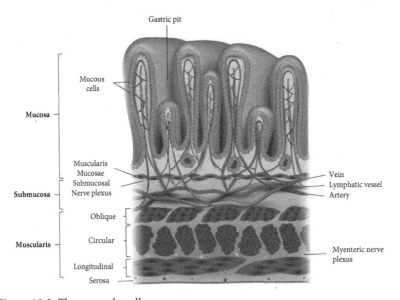

Figure 10.2 The stomach wall.

Function

The function of the GI system is to ingest and digest food, absorb nutrients, and eliminate waste (Campbell, 2011). Ingesting food begins with mastication, which breaks down the food into small pieces, or a bolus of food. In order for mastication to occur, the brain must tell the mouth to release saliva from the salivary glands (NIDDKD, 2017). Salivation is necessary to moisten the pieces of food to break them down into smaller and smaller pieces with the help of enzymes. According to Colbert and colleagues (2020), chewing food releases the enzyme salivary amylase to break down the starches before the food travels to the stomach. After food enters the stomach, normal digestion begins with the release of acidic enzymes that break the food down with a churning motion (Campbell, 2011). This action creates a partially digested food called chyme that travels to the small intestines (Colbert et al., 2020). As it passes through the first part of the small intestine (the duodenum), chyme is broken down further by chemicals secreted by the pancreas, gallbladder, and liver (Collins, 2021). Sugar in the chyme enters the bloodstream, causing the pancreas, one of the auxiliary organs in the GI system to secrete insulin, which allows the absorption of sugar by the rest of the body (Johns Hopkins Medicine, 2020). Thus, the pancreas actually has two functions: It directly secretes digestive enzymes into the duodenum, and it releases insulin into the bloodstream. Too little insulin results in elevated levels of plasma glucose, which can develop into diabetes. The chyme travels through the small intestines, where most of the nutrients are absorbed (Clemente, 1985) before the waste is sent to the large intestine and colon. The large intestine removes water from the stool and stores the final waste product before it is defecated through the anus (NIDDKD, 2017).

Illness

There are many common diseases of the GI system, including irritable bowel syndrome (IBS) as well as stomach and colon cancer. IBS, often referred to as spastic colon, is a dysfunction of the large intestine that is associated with cramping, diarrhea, and constipation (Mayo Clinic, 2020). It can be the result of certain foods, bacteria in the gut, or anxiety. IBS is a recurring disorder, and prevalence is more common among individuals who have experienced stress during childhood (Mayo Clinic, 2020). IBS afflicts at least 11% of the global population (Corsetti et al., 2018), but prevalence may be higher than reported due to patients' reluctance to seek help.

According to the IBS Global Disease Burden Report of 2018, IBS is characterized three ways: IBS–diarrhea, IBS–constipation, and IBS–mixed (constipation and diarrhea). These illnesses are responsible for a significant burden due to work-related absenteeism and reduced productivity, compared to other employees without IBS (Faresjo et al., 2016). Patients with IBS have experienced dismissive attitudes and comments from healthcare professionals who did not believe that they were ill and telling them, "It's IBS; go home and deal with it" (Corsetti et al., 2018). Patients may be affected psychologically and socially as many report reluctance to eat meals with others because of the inconsistent experience with IBS-D or IBS-M. Because of the stigma associated with the condition, many patients fail to explain their condition to friends, which causes misinterpretation of the patients' seemingly inconsistent or rude behavior.

Colon cancer is the second leading cause of cancer-related deaths in men and women in the United States (American Cancer Society [ACS], 2020), with the lifetime risk of developing colon or rectal cancer at 4.4% among men and 4.1% among women. In the United States, African Americans are more likely to be diagnosed than other ethnic groups, regardless of gender (U.S. Cancer Statistics Working Group, 2020). Colon cancer can occur anywhere on the large intestine or colon, which is a 5-foot long muscular tube (ACS, 2020). The cancer is often detected during colonoscopies, which identify abnormalities (polyps) (Stage I) on the inner lining of the colon or rectum (mucosa). If not removed early in their development, they can spread into the outer layers of the mucosa (Stages II and III) and into the blood vessels or lymph nodes.

Individuals can decrease their risk of developing colon cancer by increasing exercise, decreasing weight if they are overweight or obese, decreasing intake of red meat (especially if it is charred), and decreasing heavy drinking (ACS, 2020). Smoking tobacco products is also highly correlated with development of colon cancer. Treatment of colon cancer depends on the stage at which it was identified. Early stage cancer may be treated simply by the doctor removing polyps during a colonoscopy (Johns Hopkins Medicine, 2020). Treatment to reduce the size of the tumor may include chemotherapy with one medication or a "cocktail" of several medications. According to the Johns Hopkins Medical Center, 90% of people who receive localized surgery live 5 years or more. If the cancer metastasizes to nearby organs, the 5-year survival rate is reduced to approximately 71%.

In addition to obesity's involvement in development of colorectal cancer (Hanyuda et al., 2017), obesity is implicated in the onset of other diseases, including Type 2 diabetes mellitus, as mentioned previously in this chapter. Diabetes is the result of inadequate insulin secretion, or action, which results in persistent, excessive glucose, or hyperglycemia (American Diabetes Association, 2013). While family heredity is partially responsible for Type 2 diabetes, examination of the social determinants of health that affect the process of developing obesity is warranted. Up to 75% of cases (Costacou & Mayer-Davis, 2003) can be treated by improved diet and increased exercise (Bird et al., 2015). Type 2 diabetes can be a devastating illness as it can cause blindness, renal failure, cardiac problems, stroke, and amputation of the lower limbs and reduces longevity up to 10 years (Bird et al., 2015). In addition to obesity, several sociodemographic indicators have been shown to predict Type 2 diabetes, including household annual income below $30,000 and minority status (Bird et al., 2015).

Injuries

Traumas can cause injuries to the GI system that impair eating. A strong, organized, sucking reflex is critical for the neonate's nourishment and survival. A healthy neonate has a strong sucking reflex, which can be elicited by stroking its cheek or placing its hand to its mouth (Aby, 2020). Anomalies include the cleft lip or cleft palate; these occur between the fourth and seventh weeks of gestation when the sides of the embryonic "face" fail to come together and join at the midline (Centers for Disease Control and Prevention [CDC], 2020c). The cleft can occur solely at the upper lip or become a complete separation of the roof of the mouth, including the soft and hard palates. If the dysfunction of the cleft is extensive and the newborn is not able to suck in a coordinated way, it cannot latch on to the nipple to nurse. According to the Cleft Lip and Palate Association (CLAPA), one in 1,200 babies in the United Kingdom is born with a cleft lip and/or palate (CLAPA, 2020). In the United States, one in 1,600 babies is born with a cleft lip and cleft palate, 1 in 17,00 is born with cleft palate only, and 1 in 2,800 is born with cleft lip only (CDC, 2020c). There are no clear explanations for the disparity between the U.K. and U.S. prevalence rates of this birth defect. Prevalence in the United States is highest among Native Americans, Asians, and Hispanics and lower among African Americans. While there appears to be a genetic component, the CDC (2020a) reported that women who smoke during their pregnancy, have diabetes, or use certain medications to treat epilepsy during the first trimester have an increased risk of giving birth to a baby with a cleft lip or palate. Surgery is recommended to repair the palate, which improves positioning of teeth, eating, speech, and language development, as well as cosmetic concerns (CLAPA, 2020). Later, psychotherapy may be indicated to help the child work through problems with low self-esteem if the face is disfigured.

If a trauma affects a structure in the upper GI (i.e., esophageal) area, it may interfere with swallowing, and patients may elect liquid tube feedings (Cancer Research UK, 2020). According to Cancer Research UK, if the patient's stomach and intestines are functional, a liquid formula is delivered through a nasogastric tube that the doctor inserts directly through the nose, down the esophagus, and into the stomach or small bowel, where the nutritive liquid is digested normally. Another type of enteral feeding system entails inserting a tube through the skin into the stomach or small bowel area and delivering liquid food through the tube. This tube is called a G-tube (gastric tube) when it is placed in the stomach or J-tube (jejunal tube) when placed in the small intestine. When the method that sends nutrition through the intestines is not possible, liquid food is delivered directly into the vein that goes to the heart (Cancer Research,

UK). The nurse will need to instruct the patient and caregivers how to deliver the formula and clean the tube to prevent bacteria from entering the cardiovascular system. If patients become upset and despondent when learning how they must treat themselves, the mental health clinician may need to help the patient decide if they will continue with the treatment or refuse feedings. Clinicians may need to help the family accept the patient's right to self-determination and work through their feelings about their loved one dying if they choose to refuse nourishment.

(T) Mental health clinicians can benefit from understanding the technology used to surgically treat obesity

Treatments for obesity include several types of surgeries to physically reduce the amount of food the individual can comfortably eat. These surgeries include the original Roux-en-Y gastric bypass adjustable lap band and gastric sleeve surgeries. Each of these surgeries decreases the size of the stomach, which results in the stomach sending signals to the brain that the person is satiated even though only a small amount of food is ingested. Bariatric surgery is indicated for individuals who are at least 100 pounds more than their ideal body weight, their body mass index (BMI) is greater than 35, or they have obesity-related medical problems. The first way bariatric surgery helps the individual lose weight is by reducing the stomach size, thus restricting the amount of food that the person can comfortably eat. The second way is by reducing the calories that can be absorbed into the body by "bypassing" the stomach and sending the food directly to the small intestines (Mayo Clinic, 2020). Each of these ways has assets and detriments. The positive side to these surgeries is that they result in fast, long-term weight loss, with approximately 40%–80% of excess weight typically lost (American Society for Metabolic & Bariatric Surgery [ASMBS], 2020). A serious negative side effect is that individuals must take in enough minerals and vitamins to make up for their loss from the food (ASMBS, 2020). While these surgeries have good long-term follow-up, the patient must follow doctor's orders because these surgeries can be negated by overeating, resulting in the patient regaining the weight they have lost (Maleckas et al., 2016).

Figure 10.3 shows the gastric bypass or Roux-en-Y, which is the gold standard of weight loss surgeries and is accomplished by the surgeon creating a stomach pouch by separating a small area of the stomach and attaching it to the small intestine to let the food "bypass" the lower stomach. The gastric lap band surgery involves the surgeon placing an adjustable band around the beginning of the stomach to make it smaller. The band can be tightened or relaxed depending on the patient's weight loss. The sleeve gastrectomy is a newer surgery that restricts

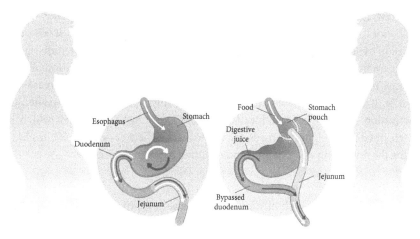

Figure 10.3 Gastric bypass.

80% of the stomach by resecting it and creating a tubular stomach in the shape of a banana, rather than a pouch. It functions by decreasing the amount of food that the stomach can fit at any one time.

(E) Mental health clinicians can benefit from understanding engineering to treat obesity

Findings indicate that a relationship of food intake and illicit or licit drug use exists, implying involvement of similar neurotransmitter systems (Corwin & Wojnicki, 2009; Volkov et al., 2013). Several medications decrease weight by affecting the dopaminergic system, which increases physical activity and metabolism. In the past, several medications contained amphetamines that placed the consumer at risk for deleterious side effects, including substance dependence. Now, the amphetamine-like substance phentermine is prescribed instead of amphetamine and can be found is several antiobesity medications. A multidrug cocktail, such as phentermine and topiramate (Qsymia®) plus naltrexone and bupropion (Contrave®), has had more success because it acts on more than one pathway (Narayanaswami & Dwoskin, 2017). Each component of the cocktail been approved in the United States and the United Kingdom.

Phentermine is an amphetamine-like substance that increases metabolism, including heart rate. While there are many debilitating side effects, one beneficial side effect is loss of taste, which is conducive to eating less. Phentermine has been shown to reduce binge eating and compulsive food cravings and has been used to treat alcohol dependence. Bupropion decreases hunger by stimulating the reward pathway. It inhibits dopamine and norepinephrine reuptake, which allows it to stimulate those receptors for an extended period of time. It has been used to treat nicotine addiction (Narayanaswami & Dwoskin, 2017). Individuals who are not candidates for surgery have benefited from administration of naloxone/naltrexone, or other opioid antagonists, which are used to decrease appetite. Based on the theory that binge eating sugary, fatty foods is related to activation of the reward pathway, an opioid antagonist (Naloxone), which is prescribed as a weight loss medication, blocks the effect of dopamine, thus limiting the rewarding effect of food and resulting in people eating less.

(M) Mental health clinicians can benefit from understanding the mathematics underlying obesity

Disease burden is defined by the CDC (2013) as considering "health, social, political, environmental and economic factors to determine the cost that disease and disability exert upon the individual and society." Obesity affects children, adolescents, and adults differently. For children and adolescents aged 2 to 19 years old, the prevalence of obesity is 18.5%, and 13.7 million of them are affected (CDC, 2019). In addition, the prevalence of obesity increases as age increases: 13.9% among children 2–5 years, 18.4% among those 6–11 years old, and 20.6% among 12- to 19-year-olds. For adults, the prevalence of obesity was 42.4% in 2017–2018, which is more than 10% higher than that in 1990–2000 (CDC, 2020a).

Obesity has generated profound health and economic consequences for U.S. society. In terms of health consequences, obesity is often related to heart disease, stroke, Type 2 diabetes, some types of cancer, and other serious diseases that reduce life expectancy. The price for that extra weight is significant. Researchers estimated the total economic cost by combining direct medical cost and indirect cost caused by lost productivity. It is estimated that the total direct medical spending attributable to obesity was about $147 billion in 2008 (CDC, 2020d). Because obesity-related diseases are correlated with more sick leaves, higher disability rate, and premature death, those days missed from work turn out to be a heavy cost to society. It is estimated that the loss of productivity has resulted in economic cost in the range between $3.38 billion and $6.38 billion (CDC, 2022).

At the individual level, people who are obese on average spend $1,429 more than those who have healthy weight. Those costs were calculated from inpatient and outpatient health services, laboratory and radiological tests, and medications.

Fuhrman (2018) reported that 71% of Americans are overweight, and the T. H. Chan School of Public Health at Harvard University (2020) stated that among African American women, 59% were obese, 41% Hispanic women were obese, and 33% of Caucasians were obese, as operationalized as a BMI of 30 or more. BMI is a composite measure of height and weight. They reported that in Canada, obesity, as defined as the average BMI score applied to 27.5 of men and 28.5 of women, which is comparable to that of the United Kingdom (27.4 of men and 26.9 of women).

Obesity carries a heavy disease burden as it is associated with the onset of other diseases, including Type 2 diabetes. While family heredity is partially responsible for Type 2 diabetes, examination of the social determinants of health that affect the process of developing obesity is warranted. Type 2 diabetes can be a devastating illness as it can cause blindness, renal failure, cardiac problems, stroke, and amputation of the lower limbs and reduces longevity by up to 10 years (Bird et al., 2015). However, up to 75% of cases can be treated by improved diet and increased exercise (Costacou & Mayer-Davis, 2003). In addition to obesity, several social determinants of health have been shown to predict Type 2 diabetes, including household annual income below $30,000 and minority status (Bird et al., 2015).

As reported by the CDC (2019), there are more than 34 million Americans, 10% of the U.S. population, who were diagnosed with diabetes. Of the total cases, Type 2 diabetes accounted for 90%–95%. In 2018, of the proportion of adults aged 18 and older living in America with diabetes (Type 1 and Type 2), 4.9 million were adults age 18–44 years old; 14.8 million were aged 45–64 years; and 14.3 million were 65 years old and older. Of the group, 17.9 million were male and 16.2 million were female. The percentage of adults with diabetes significantly increased from 9.5% in 1999–2002 to 13.0% in 2018. Figure 10.4 displays the distribution of diabetes by race/ethnicity. The Caucasian, non-Hispanic population had the highest prevalence (19.5 million), followed by Hispanic (6.4 million), then by non-Hispanic persons of African descent (5.2 million), and non-Hispanic Asians (2.3 million).

Canada is also witnessing rising rates of diabetes in the population. According to Statistics Canada (2020), there were 2.495 million Canadians who reported having been diagnosed with diabetes (Type 1 or Type 2) in 2019. Of these, 90%–95% were diagnosed with Type 2 diabetes. This accounted for 7.8% of Canadians aged 12 years and older. The proportion of Canadians aged 12 and older who reported being diagnosed with diabetes increased from 6.9% in 2015 to 7.8% in 2019.

Figure 10.5 presents the prevalence of total diabetes (in percentage) by age groups during the period 2015–2019. Diabetes increased with age, with the highest prevalence rate among older adults 65 years and over. For instance, the prevalence rate of diabetes varied among different age groups in 2019: 0.7% among children and adolescents 12 to 17 years, 1.1% among young adults 18 to

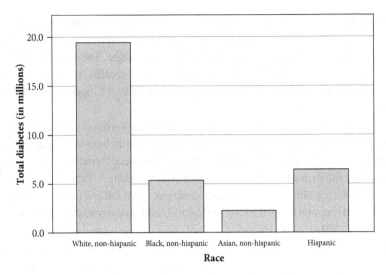

Figure 10.4 Prevalence of diabetes by race/ethnicity, United States, 2018.
Note: Data are expressed in millions.

Data source: Centers for Disease Control and Prevention. *National diabetes statistical report 2020.*
https://www.cdc.gov/diabetes/pdfs/data/statistics/national-diabetes-statistics-report.pdf. Chart
created by Dr. Liyun Wu.

34 years, 4.5% among adults 35 to 49 years, 11.2% among adults 50 to 64 years,
and 19.2% among older adults 65 years and over.

(H) Mental health clinicians can benefit from applying these STEM principles to health regarding treatment of problems with the GI tract

Mindfulness is a therapeutic adaptation of the 2,000-year-old Buddhist practice
of meditation (Mishra, 2017) that trains people to focus on the rhythm and reg-
ularity of their inhalations and exhalations. The practice of mindfulness differs
from Buddhist practice because the element of spirituality is removed in the
former, leaving a secular practice. Kabat-Zin is the primary thinker in the area
of mindfulness and developed the "mindfulness-based stress reduction" (MBSR)
program to treat stress, physical illness, and mental health problems (Shonin &
Kabat-Zinn, 2016). He clearly stated that MBSR is not about Buddhism even
though it adapts Buddhist practices, and the practice is not spiritual. The focus
of mindfulness on repetitive breathing centers the person's mind, which then
becomes detached from outside stimulation, including anxious feelings focused
on bodily sensations attributed to IBS. Mindfulness therapy applies meditation

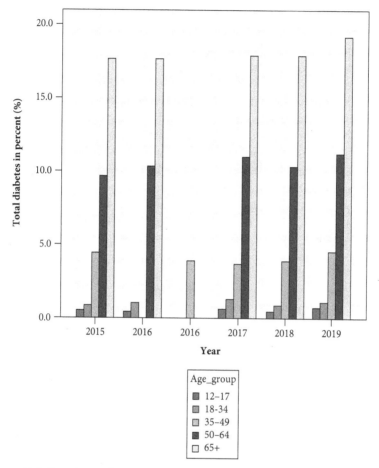

Figure 10.5 Prevalence of Type 1 and Type 2 diabetes by age group, Canada, 2015–2019.

Note: Data are expressed in percentages.

Data source: Centers for Disease Control and Prevention. *National diabetes statistical report 2020*. https://www.cdc.gov/diabetes/pdfs/data/statistics/national-diabetes-statistics-report.pdf. Chart created by Dr. Liyun Wu

and relaxation to calm the client's mind so he or she can notice and accept physical symptoms without attaching anxious feelings to them. At the same time, the sufferer is trained to remain detached from judgmental or anxious thoughts associated with the sensations in their abdomen in order to remove negative emotions that exacerbate the irritable bowel symptoms.

Mindfulness-based stress reduction is a manualized treatment that trains the therapist, who trains the client, to practice the discipline until the client can engage in meditation without a leader. It has been shown to reduce IBS symptom severity (Ballou & Keefer, 2017) and is correlated with more improved scores on a health-related quality-of-life measure and decreased scores on the Psychological Stress Questionnaire (Gaylord et al., 2011). The practice of mindfulness is also associated with reduced catastrophizing when becoming aware of abdominal pain (Garland et al., 2012) and is effective during face-to-face sessions, as well as treatment using an internet IBS intervention. MBSR has been effective in reducing burnout with baccalaureate and master of social work medical social workers in the pediatric field. Compared to baseline, social workers who received a condensed 6-week version of the MBSR showed less compassion fatigue on the Secondary Traumatic Stress subscale of the Professional Quality of Life (ProQOL), as well as higher scores on the Mindful Attention and Awareness Scale (MAAS) and on the Caring Efficacy Scale (CES) score following MBSR (Trowbridge et al., 2017).

Conclusion

In conclusion, this chapter on the GI system introduced the reader to the science, especially the structure and function, of the GI system, as well as typical diseases that afflict some patients. Cleft palate deformities were discussed as an injury to the GI system as it occurs when the embryo's face doesn't develop as it should. Technological advances in treatment of IBS and colon cancer were discussed because of their frequency. Because obesity is such a widespread problem, it is important for clinicians to understand the relationship between obesity and Type 2 diabetes. Medications for treatment of obesity, with a focus on diminishing cravings, were discussed. Finally, mindfulness was introduced as a treatment for clinicians to use with clients who are struggling with diseases of the GI tract. In summary, clinicians who understand the STEM-H model as applied to the GI system are able to work as members of a medical team that treats patients with a range of problems, as well as practice independently with clients who are struggling with symptoms of illnesses or treatments of the GI tract.

Glossary

Anorexia nervosa   An eating disorder characterized by food restriction, low body weight, and poor body image

Bulimia nervosa   An eating disorder characterized by binge eating followed by purging

Peristaltic motion   A to-and-fro motion most often used to describe the activity of the digestive system

Satiety   Satisfied feeling after eating

Websites

American Cancer Foundation: https://www.cancer.org

National Eating Disorders Association: https://www.nationaleatingdisorders.org/learn/by-eating-disorder/bulimia

Overeaters Anonymous: https://oa.org

11

How Understanding the Urogenital System Can Benefit Mental Health Clinicians

Introduction

As the term implies, the urogenital system combines the urinary and the reproductive systems. While this may seem counterintuitive, structurally, both systems are located in the lower abdomen, and in the case of the male, their functions overlap with each other. The urinary system contributes to the sexual response of the male and is critical for reproduction. In and of itself, the urinary system provides a life-giving function that is required to remove toxins from the body and regulate total body water. Inability to remove these toxins results in death. This chapter discusses, in detail, the technology inherent in artificial removal of toxins when the urinary system has failed. In addition, the technology section of the reproductive system elucidates in vitro fertilization (IVF), which includes processes and procedures that overcome infertility. This chapter informs clinicians about the two types of dialysis that their clients or their clients' families may have the occasion to work with. This chapter also presents information about gender fluidity for mental health clinicians who may work with persons who maintain a nonbinary identity. The chapter informs this material in the light of STEM-H (science, technology, engineering, and mathematics as applied to health).

STEM-H Principles Underlying the Urogenital System

(S) Mental health clinicians can benefit from understanding science for the urogenital system

The Urinary System

Structure of the urinary system. At approximately 30 days postfertilization, the cells of the embryo begin to develop into the area that will later become the urinary system (Collins, 2021). At birth, the neonatal kidney weighs around 23g (0.8 oz) and continues to grow for the first few months postpartum. In the adult, each of the two bean-shaped kidneys is approximately the size of a fist and is located in

STEM-H for Mental Health Clinicians. Marilyn Weaver Lewis, Liyun Wu, and Zachary Allan Hagen, Oxford University Press.
© Oxford University Press 2023. DOI: 10.1093/oso/9780197638514.003.0011

the abdominal cavity on either side of the spinal column. Each is surrounded by a layer of connective tissue, a layer of fatty tissue that protects the kidney, and a thin layer of fibrous tissue, called the renal capsule (Ogobuiro & Tuma, 2021). As Figure 11.1 shows, the inferior vena cava sends out up to four to five veins to each pyramidal structure in the medulla. The aortic artery branches into two renal arteries that go to each kidney (Colbert et al., 2020). Both the trunk of the aortic artery and the inferior vena cava continue to travel down to the area above the bladder, where they bifurcate and travel to each leg. These structures provide the extensive blood supply to the kidneys. In fact, from 20% to 25% of cardiac output goes to the kidneys, of which the cortex houses 90%–95% of the kidney's blood supply (Amerman, 2019).

Urine travels from the kidney through the ureters into the bladder where it remains until it receives signals from the body to be expelled. This function is controlled by two sphincters, which are circular muscles that close off the opening of the bladder to keep urine from leaking (Hubert, 2019). The sphincter

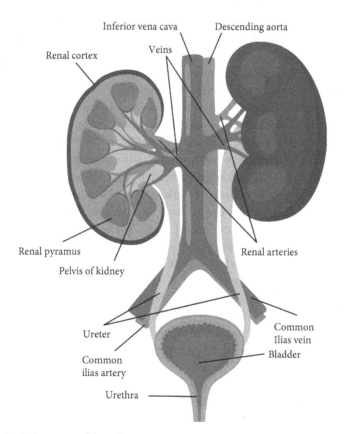

Figure 11.1 Anatomy of the urinary system.

that is closest to the bladder is the internal urethral sphincter, and its action is involuntary; it tells the bladder to release urine when it senses that the bladder is filled. The second sphincter, the external urethral sphincter, is at the pelvic floor, is voluntary, and can be strengthened by exercises (Colbert et al., 2020).

The renal cortex, which is the outer layer of the organ, is inside the renal capsule. If you look closely at the next layer, which is the medulla, you will see renal pyramids (renal pyramus) and columns of tissue that separate them. Each of these small structures comprises one pyramid and one half of a column. The other half of the column is associated with the adjoining pyramid. These structures filter the substance in the one million nephrons in each kidney. On average there are approximately 5 to 11 renal pyramids and columns that send urine down the ureter (Campbell, 2011a). At the end of the pyramids, waste is drained into funnel-like structures that drain into the pelvis of the kidney, the third layer, which then drains into the ureter (Colbert et al., 2020). The ureters are muscular tubes that send urine to the bladder using peristaltic waves. These are so forceful that even if one were to stand on their head, urine would still travel up to the bladder because of the waves (Campbell, 2014). The ureters enter the bladder from behind. The size of the bladder depends on the volume of urine present.

The filter in the body is the nephron, which has two components: the glomerulus and the tubule. The Latin word for glomerulus means ball of yarn (Davis, 2021), as shown in Figure 11.2. It is created by the very small bundle of capillaries (Pollak et al., 2014), called the afferent arterioles. These enter a semicircular space, the Bowman's capsule, which provides a cup for the arterioles to enter and become a tangled mass before exiting as the efferent arteriole. Filtration begins in the zone of filtration with the nephron and glomerulus, which are in the cortex of the kidney. The part of the tubule that is closest to the glomerulus travels from the upper cortex down into the medulla, where it becomes the descending segment of the loop of Henle. The urine releases proteins, glucose, and sometimes red blood cells into the zone of reabsorption of the tubule, where they are reabsorbed back into the bloodstream (Hisrich, 2021). The process continues with the zone of secretion in the ascending segment of the loop of Henle, which is into the renal cortex. There, more water and sodium are reabsorbed from the filtrate in the nephrons. This process leaves urea, some sodium, excreted medications, and water in the collecting ducts, which then travel through the ureters, until reaching the bladder to be stored and excreted (Hisrich, 2021).

The bladder is a holding tank for urine. In the male, it lies above the prostate, and, in the female, it lies in front of the uterus. When the bladder is empty, it lies in the pelvic area, but when it is full, it expands toward the abdominal cavity (Gomella & Chung, 2021). According to Gomella and Chung, the bladder is held

Urine formation

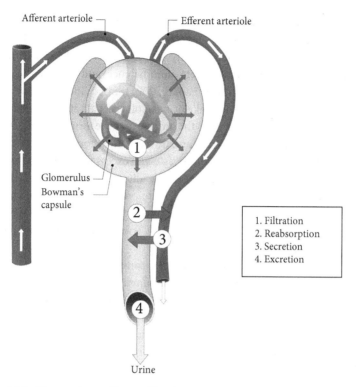

Figure 11.2 Glomerulus and loop of Henle.

in place by ligament-like fibrous muscles that attach the neck of the bladder to the side walls of the pelvis and the rectum and attach the apex of the bladder to the umbilical area. The inside of the bladder is covered by pleats created by a mucous layer that expands and lies flat when the bladder is filled (Colbert et al., 2020). The urethra extends from the bladder to exit at an external opening in the genital region. On average, it is approximately 1.57 inches in the female, but 7.47 inches in males (Gomella & Chung, 2021). In males the distal section of the urethra is surrounded by the penis and ends in a slit that allows urine to empty. During urination, the urethral opening becomes tube-like. In females, the urethra is a tube that also travels from the bladder and exits at an opening between the clitoris and the vagina. In the event this process does not work as it should, the individual could develop a urinary tract infection, which are more common in women, from bacteria that is introduced through the urethra (Greenstein et al., 2020).

Function of the urinary system. According to Campbell (2011a), the kidneys are responsible for maintaining the volume and content of the bodily fluids. They do this by filtering 52.83 gallons of fluids from renal blood flow each day (Ogobuiro & Tuma, 2021) to remove waste, maintain the balance of electrolytes in the fluid, balance acidity and alkalinity in the blood, produce hormones, maintain calcium and potassium balance, and regulate the production of red blood cells (Murray & Paolini, 2021), in addition to what we normally think of as its function, to make urine (Colbert et al., 2020). As Figure 11.2 shows, there are several functions in the process of urine formation: filtration, reabsorption, secretion, and excretion and through those four processes maintain homeostasis and rid the body of toxic waste and excess fluid. First, homeostasis is maintained by balancing the blood's pH (acidity and alkalinity) and disposing its waste products (Narayan, n.d.). The waste products are filtrated, and some materials are reabsorbed into the renal veins that then take this processed blood back to the bloodstream. The substance that is left is sent via the ureter to be excreted as urine.

The cortex of each healthy adult kidney contains approximately 1 million filtering units, called nephrons. When combined, the nephrons and glomeruli produce 1.59 quarts of liquid urine every day (National Kidney Foundation [NKF], 2021a; Pollak et al., 2014). According to the NKF, kidneys filter and return approximately 200 quarts of liquid to the bloodstream every 24 hours, with about 2 quarts voided as urine, while the other 198 quarts are returned to the system to repeat the process. Normal kidneys purify the blood 40 times per day, and according to Hisrich (2021) reabsorb 100% of the red blood cells and proteins, as well as the glucose, during that process. The end product contains 95% water, less than 5% urine, and less than 5% salts. This end product is passed down the tubule, which becomes the ureter, and then travels to the bladder, where it is stored until it is excreted as urine (Gomella & Chung, 2021). The healthy kidneys manage the sodium and potassium, pH levels in the body; release hormones and vitamin D; help regulate blood pressure; control concentrations of electrolytes; and eliminate waste products and other substances in the body (NKF, 2021a). Excreting water and nonabsorbed waste through the ureter maintains the appropriate balance between acidity and alkalinity (Iwanaga, 2021). Faulty functioning of this highly complicated filtration process accounts for 90% of renal problems and can result in end-stage renal disease (ESRD) (Wiggins, 2007).

The Reproductive System

Structure of the reproductive system . Figure 11.3 shows the male and female reproductive organs next to each other. Each of these organs is similar to the other. Both are characterized by two sexual spherical structures that contain reproductive components: The testicles are housed in the scrotal sacs at the base of

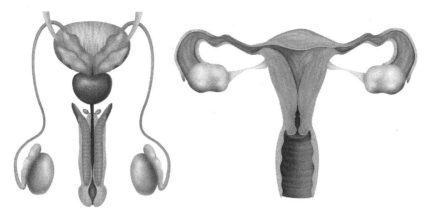

Figure 11.3 Male (*left*) and female (*right*) reproductive systems.

the external penis in the male; and the ovaries are housed at the end of the fallopian tubes at the top of the uterus. The male's and the female's system both have a long canal that extends from the midline and culminates in an opening at the end of the penis in the male and the vagina in the female.

Both the male and the female have internal as well as external structures. The female's internal structures consist of 1 fallopian, 2 ovaries, 1 uterus, and 1 cervix. The main structure in women is the uterus, which includes the fallopian tubes, which emerge at the sides at the top of the structure. The eggs in the ovaries are not visible because they are covered by the ovary's several-layer sac of fibrous connective tissue (Schober, 2021). Under the layers of the sac's outer membrane lies a cortex, where the eggs reside. At birth, a female is born with approximately 1 million immature eggs, or oocytes. These oocytes stop maturing at birth and don't resume maturing until puberty. Every month after puberty until menopause, approximately 10 eggs develop in one of the ovaries, and one is released into the fallopian tube (Heinze, 2019a) where it may be fertilized. Occasionally, in some women, more than one egg will be released and fertilized, resulting in fraternal twins, but typically more than one egg is not released until the alternate ovary releases eggs the next month (Campbell, 2011a).

Figure 11.4 depicts the fallopian tubes, which are extensions of the uterus. The uterus is a pear-shaped muscle that consists of an outer lining; a middle muscle, the myometrium; and the inner lining, the endometrium (Woodman, 2021). According to Woodman, the uterus has two sections. The muscular body is in the upper two thirds, while the cervix forms the lower one third. The uterus is normally the size of a fist until pregnancy, when it grows to the size of a basketball (Heinze, 2019a) and can accommodate a typical seven-pound, 20-inch fetus. Even though the uterus becomes enlarged and thinner during pregnancy

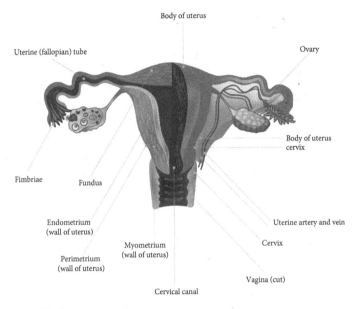

Figure 11.4 The female reproductive system.

to accommodate the size of the fetus, it retains the strength to expel the baby during labor.

The uterus is protected by the cervix, which is composed of fibers that are elastic and can open wide enough during childbirth for the baby to pass into the cervical canal (Woodman, 2021). At birth, the cervix's opening is covered by the hymen, a tissue layer in the vaginal vault that protects the uterus from the external environment. The hymen can be broken during the initial sexual act or in some cases by tampons or vigorous exercise (Campbell, 2011a). The fallopian tube comprises smooth muscle and a mucous lining and has cilia on the ends to create waves that pull in the sperm (Heinze, 2019a). If the egg travels down into the fallopian tube and is fertilized, it becomes a zygote and is implanted in the endometrium or lining of the uterus. A new mucous plug forms over the cervix to protect the zygote from the external intrauterine environment.

The female's external organs include the external genitalia, or vulva, consists of several parts. The vaginal and urethral openings are surrounded by a rim of tissue, the labia minora, and a rim of larger tissues, the labia majora, which protect the openings. At the top of the structure sits the clitoris, which is a small bulb-like structure that is covered by tissue forming the clitoral hood, or prepuce, which protects the highly sensitive structure from friction.

The male also has internal as well as external reproductive organs. As Figure 11.5 shows, the external organs include the gonads, or testes, which are housed

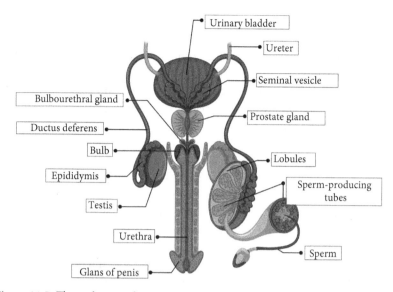

Figure 11.5 The male reproductive system.

in the scrotum (Schober, 2021). The male reproductive system differs from the female's in that the bladder and the prostate emerge at the base of the penis along with the vas deferens duct (Schober, 2021). The male reproductive system is more intertwined with the urinary system than the female's. In the male, both urine and semen are ejected from the penis, whereas the woman has two distinct outlets: the urethra (urinary) and vagina (reproductive). The testicles hang down from the male's body in order to maintain their temperature around 3 degrees cooler than the body. The male system also includes the prostate gland, a round gland that surrounds the ureter as it emerges from the bladder. It sits above the penis. The prostate is considered an accessory sex gland (Schober, 2021) and is absent in the female reproductive system. It is responsible for the production of the fluid that facilitates transportation of male sperm.

Function of the reproductive system . The human reproductive system is designed so the DNA contained in the head of the sperm mixes with the DNA in the female's ovum (Campbell, 2021). The sperm's head, or acromere, is enclosed with an enzyme that helps it penetrate the ovum. The sperm includes a middle section of mitochondria that provides energy and a tail for locomotion so it can swim to the ovum (Campbell, 2021). The female's counterpart to the sperm is the ovum and contains a nucleus that holds the genetic material of the egg and is surrounded by cytoplasm. It is the destination of the sperm's journey.

The activity of sex hormones initiates the maturation of children who develop secondary sex characteristics and become able to reproduce their genetic material. In both the male and female reproductive systems, the process begins in the hypothalamus, which informs the anterior pituitary gland to release two sex hormones, the follicle-stimulating hormone (FSH) and the luteinizing hormone (LH) (Campbell, 2011a). Without FSH and LH, the testes and ovaries remain inactive, as they are before puberty. When FSH and LH are active, they stimulate the ovaries in the female to release estrogen and progesterone and the male's testes to release testosterone.

In order for the woman to be able to become pregnant, her body goes through several hormonal phases to prepare her ovaries to release her eggs and the uterus to receive a fertilized egg. Day 1 of menses is designated as the first day of the menstrual cycle, which is divided into two phases. The follicular phase lasts roughly from Day 1 until ovulation, which is approximately 14 days later. The LH spike causes ovulation (around Day 14 of the woman's reproductive cycle). At that time, the eggs become mature and ready to be fertilized, and the uterus becomes ready to receive a fertilized egg. If the egg does not become fertilized, the uterine lining sloughs off, and menstruation, or menses, begins. Day 1 of menses is designated as the first day of the menstrual cycle, which is divided into two phases.

Figure 11.6 shows that the hormonal phase begins at menses, or menstruation, which is characterized by low levels of the reproductive hormones, estrogen

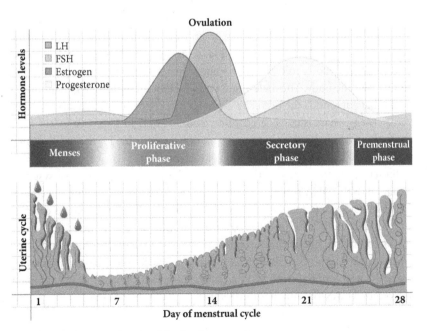

Figure 11.6 Menstrual cycle of the fertile woman.

and progesterone, and the sloughing off of the uterine lining. FSH and LH are also low. Around 7 days after the onset of menses, there is a spike in estrogen and progesterone. Several days later, a spike in LH occurs along with a smaller spike in FSH. This cluster of hormonal activities occurs during ovulation and takes place during the proliferative phase. The follicular phase lasts roughly from Day 1 until ovulation, which is approximately 14 days later. The second menstrual phase begins at the end of ovulation, typically around Day 16 (Campbell, 2011a). Following that phase, at around 21 days since menses, FSH and LH increase, which is depicted in lower but more sustained spikes of the hormones during the secretory phase. During this phase, as the lower graph of the menstrual cycle shows, the uterus is responding to the hormones by thickening. By Day 21 of the menstrual cycle, the uterine lining is thick and dense and capable of housing a fertilized zygote. When the woman's egg is released, it is drawn up into the fallopian tube by cilia, or hairs, and floats down to the uterus, where it can be fertilized by the male's sperm. If fertilization does not occur, hormones subside during the premenstrual phase, especially estrogen and progesterone, and the uterine lining sloughs off during menses until it is thin and compact by Day 5 or 6 of the postmenstruation phase. In normal females who had experienced puberty, the cycle repeats itself month after month until the females reach menopause, at which time the reproductive hormones decrease, and eggs are no longer released from the ovaries.

In the event an egg is fertilized and a zygote formed, it normally will become implanted in the uterine wall. As most women do not know when the embryo was actually conceived, which is defined as conceptual age, gestation is determine using the first day of her most recent menstrual period (Curran, 2019) and lasts on average 38 to 42 weeks (Collins et al., 2021). While it can receive the nourishment it needs from the maternal blood supply from the uterine lining while it is a zygote, as it matures it needs a different source of nourishment. To accomplish this, the fetus develops a placenta, which covers the gestational sac and is attached to the uterus to provide its oxygen and nutrition around the age of 6–12 weeks (Jauniaux & Burton, 2021). According to Jauniaux and Burton, the gestational sac, or placenta, is filled with amniotic fluid, which suspends the developing fetus in secretions from the mother and amniotic tissues and fetal urine. At its largest, the placenta weighs on average 1.1 pounds. The fetus is attached to the uterus by a yolk stalk, which is the precursor to the umbilical cord, which comprises flattened cells, and attached in the center portion of the placenta.

In the male, testosterone stimulates FSH and LH to in turn stimulate the testes to make several million sperm per day. They are reproduced in an ongoing basis and mature on average after 64 days (Schober, 2021). The testes are suspended in scrotal sacs that maintain their temperature at 3 to 4 degrees below body temperature. During the process of spermatogenesis, they make millions of sperm daily from a cell layer in the testes. Mature sperm are not mobile until they learn to swim. When they mature, they migrate down to the seminal vesicles, where sperm is stored. The sperm wait in the vesicles until the male ejaculates, when they travel down the male urethra and are ejected from the penis (Heinze, 2019b).

In order for them to leave the male, the man has to become sexually aroused, develop an erection, and ejaculate. The parasympathetic branch of the autonomic nervous system is responsible for the man's arousal. It allows the penis to become engorged with blood so it can become erect and enter the female. The sympathetic nervous system becomes activated when the man ejaculates, allowing the penis to expel the seminal fluid (Schober, 2021). Because the male urinates and ejaculates through one urethra, his body has to prevent urine from being expelled along with the semen. This is achieved by the function of the prostate gland, which squeezes off the opening from the bladder during sex so only semen travels down the urethra (Heinze, 2019b).

As the sperm are traveling from the vas deferens, they receive fluid from the seminal vesicle (Campbell, 2011a). According to Campbell, this fluid is alkaline and neutralizes the acidity in the vagina, as well as secreting sticky proteins that enter the cervix. Because the sperm can remain in the vagina for several days, the fluid from the seminal vesicles also contains fructose so the sperm can survive longer (Schober, 2021). According to Schober, the third structure that provides fluid is the bulbourethral, or Cowper's, gland, which also releases alkaline fluid before ejaculation. The millions of sperm in the 2 to 5 mL of semen (Heinze, 2019b) receive these fluids to increase the opportunity for reproductive success. After ejaculation, the sperm begin to swim steadily and typically arrive at the uterine tubes within an hour (Schober, 2021). According to Schober, after they enter the woman's reproductive tract, the sperm go through a process that enables them to fertilize the egg by increasing their mobility and changing the acrosome so it can pierce the corona of the egg.

During the female's ovulation, the cervix's sticky, mucous lining thickens in order for the sperm to adhere to it and remain close to the uterus (Heinze, 2019b). Because the mucus is alkaline, it also helps to reduce the acidity of the vagina to increase the probability the sperm will survive. The increased mucus at the cervix opening also functions to keep the sperm in the vagina so they can have longer access to the egg. Sperm deposited near the cervix survive approximately 5 days. A few hundred sperm swim up the uterus, where it can take a week to reach the egg as it floats down the fallopian tube.

If a healthy sperm fertilizes the egg, chromosomes divide and lend one half of their genetic material to the nucleus. At fertilization, the zygote receives 23 chromosomes from each parent, 2 of which are sex chromosomes that designate whether the developing organism becomes female (XX) or male (XY) (Aatsha &

Kewal, 2021). The zygote divides into many cells, as shown in Figure 11.7. By Day 2, a zygote will divide into a two-cell, to four-cell, to eight-cell stage by Day 4. As can be seen by the figure, around Day 5 the cells develop into a structure called a blastocyst, which occurs around the fourth day after fertilization. The blastocyst has more than 35 cells around Day 4, which increase to 256 cells around Day 6 (Campbell, 2021). The blastocyst travels down into the uterus approximately 72 hours before it becomes implanted, and during that time, it interacts with other cells in the uterus (Jauniaux & Burton, 2021).

The blastocyst folds in on itself and forms a tube-like structure. The structures begin to develop when the blastocyte implodes and becomes a tubelike structure called the notochord, from which the remaining layers of embryonic tissues form. During the first month of gestation, an amniotic sac forms around the fertilized egg; it grows and fills with fluid, which cushions the embryo, and a placenta develops to transfer the nutrients from the mother to the fetus and the waste from the fetus (Cleveland Clinic, 2020). By gestational age 4 weeks, the embryo is the size of a pinhead (Curran, 2019), and its heart tube beats about 65 times per minute (Cleveland Clinic, 2020). According to Curran, 1 week later, the zygote has become an embryo, and the heart has

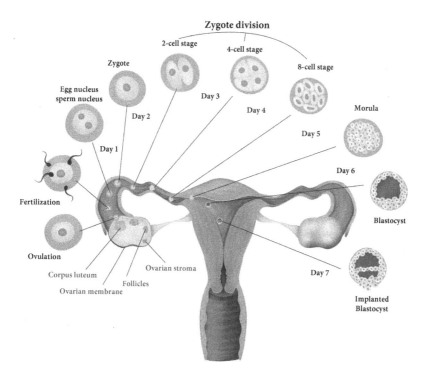

Figure 11.7 Ovulation and fertilization process.

begun to develop and, by the end of the week, has begun beating. The central nervous system (spine and brain) is also developing, and at this stage in development, birth defects can begin to develop, which have no known cause or several causes. At 6 weeks' gestation, the embryo is the size of a pea. The heart is beating at about 110 beats/minute, and the eyes, nostrils, and arms are developing, while at 8 weeks, the embryo is the size of a bean (Curran, 2019), and the neural tube that develops into the central nervous system is well formed (Cleveland Clinic, 2020). The zygote continues to develop into an embryo, and after 9 weeks, it more closely resembles a fetus. It is incorrect to refer to the fetus as an unborn baby, which is reserved for the offspring when it is born. By 10 weeks, the embryo's tail has receded, and it is now called a fetus. It typically weighs 1.2 ounces and is 1.2 inches. By 13 weeks, the heartbeat is detectable, the genitalia are fully developed, and the sex of the fetus is discernible; its nervous system starts to function, and its facial features are discernible (Cleveland Clinic, 2020), and all the organs are formed but unable to sustain life (Curran, 2019). By 15 weeks, the mother may feel fluttering, or quickening, when the fetus is active. Quickening has been identified as a major time during pregnancy when the mother develops the maternal–fetal bond (Lewis, 2008). At around 18 gestational weeks, the fetus can respond to sounds and on average is 8.6 inches long and 7.9 ounces. Two months later, it is having rapid eye movements during sleep. If the fetus is female, all her eggs are in her ovaries, and if male, his testicles have begun to move from the abdomen to the scrotum (Office on Women's Health [OWH], 2019b) around 24 weeks. Survival outside the womb, with intensive care (Cleveland Clinic, 2020), would be around 9% at 5.1 months, 33% at 5.3 months, 65% at 5.5 months, 81% at 5.8 months, and 87% at six months (Curran, 2019). During the third trimester, the fetus forms muscles and stores body fat, and by 40 weeks is 20.2 inches long and weighs eight pounds (Curran, 2019). It is the third trimester when the fetus' organs mature, and it develops weight at approximately one-half pound each week (OWH, 2019b).

Childbirth is the objective of conception and gestation. It is signaled by a rush of hormones that initiate labor, the rhythmic contractions of the uterus that expel the fetus from the vaginal canal. The vagina, made of muscles and tendons, is capable of widening to a great degree to allow the baby to exit (Woodman, 2021). Labor has several stages: dilation (uterine contractions cause the cervix to open to allow the baby to exit from the mother); expulsion (onset is when the cervix is totally open and the baby is delivered); crowning (when the baby's head leaves the mother); and the placental stage, when the afterbirth or placenta is expelled (Colbert et al., 2020). When the baby is born, it is attached to the placenta, and the physician or midwife must cut the umbilical cord to detach it. Oxytocin is a hormone that has been attributed to maternal bonding and is released during pregnancy when the contractions put pressure on the cervix (Prior, 2013).

Illnesses of the Urinary System

Kidney stones. Passing a kidney stone is an extremely painful condition because there are many pain receptors in the kidneys and ureters (Campbell, 2014). It is also relatively common. According to Litwin and Saigal (2012), among men living in the United States, lifetime prevalence of having at least one episode of kidney stones is 11.39% and, among women, 6.44%, with a 5-year risk of recurrence as high as 50% (Khan et al., 2017). According to Khan and colleagues, risk factors for developing kidney stones include weight gain, obesity, and diabetes, as well as gender, non-Hispanic Caucasian race, and living in the southern United States. A kidney stone develops because of excessive levels of calcium and other minerals in the body and may be jagged or smooth and as small as a grain of sand or as large as a golf ball (National Institute of Diabetes and Digestive and Kidney Diseases [NIDDKD], 2017). Eighty percent of stones are composed of calcium (Khan et al., 2017; Ogobuiro & Tuma, 2021). They can vary in size from very small to too large to travel down the ureter. According to the NIDDKD (2017), symptoms include sharp pains in the back; discolored, nonproductive, and odiferous urine; and sometimes nausea, vomiting, fever, and chills. While in the past surgery was the only choice for treatment of kidney stones, a newer process, lithotripsy, is now used to break up the stones into small pieces that can pass through the ureter and is the most prevalent treatment for kidney stones.

End-stage renal disease . End-stage renal disease (ESRD) is diagnosed when the glomerular filtration rate is 15% or less than the optimal capacity and the kidneys can no longer remove urea from the blood and maintain equilibrium between acidity and alkalinity (Campbell, 2011b). Without removal, toxins build up in the body and create a medical crisis. The most common causes of ESRD in the United States are diabetes and high blood pressure.

The treatment for ESRD is either kidney transplant, which is difficult to arrange, or dialysis. There are two types of dialysis: hemodialysis and peritoneal dialysis. The latter can be performed at home either several times during the day or once at night. In addition to the technical aspect of the treatment, the process is complicated by food restrictions and a complicated medication regimen. While this treatment of ESRD is burdensome, it extend one's life for several years. O'Hare and colleagues (2019) found that even though the average life expectancy for dialysis patients is less than five years, one-third of a large survey of 993 dialysis patients predicted that they would live for more than 10 years. Even though the actual average life expectancy for people receiving dialysis was 5 years or fewer, although 20.7% lived more than 10 years. On the other hand, 73.3% of the patients who received a kidney transplant lived longer than 10 years.

Illnesses of the Reproductive System

Sexually transmitted diseases . There are many sexually transmitted diseases that can negatively impact reproductive health (Centers for Disease Control and Prevention [CDC], 2018). According to the World Health Organization (WHO, 2021), in 2020 approximately 374 million new sexually transmitted infections (STIs) of chlamydia (129 million), gonorrhea (82 million), syphilis (7.1 million), and trichomoniasis (156 million) were contracted, many of which had no discernible symptoms. Several STIs infect the woman's upper reproductive tract and can affect the ovaries, endometrium, and fallopian tubes and cause misplaced or ectopic pregnancies, infertility, and chronic pelvic pain (Das et al., 2016) and pelvic inflammatory disease (PID), which increases at the cervix and travels up through the female reproductive system, resulting in infertility (WHO, 2021).

The infections can be the result of bacteria, viruses, protozoans, fungi, and parasites. *Chlamydia trachomatis* is an example of a common bacteria-related sexually transmitted disease and is the most frequently reported STD. *Chlamydia trachomatis* can cause inflammation of the cervix and PID. Women may not discover they have the illness unless alerted by their male sexual partner, as men are more likely to experience symptoms, including discharge from penis, painful urination, itching and burning sensation at urethral opening, swelling and pain around the testicles (Planned Parenthood, n.d.). Babies whose mothers had untreated chlamydia could be born with congenital blindness or develop pneumonia (Children's Minnesota, 2015). Because it is easy to treat, prenatal care can prevent prematurity and miscarriages. *Gonorrhea* is another bacterial STD that can attack the urethra, penis, vagina, fallopian tubes, cervix, and anus. In addition to PID and scarring of the fallopian tubes, gonorrhea can result in an ectopic pregnancy, which is a pregnancy that occurs in the fallopian tube or at another location outside of the uterus (Colbert et al., 2020). Because gonorrhea is a bacterial illness, it is treatable with antibiotics.

Herpes is a very common viral infection that impacts the reproductive system. There are two types of herpes viruses. Herpes simplex virus 1 is generally associated with cold sores of the mouth, while herpes simplex virus 2 is associated with the genitals, and an active episode during pregnancy can cause miscarriage or premature birth. According to WHO (2021), in 2016 more than 490 million people were infected with herpes 2. Herpes can never be cured, but episodes can be treated with an antiviral medication to shorten outbreaks and ameliorate symptoms. Treatment is ongoing throughout life as episodes are more likely to reoccur when the individual is under stress, is sick, or is tired.

Human papillomavirus (HPV) is another infection that is viral and can have a negative impact on reproductive health. HPV is incurable and common. Approximately 80% of women will develop some form of HPV during their lifetime. Not all forms cause genital warts, as common planter warts are a form of

HPV. According to WHO (2021), HPV was associated with 570,000 cases of cervical cancer in 2018 and over 311,000 cervical cancer deaths annually. While it is incurable, a vaccine has been developed to protect individuals from contracting HPV, or genital warts, and teenagers are encouraged to be vaccinated. HPV does not require intimate sexual contact to be transmitted. When an individual is affected, warts can occur on the cervix, vulvar area, and genitals and proliferate and block the vaginal canal. Of the many subtypes of HPV, two subtypes are commonly associated with cervical cancer.

Trichomonas vaginalis, or trich, is a parasitic, protozoal infection that can cause PID, infection of the urethra, and infertility and increase the risk for HIV and developing other STDs. According to the CDC (2021c), symptoms can include burning and itching of the genitals and odor. If a pregnant woman develops trich, her baby may be born prematurely and have a low birth weight (CDC, 2021c).

Parasitic sexually transmitted diseases include *pubic lice*, which can be acquired by skin-to-skin contact or sharing clothes or bedding of a person who is infested (CDC, 2019b). These parasites can be treated with over-the-counter lice medication, although care has to be taken because of its toxicity. Medication to kill lice should not be used during pregnancy without talking to the obstetrician.

Injuries of the Urinary System

Each year in the United States there are approximately 245,000 injuries to the genitourinary system (Patel et al., 2015). Injuries to the kidneys are classified as Grade I through Grade IV: Grade I indicates a kidney that is bruised and cut/lacerated; Grade II indicates deeper lacerations; III indicates deep lacerations or a shattered kidney, which often requires surgery; and IV indicates that the kidney is torn away from its source and often requires removal (Itagaki & Knight, 2004). However, most injuries are managed with noninvasive treatment (Erlich & Kitrey, 2018). In a systematic review of 9,119 adults who received trauma-related care from blunt force injuries to the renal systems, 63% of the injuries were related to vehicular accidents, followed by falls (43%), sports injuries (11%), and pedestrian accidents (4%) (Voelzke & Leddy, 2014). Patel and colleagues (2015) reported that vehicular accidents most often resulted in Grades III–IV injuries, whereas sports-related injuries resulted in lower grade injuries. They found that most sports injuries to the renal system were isolated, did not involve other systems, and had lower mortality rates. Injuries from vehicular accidents were more likely to involve several bodily systems, while sports-related injuries to the urinary system were more often the result of focused trauma (Bagga et al., 2015). Lai and colleagues (2016) compared 78 patients with acute kidney injury (AKI) with 14,504 patients without AKI. Although they did not indicate the cause of the injuries, they found that patients with AKI suffered from abdominal injuries, hepatic injuries, as well as brain injuries and had higher injury severity, were older, and had more comorbidities than those without an AKI. The AKI patients remained in the hospital longer, were more likely to receive intensive care, and had higher rates of mortality. Clearly, survivors of vehicular accidents are at an elevated risk for poor outcomes.

On the other hand, as reported by Patel and colleagues (2015), patients who experienced sports injuries were less at risk for poor outcomes. They identified skiing, snowboarding, and contact sports as the most common source of sports-related injuries, while Osterberg and colleagues (2017) identified bicycle accidents as the most common source. They determined that among bicyclists admitted to a Level 1 trauma center injuries were more often to the kidneys (75.0%), bladder (14.6%), testis (12.5%), adrenals (8.3%), and urethra (6.3%), even though some patients suffered injuries to more than one organ. The falls associated with bicycle accidents may be the cause of the injuries because falls are second only to vehicular accidents as a common cause of injuries to the genitourinary system. Itagaki and Knight (2004) studied kidney injury in a case study of a young man who experienced sports-related falls while practicing jujitsu. Jujitsu is a form of unarmed combat that was developed in Japan and uses "throwing" techniques that require the athlete to have mastered falling safely. In spite of good technique, according to Itagaki and Knight, injury can occur because it is not uncommon for the combatant to be thrown over 100 times during one session. De Meersman and Wilkerson (1982) studied nine judo players who practiced on a thin versus a thick mat and found that the sessions using the thin mat resulted in blood in the urine and abnormal glomerular filtration rates, but not the sessions on the thick mat, even though the men were thrown 100 times on each mat. They concluded it was the trauma from the mechanical impact rather than the body's reaction to the "throwing" technique that resulted in the renal trauma.

Injuries to the Reproductive System
Circumcision is an injury to the genitalia in the male and female. Male circumcision is often practiced for medical and social reasons because it is easier to clean the penis and is related to fewer urinary tract infections, fewer sexually transmitted diseases, and penile cancer (Mayo Clinic, 2021). Historically, each culture that practices circumcision of the male uses scripture, the Koran in the Muslim culture and the Old Testament of the Bible in the Jewish culture, as dogma that requires these practices. Circumcision is also practiced by the people of the Muslim faith, and today, in most Muslim countries in the world including Morocco, Tunisia, Afghanistan, Iran, and Iraq, approximately 100% of the males are circumcised. According to the National Center on Biotechnology Information (2021), male circumcision is accepted by the majority in America (71.2%), but it is not accepted as widely in Canada (31.9%) or many European

countries, where few males are circumcised: United Kingdom (20.7%); France (14.0%); Germany (10.9%); Switzerland (5.9%); Austria (5.8%); Denmark (5.3%); and Greece (4.7%). Other areas of the world where circumcision rates are low include South America (Columbia, 4.2%; Brazil 1.3%; Uruguay, 0.6%; Venezuela, 0.3%) and Asia (China, 14.0%; Japan, 9.0%; Cambodia, 3.5%; Vietnam, 0.2%; and North Korea, 0.1%).

In the Muslim culture, female circumcision, or as it is sometimes called in the western European culture, female genital mutilation (FGM), is frequently done before girls are 8 years old and often in a ritualistic ceremony (Horowitz & Jackson, 1997). There are several types of female circumcision practices (WHO, 2020). In the most traditional form, the Sunna circumcision, the clitoris is either partially or totally removed with, or without, removal of the clitoral hood. According to Peabody (2015), 97% of Egyptian girls have undergone this form of circumcision. As the clitoris is the most sensitive part of the woman's external genitalia, this type of circumcision removes the major source of the woman's sexual pleasure, which is often the objective of the practice. According to WHO, this practice is carried out to ensure that the girl is a virgin at marriage and faithful during marriage because it is believed to reduce her libido. A more extreme version of female circumcision, the clitoridectomy, removes the entire clitoris and clitoral hood as well as the inner folds of the vulva, or the labia minora. Among some African cultures, it is practiced as a female initiation rite (Peabody, 2015) and to remove sexual desire in other cultures. In this version, the labia majora may also be removed. Cultural norms have developed that promote this practice as increasing a woman's femininity because her body parts that are considered "unclean" or "male" are removed (WHO, 2020). WHO recorded that the most extreme form of female circumcision removes the clitoris, the clitoral hood, and the labia minora and sews the labia majora together to close the vagina, leaving only a small hole for urine and menstrual blood to be expelled. However, this practice of infibulation, or pharaonic circumcision, may be performed in some cases without removing the clitoris. In order to have sex, the vagina is surgically opened to accommodate the penis and for her to give birth. After birth, the vagina may be sewn together again, or "closed." A fourth group of practices that are carried out in addition to the ones previously mentioned include scraping, cauterizing, pricking, and piercing the genital areas (Peabody, 2015). Unfortunately, this practice is often carried out at home in unsanitary, nonsurgical rituals because it has been outlawed by several societies after women's rights groups and international medical associations protested and brought the practice to light.

Female circumcision, often referred to as female genital mutilation, is controversial; Horowitz and Jackson (1997) have reported that some women who have been circumcised have voiced that they are offended by the term FGM

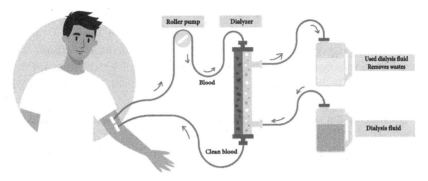

Figure 11.8 Hemodialysis.

because they do not consider their bodies mutilated. Horowitz and Jackson, both physicians, wrote that a more neutral term is ritual female genital surgery. They reported that one of the patients in their study with East African women who had experienced circumcision stated that she didn't understand the controversy because her brother was circumcised as well. They go on to write that it is critical to not pathologize the practice, as many of the women they interviewed were satisfied with the way they looked and planned to circumcise their daughters to keep them "pure and safe."

(T) Mental health clinicians can benefit from understanding technology related to the urogenital system

Urinary System

There are three ways to remove toxic waste when the kidneys are no longer able: kidney transplants and two types of dialysis (hemodialysis and peritoneal dialysis). There are long waiting lists for kidney transplants, but dialysis is common. According to the United States Renal Data System (2020), in 2017, there were 124,369 patients in the United States who suffered from ESRD, 108,131 were receiving hemodialysis, 12,572 were receiving peritoneal dialysis, while 3,666 were waiting for a kidney transplant. Because the proportion of patients receiving dialysis far outstrips kidney transplant hopefuls, this chapter focuses on hemodialysis. As Figure 11.8 shows, hemodialysis routes the individual's blood through a dialyzer machine, where the toxins are removed and the blood is returned to the body as healthy blood. To begin the process, the surgeon creates a fistula by suturing a vein and an artery together, often in the arm. This connection between artery and vein is known as a fistula. A second way to prepare the body for hemodialysis is by implanting a tube that has one end attached to the vein and the other end attached to the artery. This is called a graft. Two tubes are attached to the patient's arm, which are then attached to a dialyzer in a dialysis machine. The arrows in the figure indicate the direction of the flow of the fluids. In this schematic, the top arrows are flowing toward the dialysis machine, and based on what we know about the heart, that tube must be attached to the artery because arterial blood flows away from the heart. The figure also demonstrates that the dialyzer removes toxic waste from the blood. The bottom tube in the schematic is flowing away from the dialysis fluid toward the dialyzer. The dialysis fluid is pumped through the dialyzer to clean the blood, which is then sent back to the body. In hemodialysis, this process takes 4 hours and is done three times weekly (NKF, 2021a), most often at an outpatient dialysis clinic, although Mendonca and colleagues (2021) reported that data from developing countries with limited resources demonstrated that providing hemodialysis only twice weekly with longer session times was adequate, depending on patient characteristics.

The second type of dialysis is called peritoneal dialysis and rather than being administered externally by a machine, it is performed inside the patient's peritoneal cavity, located in the abdomen. The individual is fitted with an indwelling catheter, and about 2 quarts of dialyzing fluids are introduced through a small tube. The solution remains in the individual's peritoneal cavity for several hours in order to neutralize the toxins in the blood and then is drained into a disposable bag (NKF, 2021a). The procedure is conducted four times daily. The benefit of this type of dialysis is that individuals can be ambulatory and carry out their normal routine. Another way to receive peritoneal dialysis is to conduct the dialysis during sleep. According to Evans (2021), peritoneal dialysis is the preferred method of dialysis because the individual is not relegated to the clinic for long periods of time. A caveat is that the procedure may be too cumbersome for some clients without assistance and puts the patient at risk for infection if proper infection control measures are not followed. Traditionally peritoneal dialysis has better outcomes than hemodialysis as it occurs daily. Ideally dialysis is simply used as a temporizing measure while waiting for a kidney transplant; however, many patients who are not transplant candidates require dialysis for many years.

Reproductive System

In vitro fertilization . Infertility is defined as the failure to become pregnant, carry a pregnancy to term, and deliver a live baby within 12 months of having regular, unprotected, sexual activity (CDC, 2019a). Infertility can be attributed to the male (30%), the female (30%), or a combination of both the male and female (30%) (Hull et al., 1985). In a classic study by Hull and colleagues, among 708 infertile couples attending a fertility clinic, failure to ovulate occurred in 21% of couples, tubal damage was found to be responsible in 14% of cases, and endometriosis was found in 6% of the couples. Among 24% of the men, infertility was caused by a deficit in sperm count, distorted sperm shape, or problems with motility. Infertility remained unknown in 28% of cases (Hull et al., 1985). Risk factors for infertility include genetic makeup, hormonal irregularities, abuse of alcohol, drug use (including steroids), smoking, and being exposed to other toxins, such as from radiation. Among women attending fertility clinics, infertility was due to failure to ovulate (21%), damaged fallopian tubes (14%), and endometriosis (6%) (Hull et al., 1985).

Maternal age contributes to infertility (Grondahl et al., 2017) in part because a woman is born with a certain number of eggs that are released every month. Therefore, as the years go by, she has fewer eggs to release in ovulation (Yan et al., 2012). Other women are infertile because they have endometriosis, which is a disease where uterine tissue grows outside the uterus and can cause inflammatory reactions and scarring (Bulletti et al., 2010). Fibroid tumors, which are the most common benign tumors in women of child-bearing age (Eunice Kennedy Shriver National Institute of Child Health and Human Development, 2018) are also common contributors to infertility, especially among African American women, who were more likely to experience severe or very severe symptoms, including heavy or prolonged bleeding during their menstrual cycle, and anemia (Stewart et al., 2013). These tumors affect the embryo's ability to implant in the wall of the uterus.

In vitro fertilization is a technological process to treat infertility; a sperm fertilizes an egg using technological procedures rather than sexual intercourse. At the onset of IVF, the woman takes hormones to initiate maturation of 10 or more eggs, which are recruited, matured, and incubated overnight with live sperm (Campbell, 2021). After the egg is fertilized it is transferred into the woman's uterus with the hope that it will become implanted into the uterine wall. Eggs that are not used can be frozen and stored for potential future use by the donor or by another woman whose eggs are not viable. In cases when the problem is that there are not enough male sperm to naturally reach an egg, individual sperm can be injected into the oocyte using a process known as intracytoplasmic injection (Campbell, 2021).

In vitro fertilization allows the scientist to assess the health of the chromosomes and to evaluate the health of the embryo with genetic testing. This method also allows the parents to determine if the fetus will be male or female, giving parents the opportunity to choose the sex of their child. Fetuses that are not of the preferred sex can be prevented from developing. The ethics of this practice is under debate because people who think that human life begins at conception often believe that destroying any fertilized oocyte is paramount to murder. Other cultures that are limited in the number of children they can have can use this process to choose the sex of the child they prefer.

(E) Mental health clinicians can benefit from understanding engineering to treat the urogenital system

Urinary System

Nonpharmacological treatments are the first choice of treatment for children who have a problem staying dry at night. However, when they do not solve the problem of bedwetting, or nocturnal enuresis, there are several pharmacological options that are the second line of intervention. Desmopressin (vasopressin) is an antidiuretic medication that decreases urine production at night. Many patients are able to cease bedwetting when taking the medication, but gains disappear when the medication is discontinued (Maternik et al., 2015). Anticholinergic drugs are also used, although they aren't the first choice of medication (Maternik et al., 2015). Oxybutynin, an antagonist of the muscarinic receptor, targets the overactive bladder muscle (detrusor) by blocking acetylcholine. However, its anticholinergic side effects, such as dry mouth and blurred vision, are well known and are related to the patient's discontinuation of treatment (31% of the treatment group by 12 weeks) (Allison & Gibson, 2018). Friedman and colleagues (2011) advised that it is not recommended for children who only wet the bed at night rather than daytime as well, in part because of serious central nervous system symptoms, including hallucinations, agitation, sedation, confusion, and nightmares. Beta-3-adrenergic agonists such as Mirabegron, which relax the smooth detrusor muscle of the bladder, have been used with success for urge incontinence that is mixed (Schiavi et al., 2018) and severe (Yoshida et al., 2020). In addition, this medication has fewer side effects than oxybutynin. Tricyclic antidepressants have also been prescribed, the most common of which is imipramine. Although their results are better than a placebo, tricyclics aren't as commonly prescribed as they were in the past because they are minimally effective (Caldwell et al., 2016), and newer medications are less toxic. Botulin toxin A is a third line of intervention, but only when noninvasive procedures have not been successful (Maternik et al., 2015). The medication appears to be successful when given at the proper dose, but each treatment requires from 20 to 50 injections into the muscle of the bladder (Maternik et al., 2015), and in some cases, they only last from 6 to 9 months, and additional treatment episodes are needed (McDowell et al., 2012). While the treatment is done under local or general anesthesia (Talley et al., 2017), some patients need frequent catheterizations, which are painful and urinary tract infections are common (Gormley et al., 2012).

Reproductive System

There are several forms of birth control, which range from pharmaceutical medications, to surgeries, and to mechanical devices. Although abstinence is the only noninvasive birth control method that is 100% effective, its efficacy in preventing pregnancy depends on the ability of the woman to avoid sexual activity. This is often difficult because of natural sexual desire, or coercion, and other types of birth control are often encouraged. The least invasive method of birth control is the "rhythm method," which uses knowledge of the woman's menstrual cycle to estimate when she is ovulating and able to conceive. According to Trussell and colleagues (2018), this method is only 76% effective. Another noninvasive birth control method is the condom. Both male and female condoms have been used to thwart pregnancy but must be used correctly and are only 82% and 79% effective, respectively. Short- and long-acting pharmaceutical hormonal medications are effective, when taken as prescribed, according to OWH (2019a).

A "morning after pill" can be taken to inhibit ovulation after unintended sexual activity. Another morning after solution is implanting an intrauterine device, the Cu-IUD, within 5 days of unprotected sex (CDC, 2016). According to the CDC, other types of emergency contraception include emergency contraception pills, of which there are three: levonorgestrel; a combination of estrogen and progestin; and ulipristal acetate (UPA). Rosato and colleagues (2016) reported that UPA is the first choice in emergency contraception and has no effect on postfertilization. Invasive techniques include devices such as diaphragms and cervical caps, while long-acting intrauterine devices that are almost 100% effective (99.995% to 99.992%) (Trussell et al., 2018). Intrauterine devices are reversible, which increases their popularity. The most invasive method of birth control is sterilization of the male or female, which, according to Trussell and colleagues, is 99.999% and 99.992% effective, respectively. However, sterilization, for all intents and purposes, is often irreversible. According to Trussell and colleagues (2018), while the odds of a man impregnating a female after male sterilization is only 0.15%, the odds of a woman becoming pregnant after having her fallopian tubes severed is only 0.5%.

(M) Mental health clinicians can benefit from understanding mathematics

Urinary System

Chronic kidney disease (CKD) is a medical condition in which the kidneys are damaged and cannot filter blood as well as they should. Due to this failure, excess waste and fluid from blood may result in a wide array of health consequences, including anemia or a low number of red blood cells, increased occurrence of infections, depression, heart diseases, or stroke. By estimation, there are 37 million U.S. adults with CKD, which is every one of seven adults (CDC, 2021a). The proportion of CKD increases as individuals age. The proportion of CKD among people aged 65 and older is 38.1%, while the proportion of adults 45–64 years is 12.4%, and 6.0% among adults 18–44. When comparing CKD among genders, there are slightly more women than men: 14.3% of women are diagnosed with CKD versus 12.4% of men (CDC, 2021b). Non-Hispanic adults of African descent are most likely to develop CKD (16.3%), followed by Hispanics (13.6%), non-Hispanic Asians (12.9%), and non-Hispanic Caucasians (12.7%).

Figure 11.9 depicts data extracted from the (CDC, 2021b) that represent CKD in the United States. The CKD conditions progress at varying levels and are classified into four stages, 1–4. According to the CDC (2020b), the prevalence of CKD by stage during the period 1988–2016 was based on data from the National Health and Nutrition Examination Survey and shows that during the period 1988–1994 in the United States, the prevalence of patients with CKD was highest in Stage 1 (4.09%) and Stage 3 (4.45%), with the least in Stage 4 (0.24%). During the period 1999–2006, more evidence of CKD occurred, but the same relationship remained: the most in Stage 1 (5.22%) and Stage 3 (6.27%) and the fewest in Stage 4 (0.39%). During the period 2015–2016, the prevalence of CKD

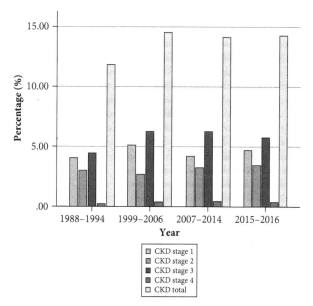

Figure 11.9 Prevalence of chronic kidney disease by stage and year, 1988–1994 to 2015–2016.

Note: CKD, chronic kidney disease. Data: Prevalence of CKD in the general population: CKD stages among U.S. adults, 1988–1994 vs. 1999–2006 vs. 2007–2014 vs. 2015–2016.

Data source: National Health and Nutrition Examination Survey (NHANES). Centers for Disease Control and Prevention. (2020). https://nccd.cdc.gov/CKD/detail.aspx?QNum=Q8. Chart created by Dr. Liyun Wu.

Stage 1 decreased to 4.68%, but increased in Stage 3 (5.79%) and 0.36% in Stage 4. Overall, the prevalence of all CKD Stages 1–4 remained in the range from 11.79% during the period of 1988–1994 to 14.23% during the period 2015–2016. (CDC, 2020a).

Figure 11.10 displays the prevalence of treated ESRD per million U.S. residents during the period 2000–2018 (CDC, 2020b). The chart reports not only total cases, but also cases of functioning kidney transplants as well as dialysis treatment. During the period 2000–2018, the prevalence of kidney transplantation increased from 353.225/million residents to 696.784/million residents from 2000 to 2018 respectively. During the same period, the prevalence of dialysis treatment rose from 927.375/million residents to 1,685.216/million residents,

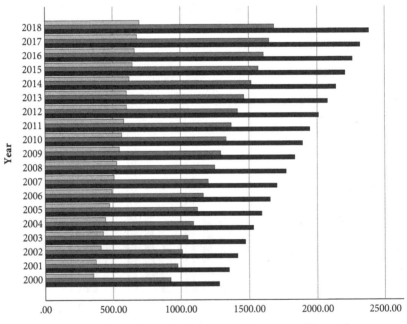

Prevalence of treated end-stage renal disease per million residents

■ Total cases
▨ 2=Dialysis
▨ 3=Transplant

Figure 11.10 Prevalence of treated end-stage renal disease (ESRD), United States, 2000–2018.

Note: Data are expressed in millions.

Data source: Centers for Disease Control and Prevention. (2020). *Chronic kidney disease (CKD) surveillance system.* https://nccd.cdc.gov/ckd/detail.aspx?Qnum=Q67. Chart created by Dr. Liyun Wu.

respectively. In sum, there were 1,280.6 patients/million residents receiving ESRD treatment in 2000 and 2,382 patients/million residents under treatment in 2018 (CDC, 2020b).

Reproductive System

According to the National Survey of Family Growth 2017–2019, only 38.7% of females aged 15–19 used any contraceptive method. For other age groups, the proportion of women using any contraceptive method significantly increased: 60.9% among women aged 20–29, 72.3% among women aged 30–39, 74.8% among women aged 40–49. Using the same data from the National Survey of Family Growth, non-Hispanic Caucasian women had the highest utilization of contraception (69.2%), followed by non-Hispanic women of African descent (61.4%), and Hispanic women (60.5%).

Utilization of contraception was similar across educational attainment. For women without a high school degree, their proportion of using any contraceptive method is 71.2%. Contraception was used by 70.0% of women with a high school degree or GED (General Equivalency Degree, 71.3% of women with some college education, and 69.1% of women with a baccalaureate degree or above.

Currently, adults utilize four common conceptive methods: female sterilization, birth control pills, male condoms, and long-acting reversible contraceptives (LARCs). As can be seen in Figure 11.11, among women who choose sterilization, those aged 40–49 had the highest rate (39.1%), women aged 30–39 had the second highest rate (21.2%), women aged 20–29 had the third highest rate (2.9%) (CDC, 2021b). Young women were more likely to use birth control pills than older women. The percentage of women using pills varied by age group: 19.5% of females aged 15–19 used birth control pills; 21.6% of women aged 20–29; 10.9% among women aged 30–39; and 6.5% among women aged 40–49. The proportion of women who partnered with men using male condoms also varied by age group: 5.1% of female respondents aged 15–19, 10.4% of female respondents aged 20–29, 9.7% of female respondents aged 30–39, and 6.5% of female respondents aged 40–49. In terms of LARC status, women aged 20–29 had the highest utilization (13.7%), women aged 30–39 had the second highest utilization (12.7%), women aged 40–49 had the third highest utilization (6.6%), and last the percentage was 5.8% among females aged 15–19.

As Figure 11.12 shows, among women who used female sterilization, the percentage was 18.5% among non-Hispanic Caucasian women, 17.6% among non-Hispanic women of African descent, and 19.9% among Hispanic women (CDC, 2021b). There were more non-Hispanic Caucasian women using pills (17.8%) than non-Hispanic women of African descent (8.1%) and Hispanic women (7.9%). Among women respondents who reported male condom use, the percentage was 7.0% among non-Hispanic Caucasian women, 11.0% among

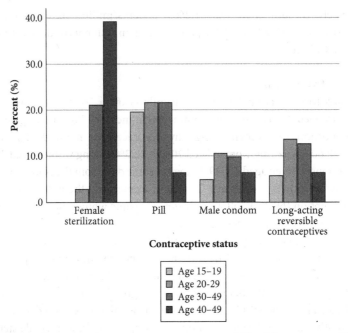

Figure 11.11 Contraceptive status among women aged 15–49 by age group, United States, 2017–2019.

Note: Data are expressed in percent.

Data source: Centers for Disease Control and Prevention. (October 20, 2020). *Current contraceptive status among women aged 15–49: United States, 2017–2019*. https://www.cdc.gov/nchs/products/dat abriefs/db388.htm. Chart created by Dr. Liyun Wu.

non-Hispanic women of African descent, and 10.5% among Hispanic women. Last, among women who used the LARC method, the percentage is very similar across race/ethnicity: 10.9% among non-Hispanic Caucasian women, 10.9% among non-Hispanic women of African descent, and 10.3% among Hispanic women.

(H) Mental health clinicians can benefit from applying STEM to health

Urinary System

Women are more likely to suffer from incontinence than men (Nitti, 2001). In addition to gender, risk factors include history of pelvic trauma, urinary tract infections, smoking, diabetes mellitus (Pansota et al., 2019), obesity, having had a child (Swanson et al., 2005), and menopause (Ogobuiro, & Tuma, 2021; Pansota

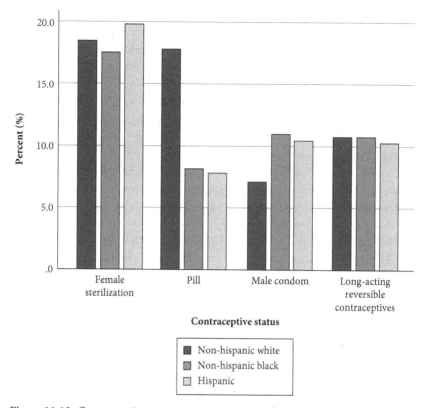

Figure 11.12 Contraceptive status among women aged 15–49 by race/ethnicity, United States, 2017–2019.

Note: Data are expressed in percent.

Data source: Centers for Disease Control and Prevention. (October 20, 2020). *Current contraceptive status among women aged 15–49: United States, 2017–2019.* https://www.cdc.gov/nchs/products/databriefs/db388.htm. Chart created by Dr. Liyun Wu.

et al., 2019). As you can see, many of these risk factors are gender specific. Aoki and colleagues (2017) reported that stress incontinence peaks at around age 50, and according to Swanson and colleagues (2005) prevalence does not increase with age.

There are several types of incontinence. Stress incontinence occurs when urine is involuntarily voided when the individual sneezes or coughs or during strenuous activity (Ogobuiro & Tuma, 2021), including sex. This kind of incontinence occurs when the pelvic floor muscles are weak and can occur among postmenopausal women (Aoki et al., 2017). Urge incontinence occurs when the bladder contracts involuntarily without a trigger. This can occur when the individual stands or bends over (postural incontinence), which inadvertently puts pressure on the bladder. In some cases, the inadvertent loss of urine occurs because the individual, especially among seniors, has a strong urge to urinate and is unable to reach the bathroom in time (MedlinePlus, 2021). Overflow incontinence occurs when there is blockage in the urethra, the bladder does not empty completely, and urine remains in the bladder, which becomes too full. Once the bladder is completely full, it overflows in the form of inadvertent urination. According to MedlinePlus, this problem is more common among men. Prostate surgery is correlated with incontinence among men (Aoki et al., 2017). Neurogenic incontinence occurs because of problems in the nervous system, although some individuals suffer from mixed incontinence, which is the result of two types of the illness, often urge and stress incontinence. Incontinence is a hidden problem, and clinicians may treat individuals and families for a different presenting problem but find that they struggle with incontinence. Clinicians may have clients whom they treat for incontinence that are young and older individuals. These clients may include postmenopausal women, men with prostate problems, and children who wet the bed at night and their underpants during the day.

Despite the several types of urinary incontinence, it can be shameful and interfere with help seeking because of embarrassment and the belief that incontinence is an inevitable burden of aging (Horrocks et al., 2004). Caregivers of family members with incontinence may be the ones to seek help because of the burden of responsibilities for washing bedsheets, maintaining the incontinent person's hygiene, the expense of pads and incontinence underwear, as well as the social isolation, reduced quality of life, and increased depression and anxiety (Kirli et al., 2021). Indeed, incontinence was a risk factor for nursing home placement (Leung & Schnelle, 2008).

There are several treatments that are attempted as first-line interventions. The initial treatment is to recommend that the client make a medical appointment to discuss their problem. Often the medical advice will be to learn exercises to strengthen the pelvic floor musculature. In addition to supporting the client's adherence to the pelvic floor muscle exercise regimen, the clinician may support the adult patient or caregiver by helping to institute a noninvasive behavioral treatment program (Stover et al., 2008). The behavioral program's initial phase may require the client to maintain a "bladder log" (Gormley et al., 2012) of the amount of and time when liquid was drunk on a daily basis. Clinicians may find it helpful to create a chart that provides behaviors as well as days of the week. For example, let's assume that the client is a 10-year-old-child who has never gone seven consecutive nights without wetting the bed. The caregiver helped the child create a chart on which behaviors were recorded. In this chart, the caregiver will help the child identify favorite reinforcers (toys, food, activities) which they contract to earn. A contingency contract is a written contract that identifies the child's behavior and the reinforcers they receive at the end of the time period. Because the child is older, they can be expected to work for a reinforcer for a week. Punishing statements are not included in the contract. Bedwetting is indicated by a message to "try again" the following night. For example, on Sunday at breakfast, the child drank a 6-oz glass of milk and 1 oz of milk with oatmeal. These data would be recorded on the chart under the heading liquid consumed. The time of day would also be recorded. Everything else the child drank during the day would be recorded. The caregiver would also record each time the child urinated. Then, the caregiver indicates whether the child wet the bed during the night. This is repeated for each day of the week. Each night the child stayed dry they would earn a star on the chart, which would be a positive reinforcer. Successes would be recorded every night, but nothing would be placed on the chart the nights the child wet the bed. The mornings that the sheets were wet, the child was expected to wash their own sheets. At the end of the week, the child would earn a larger positive reinforcer if they were able to stay dry the entire week. Stover and colleagues (2008) reduced the reinforcement schedule after 14 dry mornings, and eventually the child received one reinforcer per month. Their program resulted in no bedwetting at 3-month follow-up after 16 weeks of treatment. If the physician recommended medications, the clinician can instruct the family to include a box on the chart that indicates whether the child takes the medication as directed. Sometimes, the child may need additional help to wake up to urinate, and the parent may decide to purchase an alarm system that alerts the child if their underpants become wet (Vande Walle et al., 2012). Enuresis alarms have sensors that emit an auditory alarm when the bedclothes or sheets become wet. According to Vande Walle and colleagues, use should be continued for 2 to 3 months or until the child is dry for 14 consecutive nights.

Reproductive System
Nonbinary is a term that is sometimes used as an umbrella term to refer to individuals who do not identify with their sexual characteristics. Nonbinary individuals may claim sexual identities that are nonconforming and not based on their genitalia. While some may identify as a man or a woman, they are still able to indicate whether they are comfortable with their sex (cis) or have identified as non-cis or transgender. Some individuals do not claim binary terms and refer to themselves as genderqueer or as gender fluid. Others indicate that they are intersex and retain sex organs of both male and female, while others state that they are asexual and do not claim a sex (Tinder, n.d.).

In an analysis by the Williams Institute of the Generations and TransPop studies, Wilson and Meyer (2021) reported that at the time of the cross-sectional studies, there were over 1.2 million individuals living in the United States who self-identified as transgendered, or cisgender, nonbinary lesbian, gay, bisexual, transgender, or queer (LGBTQ) adults. Of this group, 7.5% (confidence interval [CI] = 5.9–9.5) were cisgender, and 32.1% (CI = 24.8–40.4) were transgender. When identifying their gender identity, 39% of the population self-reported their gender identity as an LBQ cis woman, while 19% identified as a GBQ cis man, and 42% identified as transgender. When identifying their sexual orientation, 31% identified their orientation as queer, 17% as bisexual, 17% as pansexual, 14% as on the asexual spectrum, 10% as gay, 6% as lesbian, 3% as same-gender loving, and 2% as another identity.

Society's acceptance of LGBTQ minority sexual status has changed over time according to Flores (2019). In a study of 174 countries from 1981 to 2017, Flores found that the rank of a country's score on social acceptance of LGBT people was compared by time intervals. Overall, countries that were more tolerant in earlier time periods remained tolerant, and those that were least tolerant remained less tolerant, resulting in polarization. In the interval from 2014 to 2017, the highest rank of 1 (as the most accepting) in a measure of social acceptance among 174 countries was Iceland during 2014–2017, up from the fourth rank in 2000–2003. Canadians were ranked fourth in the world in social acceptance during 2014 to 2017, up from 13th during 2000 to 2003; Great Britain ranked 11th, up from 21st; while the United States ranked 21st, up from 29th. Some countries showed little to no movement. For example, Mexico ranked 32nd during 2000 to 2003 as well as during 2014 to 2017, while China only changed in rank to 101st from 103rd. On the other hand, Egypt improved to 169th from 174th (the lowest rank), Jordan improved to 114th rank from 164th, and Ghana improved to 141st from 152nd. In spite of relaxed laws concerning homosexual behavior, personal attacks are prevalent. As can be seen from Wilson and Meyer's data (2021), in the nonbinary group of LGBQ adults age 18 to 60, many individuals (55%) had been assaulted, considered suicide (94%), and had attempted suicide (39%). Similarly, over half self-reported that as children they were often bullied (53%) or had experienced emotional abuse (82%), physical abuse (40%), and sexual abuse (41%). These findings are of great concern to clinicians because, in addition to those experiences, 51% self-reported having a serious mental illness.

According to the 2015 "Guidelines for Psychological Practice With Transgender and Gender Non-conforming People" (American Psychological Association [APA], 2015), when making the first assessment of a binary client, one should interview them about their past experiences of prejudice or discrimination, what notions of shame they have internalized, and expectations of future victimization. In addition to these experiences and concerns, the clinician must explore coping strategies and resilience (APA, 2015). According to the APA, clinicians must develop a trans-affirming practice when working with clients who are nonbinary. The APA's first guideline is that psychologists must understand that gender is a nonbinary construct that includes a range of gender identities. The APA also states that one's gender identity is not dependent on the sex one is assigned at birth. This acknowledgment is fundamental because other entities, including religious organizations, maintain that gender dysphoria is delusional unless there is discrepancy between secondary sexual characteristics of an intersex individual with physical anomalies (Furton, 2017). Past pathologizing of homosexuality, transvestism, and gender fluidity by the APA, as documented in the *Diagnostic and Statistical Manual of Mental Disorders* (*DSM*), caused untoward suffering among children and adults who reached out for help or were forced to receive an intervention because of their nonbinary sexual identity.

It's critical to note that now the APA states that clinicians must be aware of any biases they have that can cause the client to be victimized by the therapist. Clinicians must cultivate cultural competence when interviewing an individual who has identified as nonbinary. Mental health is not limited to people who are cis assigned. Simbar and colleagues (2018) found that patients who were receiving gender reassignment surgery had higher scores on scales of quality of life, as well as scales of body image, compared to those who were not receiving treatment or were only receiving hormonal therapy. They also found that higher scores on a body image scale were related to better scores on an index of mental health. Colvin and colleagues (2019) compared ways 1,504 cisgender, transgender, or gender-diverse Canadian youth were referred to a mental health clinic. They found that cisgender men (42.6%) and cisgender women (40.9%) were more likely to have been referred to the clinic by a provider compared to transgender (28.6%) or gender-diverse (30.8%) youth, who referred themselves (60.7% and 56.4%, respectively). These findings may indicate that the youth were not comfortable discussing their mental health issues with healthcare providers (Colvin et al., 2019), perhaps because of the medicalization of nonconforming gender identities by the psychiatric profession.

This information is important for clinicians to understand because in a study of 376 adults, lower scores on well-being were related to healthcare providers seeming to be uncomfortable with their nonbinary clients' sexual identity (29%) (Stanton et al., 2017), although ignoring their sexual identity did not predict lower well-being. Bowling and colleagues (2020) reported that anxiety was related to gender-diverse individuals' ability to access services from a community provider, as it was related to reduced community social support. On the other hand, they reported that professional and interpersonal support from the community they did receive was an external strength that was related to resilience. Bowling and colleagues discussed mutual aid support groups and group therapy as methods to increase well-being and resilience among nonbinary individuals. One component of this was related to the ability of the groups to provide tangible as well as emotional support. Overall, these data seem to indicate that nonbinary individuals who are expressing dysphoria may be reacting to their clinician's negative reactions, rather than the client's reactions to their gender fluidity.

Conclusion

Chapter 11 presented the basic scientific information about the body's structure and function of the urinary system, which is critical for filtration of toxic material and elimination of waste. Illnesses and injuries to the urinary system were introduced, as were the technological and engineering advances that treat them. Because treatment of ESRD can be an extended process, the role of the clinician in supporting patients and family members was included in the chapter. The basic scientific information regarding the reproductive system is fascinating and germane, as it impacts everyone. This chapter presented familiar topics that included sexually transmitted diseases, in vitro fertilization, and sexual identity and expression. Because clinicians are called on to work with a variety of clients who have issues pertaining to the reproductive system, it's incumbent on us to become familiarized with our own biases, which may impact our treatment of clients who identify as nonbinary.

Glossary

Alkalinity A component of water that neutralizes acidic properties; contains calcium carbonate

Bifurcate To split or branch off

Cis female, cis male A female or male who identifies with their gender at their birth

Enuresis Passing urine without control, especially while asleep

Fistula Abnormal opening connecting two organs or leading from an organ to outside the body

Glomerulus The filtration unit in the kidney

Oogenesis Development of female reproductive cells

Prepuce Loose skin around the head of the penis or clitoris

Vulva Woman's external genitalia

Websites

National Institute on Aging: https://www.nia.nih.gov/
National Kidney Foundation: https://www.kidney.org
Office on Women's Health: https://www.womenshealth.gov
World Health Organization (WHO), International: https://www.who.int

References

Chapter 1

Agrawal, A., Hinrichs, A. L., Dunn, G., Bertelsen, S., Dick, D. M., Saccone, S. F., Saccone, N. L., Grucza, R. A., Wang, J. C., Cloninger, C. R., Edenberg, H. J., Foroud, T., Hesselbrock, V., Kramer, J., Bucholz, K. K., Kuperman, S., Nurnberger, J. I., Jr., Porjesz, B., Schuckit, M. A., . . . Bierut, L. J. (2008). Linkage scan for quantitative traits identifies new regions of interest for substance dependence in the Collaborative Study on the Genetics of Alcoholism (COGA) sample. *Drug & Alcohol Dependence, 93*(1–2), 12–20. https://doi.org/10.1016/j.drugalcdep.2007.08.015

American Counseling Association (ACA). (2014). *2014 ACA code of ethics* (Section G: Research & Publications). Retrieved December 10, 2020, from https://www.counseling.org/resources/aca-code-of-ethics.pdf

American Psychological Association (APA). (2017). Boundaries of competence 2.01. In *Ethical principles of psychologists & code of conduct.* Retrieved November 24, 2020, from https://www.apa.org/ethics/code?item=5#2030

Barnes, J. L., Zubair, M., John, K., Poirier, M. C., & Martin, F. L. (2018). Carcinogens and DNA damage. *Biochemical Society Transactions, 46*, 1213–1224. https://doi.org/10.1042/BST20180519

Begleiter, H., Reich, T., Hesselbrock, V., Porjesz, B., Li, T.-K., Schuckit, M. A., Edenberg, H. J., & Rice, J. P. (1995). The collaborative study on the genetics of alcoholism. *Alcohol, Health, & Research World, 19*(3), 228–236. Retrieved June 6, 2020, from https://www.ncbi.nlm.nih.gov/pmc/articles/PMC6875768/pdf/arhw-19-3-228.pdf

Boss, P. (1999). Goodbye without leaving. In *Ambiguous loss: Learning to live with unresolved grief* (location 433–591 or 1483 [Kindle]). Harvard University Press.

Brooks, P. J., Enoch, M.-A., Goldman, D., Li, T.-K., & Yokoyama, A. (2009). The alcohol flushing response: An unrecognized risk factor for esophageal cancer from alcohol consumption. *PLoS Medicine, 6*(3), e1000050. https://doi.org/10.1371/journal.pmed.1000050

Bryant, P. E., Riches, A. C., & Terry, S. Y. A. (2010). Mechanisms of the formation of radiation-induced chromosomal aberrations. *Mutation Research, 701*(1), 23–26. https://doi.org/10.1016/j.mrgentox.2010.03.016

Campbell, J. (2011). Nature and aetiology of disease. In *Campbell's pathophysiology notes* (location 920 of 14135 [Kindle]). Lorimer Press.

Carneiro, I. (2017). Understanding epidemiology. In *Introduction to Epidemiology* (3rd ed., pp. 3–21). McGraw Hill, Open University Press.

Centers for Disease Control and Prevention (CDC). (2021). *Contact tracing.* Retrieved October 7, 2021, from https://www.cdc.gov/coronavirus/2019-ncov/daily-life-coping/contact-tracing.html

Chen, Y.-C., Yang, L.-F., Lai, C.-L., & Yin, S.-J. (2021). Acetaldehyde enhances alcohol sensitivity and protects against alcoholism: Evidence from alcohol metabolism in subjects with variant ALDH2*2 gene allele. *Biomolecules, 11,* 1183. https://doi.org/10.3390/biom11081183

Council of Social Work Education (CSWE). (2015). *Educational & policy accreditation standards (EPAS).* Retrieved June 3, 2020, from https://www.cswe.org/getattachment/Accreditation/Standards-and-Policies/2015-EPAS/2015EPASandGlossary.pdf.aspx

Goffman, E. (1963). Stigma and social identity. In *Stigma: Notes on the management of spoiled identity* (pp. 1–40). Simon and Schuster Publishing.

Goodwin, D. W., Schulsinger, F., Moller, N., Hermansen, L., Winokur, G., & Guze, S. B. (1974). Drinking problems in adopted and nonadopted sons of alcoholics. *Archives of General Psychiatry, 31*(2), 164–169.

Hesselbrock, M. N., Hesselbrock, V. M., & Chartier, K. G. (2013). Genetics of alcohol dependence and social work research: Do they mix? *Social Work in Public Health, 28*(3–4), 178–193. https://doi.org/10.1080/19371918.758999

Hrubec, Z., & Omenn, G. S. (1981). Evidence of genetic predisposition to alcoholic cirrhosis and psychosis: Twin concordances for alcoholism and its biological points by zygosity among male veterans. *Alcoholism: Clinical & Experimental Research, 5*(2), 207–215. https://doi.org/10.1111/j.1530-0277.1981.tb04890.x

Jin, F., Thaiparambil, J., Donepudi, S. R., Vantaku, V., Piyarathna, D. W. B., Maity S., Krishnapuram, R., Putluri, V., Gu, F., Purwaha, P., Bhowmik, S. K., Ambati, C. R., von Rundstedt, F.-C., Roghmann, F., Berg, S., Noldus, J., Rajapakshe, K., Godde, D., Roth, S., . . . Putluri M. (2017). Tobacco-specific carcinogens induce hypermethylation, DNA adducts and DNA damage in bladder cancer. *Cancer Prevention Research (Philadelphia), 10*(10), 588–597. https://doi.org/10.1158/1940-6207.CAPR-17-0198

Lewis, M. W. (2016). The intersection of genetics and social work: An interview with Michie Hesselbrock, PhD. *Journal of Social Work in the Addictions, 16*(3), 325–331. https://doi.org/10.1080/1533256X.2016.1201371

National Human Genome Research Institute (NHGRI). (2019). Chromosome abnormalities fact sheet. Retrieved October 10, 2021, from Chromosome Abnormalities Fact Sheet (genome.gov).

National Human Genome Research Institute (NHGRI). (2020). Human genome project FAQ. Retrieved October 10, 2021, from https://www.genome.gov/human-genome-project/Completion-FAQ

National Institute on Alcohol Abuse and Alcoholism (NIAAA). (2016). *Collaborative studies on Genetics and Alcoholism (GOGA) study.* Retrieved June 6, 2020, from https://www.niaaa.nih.gov/research/major-initiatives/collaborative-studies-genetics-alcoholism-coga-study

Oh, S. S., Ju, Y. J., Lee, S., & Park, E.-C. (2019). Primary reason for drinking among current, former, and never flushing college students. *International Journal of Environmental Research & Public Health, 16*, 211. https://doi.org/10.3390/ijerph16020211

Ozasa, K. (2016). Epidemiological research on radiation-induced cancer in atomic bomb survivors. *Journal of Radiation Research, 57*(S1), i112–i117. https://doi.org/10.1093/jrr/rrw005

Suddendorf, R. F. (1989). Research on alcohol metabolism among Asians and its implications for understanding causes of alcoholism. *Public Health Reports, 104*(6), 615–620.

Thys, R. G., Lehman, C. E., Pierce, L. C. T., & Wang, Y.-H. (2015). Environmental and chemotherapeutic agents induce breakage at genes involved in leukemia-causing gene rearrangements in human hematopoietic stem/progenitor cells. *Mutation Research*, *779*, 86–95. https://doi.org/10.1016/j.mrfmmm.2015.06.011.

Turnpenny, P. D., Ellard, S., & Cleaver, R. (2022). *Emery's elements of medical genetics and genomics* (16th ed., pp. 67–83). Elsevier.

U.S. Department of Energy (USDE). (2019). Human genome project. Retrieved October 10, 2021, from https://web.ornl.gov/sci/techresources/Human_Genome/index.shtml

Chapter 2

Advokat, C. D., Comaty, J. E., & Julien, R. M. (2019). *Julien's primer of drug action: A comprehensive guide to the actions, uses, and side effects of psychoactive drugs* (14th ed., pp. 39–68). Worth Publishers.

Algattas, H., & Huang, J. H. (2013). Traumatic brain injury pathophysiology and treatments: Early, intermediate, and late phases post-injury. *International Journal of Molecular Sciences*, *15*(1), 309–341. https://doi.org/10.3390/ijms15010309

Andresen, M., Gazmuri, J. T., Marin, A., Regueira, T., & Rovegno, M. (2015). Therapeutic hypothermia for acute brain injuries. *Scandinavian Journal of Trauma, Resuscitation and Emergency Medicine*, *23*, 42. https://doi.org/10.1186/s13049-015-0121-3

Baron, E., & Solanki, G. (2021). Spinal cord and spinal nerves: Gross anatomy. In S. Standring (Ed.), *Gray's anatomy* (42nd ed., pp. 856–871). Elsevier.

Bhangoo, R. S., Vergani, F., & Fernandez-Miranda, J. C. (2021). Meninges and ventricular system. In S. Standring (Ed.), *Gray's anatomy* (42nd ed., pp. 398–414). Elsevier.

Campbell, J. (2011). The nervous system. In *Campbell's physiology notes* (pp. 109–138). Lorimer Press.

Catani, M., & Zilles, K. (2021). Cerebral hemispheres. In S. Standring (Ed.), *Gray's anatomy* (42nd ed., pp. 512–539). Elsevier.

Centers for Disease Control & Prevention (CDC). (2017). Surveillance indicators. In Manual for the surveillance of vaccine-preventable diseases (Chap. 18). Retrieved November 4, 2020, from https://www.cdc.gov/vaccines/pubs/surv-manual/chpt18-surv-indicators.html

Centers for Disease Control & Prevention (CDC). (2018). *Introduction to public health surveillance*. Retrieved November 3, 2020, from https://www.cdc.gov/publichealth101/surveillance.html

Centers for Disease Control and Prevention. (2019). *Surveillance report of traumatic brain injury-related emergency department visits, hospitalizations, and deaths—United States, 2014*. Retrieved January 22, 2022, from https://stacks.cdc.gov/view/cdc/78062

Centers for Disease Control & Prevention (CDC). (2020). *Explosions and Blast Injuries: A Primer*. Retrieved May 22, 2020, from https://www.cdc.gov/masstrauma/preparedness/primer.pdf

Chen, H., Wu, F., Yang, P., Shao, J., Chen, Q., & Zheng, R. (2019). A meta-analysis of the effects of therapeutic hypothermia in adult patients with traumatic brain injury. *Critical Care*, *23*(396), 1–12. https://doi.org/10.1186/s13054-019-2667-3

Chhetri, K. P., & Das, J. M. (2020). Neuroanatomy, neural tube development, and stages. In StatPearls. StatPearls Publishing. https://www.ncbi.nlm.nih.gov/books/NBK557414/

Cleveland Clinic. (n.d.). *Spine structure & function*. Retrieved October 15, 2021, from https://my.clevelandclinic.org/health/articles/10040-spine-structure-and-function

Colbert, B. J., Ankney, J., & Lee, K. T. (2020). The nervous system, part I. In *Anatomy & physiology for health professions* (4th ed., pp. 171–192). Pearson Publishing.

Crossman, A. R., & Catani, M. (2021). Overview of the nervous system. In S. Standring (Ed.), *Gray's anatomy* (42nd ed, pp. 386–397). Elsevier.

Haselsberger, K., Pucher, R., & Auer, L. M. (1988). Prognosis after acute subdural or epidural hemorrhage. *Acta Neuochirurgica, 9,* 111–116. https://doi.org/10.1007/BF0 1560563

Hillis, A. E. (2014). Inability to empathize: Brain lesions that disrupt sharing and understanding another's emotions. *Brain: The Journal of Neurology, 137,* 981–997. https://doi.org/10.1093/brain/awt317

Hodge, C. W., McGurk, D., Thomas, J. L., Cox, A. L., Engel, C. C., & Castro, C. A. (2008). Mild traumatic brain injury in U.S. soldiers returning from Iraq. *New England Journal of Medicine, 358*(5), 453–463. https://doi.org/10.1056/NEJMoa072972

Hoffman, O., & Weber, J. R. (2009). Pathophysiology and treatment of bacterial meningitis. *Therapeutic Advances in Neurological Disorders, 2*(6), 401–412. https://doi.org/10.1177/1756285609337975

Huang, L., & Obenaus, A. (2011). Hyperbaric oxygen therapy for traumatic brain injury. *Medical Gas Research, 1*(1), 21. https://doi.org/10.1186/2045-9912-1-21

Human Origin Project. (n.d.). Functional areas of the brain. Retrieved October 15, 2021, from https://humanoriginproject.com/functional-areas-of-brain/

Jimsheleishvili, S., & Dididze, M. (2021). Neuroanatomy, cerebellum. In StatPearls. StatPearls Publishing.

Koehmstedt, C., Lydick, S. E., Patel, D., Cai, X., Garfinkel, S., & Weinstein, A. A. (2018). Health status, difficulties, and desired health information and services for veterans with traumatic brain injuries and their caregivers: A qualitative investigation. *PLoS One, 13*(9), e0203804. https://doi.org/10.1371/journal.pone.0203804

Koelman, D. L. H., Brouwer, M. C., & van de Beek, D. (2019). Targeting the complement system in bacterial meningitis. *Brain, 142,* 3325–3337. https://doi.org/10.1093/brain/awz222

Kratz, A. L., Sander, A. M., Brickell, T. A., Lange, R. T., & Carlozzi, N. E. (2017). Traumatic brain injury caregivers: A qualitative analysis of spouse and parent perspectives on quality of life. *Neuropsychological Rehabilitation, 27*(1), 16–37. https://doi.org/10.1080/09602011.2015.1051056

Lee, B., & Newberg, A. (2005). Neuroimaging in traumatic brain imaging. *NeuroRx, 2,* 372–383. https://doi.org/10.1602/neurorx.2.2.372

Lin, J. W., Tsai, J. T., Lee, L. M., Lin, C. M., Hung, C. C., Hung, K. S., Chen, W. Y., Wei, L., Ko, C. P., Su, Y. K., & Chiu, W. T. (2008). Effect of hyperbaric oxygen on patients with traumatic brain injury. *Acta Neurochirurgica, Supplements, 101,* 145–149. https://doi.org/10.1007/978-3-211-78205-7_25

Logan, S. A. E., & MacMahon, E. (2008). Viral meningitis. *BMJ, 336,* 36–40. https://doi.org/10.1136/bmj.39409.673657.AE

Mayo Clinic. (2020). *Hyperbaric Oxygen Therapy.* Retrieved September 12, 2021, from https://www.mayoclinic.org/tests-procedures/hyperbaric-oxygen-therapy/about/pac-20394380

Mayo Foundation for Medical Education & Research (MFMER). (2020). *Traumatic brain injury: Diagnosis.* Retrieved May 20, 2020, from https://www.mayoclinic.org/diseases-conditions/traumatic-brain-injury/diagnosis-treatment/drc-20378561

McGill, F., Griffiths, M. J., Bonnett, L. J., Geretti, A. M., Michael, B. D., Beeching, N. J., McKee, D., Scarlett, P., Hart, I. J., Mutton, K. J., Jung, A., Adan, G., Gummery, A., Sulaiman, W. A. W., Ennis, K., Martin, A. P., Haycox, A., Miller, A., Solomon, T., & UK Meningitis Study Investigators. (2018). Incidence, aetiology, and sequelae of viral meningitis in UK adults: A multicentre prospective observational cohort study. *Lancet, Infectious Diseases, 18*(9), 992–1003. https://doi.org/10.1016/S1473-3099(18)30245-7

Medicine Libre/Texts. (2020). *Functions of the brain stem.* Retrieved October 15, 2021, from https://med.libretexts.org/@go/page/7619

Meningitis Research Foundation. (n.d.). *Viral meningitis.* Retrieved July 25, 2021, from https://www.meningitis.org/meningitis/causes/viral-meningitis

Mercadante, A. A., & Tadi, P. (2020). Neuroanatomy, gray matter. In StatPearls. StatPearls Publishing. Retrieved July 24, 2021, from https://www.ncbi.nlm.nih.gov/books/NBK553239/?report=reader

Molnar, Z., & Collins, P. (2021). Development of the nervous system. In S. Standring (Ed.), *Gray's anatomy* (42nd ed., pp. 233–263). Elsevier.

Northern Brain Injury Association (NBIA). (2020). *The structure and function of the human brain.* Retrieved June 24, 2020, from https://www.nbia.ca/brain-structure-function/

Pirau, L., & Lui, F. (2020). Frontal lobe syndrome. In StatPearls. StatPearls Publishing. Retrieved December 3, 2020, from https://www.ncbi.nlm.nih.gov/books/NBK532981/#:~:text=Frontal%20lobe%20syndrome%20is%20a,%2C%20and%20language%2Fspeech%20production

Schiess, N., Groce, N. E., & Dua, T. (2021). The impact and burden of neurological sequelae following bacterial meningitis: A narrative review. *Microorganisms, 9*(5), 900. https://doi.org/10.3390/microorganisms9050900

Schmahmann, J. D. (2021). *Cerebellum.* In S. Standring (Ed.), *Gray's anatomy* (42nd ed., pp. 465–488). Elsevier.

Schumacher, R., Walder, B., Delhumeau, C., & Muri, R. M. (2016). Predictors of inpatient (neuro)rehabilitation after acute care of severe traumatic brain injury: An epidemiological study. *Brain Injury, 30*(10), 1186–1193. https://doi.org/10.1080/02699052.2016.1183821

Seladi-Schulman, J. (2019). *Hippocampus.* Retrieved October 15, 2021, https://www.healthline.com/human-body-maps/hippocampus#1

Sinclair, H. L., & Andrews, P. J. D. (2010). Bench-to-bedside review: Hypothermia in traumatic brain injury. *Critical Care, 14*(1), 204–214. https://doi.org/10.1186/cc8220

Sokhi, J., & Reddy, U. (2019). Therapeutic hypothermia and acute brain injury. *Anaesthesia & Intensive Care Medicine, 21*(1), 13–15. https://doi.org/10.1016/j.mpaic.2019.10.019

Teasdale, G., & Jennett, B. (1974). Assessment of coma and impaired consciousness. A practical scale. *Lancet, 2,* 81–84. https://doi.org/10.1016/S0140-6736(74)91639-0

Thompson, K., Pohlmann-Eden, B., Campbell, L. A., & Abel, H. (2015). Pharmacological treatments for preventing epilepsy following traumatic head injury. *Cochrane Systematic Review, 2015*(8), CD009900. https://doi.org/10.1002/14651858.pub2

Chapter 3

Advokat, C. D., Comaty, J. E., & Julien, R. M. (2019). *Julien's primer of drug action* (pp. 39–68). Worth Publishers.

Afghani, E., Pandol, S. J., Shimosegawa, T., Sutton, R., Wu, B. U., Vege, S. S., Gorelick, F., Hirota, M., Windsor, J., Lo, S. K., Freeman, M. L., Lerch, M. M., Tsuji, Y., Melmed, G. Y., Wassef, W., & Mayerle, J. (2015). Acute pancreatitis—progress and challenges: A report on an international symposium. *Pancreas, 44*(8), 1195–1210. https://doi.org/10.1097/MPA.0000000000000500

American Cancer Society. (2022). *Key statistics for pancreatic cancer.* Retrieved January 15, 2022, from https://www.cancer.org/cancer/pancreatic-cancer/about/key-statistics.html

Aulinas, A. (2019). *Physiology of the pineal gland and melatonin.* In K. R. Feingold (Ed.), Endotext. MDtext.com. Retrieved September 30, 2021, from https://www.ncbi.nlm.nih.gov/books/NBK550972/

Ayuk, J., & Sheppard, M. C. (2006). Growth hormone and its disorders. *Postgraduate Medical Journal, 82*(963), 24–30. https://doi.org/10.1136/pgmj.2005.036087

Bancos, I. (2018). *Thyroid hormones.* Hormone Health Network. Retrieved August 20, 2021, from https://www.hormone.org/your-health-and-hormones/glands-and-hormones-a-to-z/hormones/thyroid-hormones

Berg, J. M., Tymoczko, J. L., & Stryer, L. (2002). Glycogen metabolism. In Biochemistry (5th ed., Ch. 21). W. H. Freeman. https://www.ncbi.nlm.nih.gov/books/NBK21190/

Blythe, B. J., & Bazarian, J. J. (2010). Traumatic alterations in consciousness: Traumatic brain injury. *Emergency Medicine Clinics of North America, 28*(3), 571–594. https://doi.org/10.1016/j.emc.2010.03.003

Bullock, G. (2018). *Ten symptoms of moderate or severe traumatic brain injury (TBI).* Retrieved May 20, 2020, from https://www.theraspecs.com/blog/symptoms-moderate-severe-traumatic-brain-injury-tbi/

Bulthuis, M. C., Boxhoorn, L., Beudel, M., Elbers, P. W. G., Kop, M. P. M., van Wanrooij, R. L. J., Besselink, M. G., & Voermans , R. P. (2021). Acute pancreatitis in COVID-19 patients: True risk? *Scandinavian Journal of Gastroenterology, 56*(5), 585–587. doi: 10.1080/00365521.2021.1896776.

Campbell, J. (2011). The endocrine system. In Campbell's *physiology notes* (pp. 139–166). Lorimer Publications.

Campbell, J. (2014). *Endocrine lesson 2: Endocrine glands & hormones.* Retrieved August 28, 2021, from https://www.youtube.com/watch?v=-GzANNVFznw&t=786s

Center for Disease Control and Prevention (CDC) (October 7, 2011). Morbidity and Mortality Weekly Report (MMWR)—Nonfatal Traumatic Brain Injuries Related to Sports and Recreation Activities among Persons Aged ≤19 Years, United States, 2001–2009. *60*(39), 1337–1342.

Cleveland Clinic. (2021). *Insulin pumps.* Retrieved September 6, 2021, from https://my.clevelandclinic.org/health/articles/9811-insulin-pumps?view=print

Centers for Disease Control and Prevention (CDC). (2011). Nonfatal traumatic brain injuries related to sports and recreation activities among persons aged ≤ 19 years—United States, 2001—2009. *Morbidity and Mortality Weekly, 60*(39), 1337–1342. https://www.cdc.gov/mmwr/preview/mmwrhtml/mm6039a1.htm

Chanson, P., & Salenave, S. (2008). Acromegaly. *Orphanet Journal of Rare Diseases, 3*, 17. https://doi.org/10.1186/1750-1172-3-17

Colbert, B. J., Ankney, J., & Lee, K. T. (2020). The endocrine system. In *Anatomy & Physiology: for Health Professions* (4th ed., pp. 236–258). Pearson.

Conrad, C. (2021). Pancreas. In S. Standring (Ed.), *Gray's anatomy: The anatomical basis of clinical practice* (pp. 1223–1231). Elsevier.

Davis, E. P., Glynn, L. M., Waffarn, F., & Sandman, C. A. (2011). Prenatal maternal stress programs infant stress regulation. *Journal of Child Psychology & Psychiatry, 52*(2), 119–129. https://doi.org/10.1111/j.1469-7610.2010.02314.x

Figueiredo, M., Zilhao, R., & Neves, H. (2020). Thymus inception: Molecular network in the early stages of thymus organogenesis. *International Journal of Molecular Sciences, 21*, 5765. https://doi.org/10.3390/ijms21165765

Geenen, V. (2021). The thymus and the science of self. *Seminars in Immunopathology, 43*, 5–14. https://doi.org/10.1007/s00281-020-00831-y

Herreros-Villanueva, M., Hijona, E., Banales, J. M., Cosme, A., & Bujanda, L. (2013). Alcohol consumption on pancreatic diseases. *World Journal of Gastroenterology, 19*(5), 638–647. https://doi.org/10.3748/wjg.v19.i5.638

Javed, Z., Qamar, U., & Sathyapalan, T. (2015). Pituitary and/or hypothalamic dysfunction following moderate to severe traumatic brain injury: Current perspectives. *Indian Journal of Endocrinology & Metabolism, 19*, 753–763.

Johns Hopkins Medicine. (n.d.). *Adrenal gland.* Retrieved August 15, 2021, from https://www.hopkinsmedicine.org/health/conditions-and-diseases/adrenal-glands

Khuroo, M. S., Rather, A. A., Khuroo, N. S., & Khuroo, M. S. (2016). Hepatobiliary and pancreatic ascariasis. *World Journal of Gastroenterology, 22*(33), 7505–7517. https://doi.org/10.3748/wjg.v22.i33.7507

Mayo Clinic. (2021a). *Acromegaly.* Retrieved September 9, 2021, from https://www.mayoclinic.org/diseases-conditions/acromegaly/diagnosis-treatment/drc-20351226?&mc_id=google&campaign=329764201&geo=66801&kw=How%20to%20Diagnose%20Acromegaly&ad=&network=o&sitetarget=&adgroup=1278732215644737&extension=&target=kwd-79920890311218:loc-4129&matchtype=e&device=c&account=1733789621&invsrc=neuro&placementsite=enterprise&gclid=5b411b9c2e5c1c2ff3047aa6342b46b4&gclsrc=3p.ds&msclkid=5b411b9c2e5c1c2ff3047aa6342b46b4&gclid=5b411b9c2e5c1c2ff3047aa6342b46b4&gclsrc=3p.ds

Mayo Clinic. (2021b). *Acromegaly overview.* Retrieved September 9, 2021, from Acromegaly—symptoms and causes, Mayo Clinic.

MedTronic. (2021). *The MiniMed bluetooth application.* Retrieved September 18, 2021, from https://www.medtronicdiabetes.com/minimed-770g-system-kids/?utm_source=bing&utm_campaign=Pumps+-+NB+-+Core+-+Exact&utm_medium=text&&msclkid=135b93da421f11bab9b3f29c702d6f98&gclid=135b93da421f11bab9b3f29c702d6f98&gclsrc=3p.ds)

Miller, K. (2019). *Endocrine disorders.* Retrieved August 14, 2021, from https://webmd.com

Mount Sinai. (n.d.). *Continuous blood glucose testing: How do sensors work?* Retrieved September 6, 2021, from https://www.mountsinai.on.ca/care/lscd/sweet-talk-1/continuous-blood-glucose-testing-how-do-sensors-work

National Cancer Institute. (2021). *Cancer stat facts: Pancreatic cancer.* Retrieved December 20, 2021, from https://seer.cancer.gov/statfacts/html/pancreas.html

National Institute of Child Health & Human Development (NICHD). (n.d.). *About adrenal gland disorders.* Retrieved from August 20, 2021, from https://www.nichd.nih.gov/health/topics/adrenalgland/conditioninfo)

National Institute of Diabetes and Digestive and Kidney Diseases (NIDDK). (n.d.). *Endocrine disease.* Retrieved August 14, 2021, from https://www.niddk.nih.gov/health-information/endocrine-diseases

Nazario, B. (2004). *Diabetes: Type I diabetes*. Retrieved August 16, 2021, from https://www.medicinenet.com/script/main/art.asp?articlekey=42943#toca

Petry, N. M., Martin, B., Cooney, J. L., & Kranzler, H. R. (2000). Give them prizes, and they will come: Contingency management for treatment of alcohol dependence. *Journal of Consulting & Clinical Psychology, 68*(2), 250–257. https://doi.org/10.1037//0022-006x.68.2.250

Rhys, J. (2013). Thyroid. In D. Wild (Ed.), *Thyroid stimulating hormone—An overview, ScienceDirect Topics*. Elsevier. Retrieved August 20, 2021, from https://www.sciencedirect.com/topics/chemistry/thyroid-stimulating-hormone

Rytter, M. J. H., Namusoke, H., Ritz, C., Michaelsen, K. F., Briend, A., Friis, H., & Jeppesen, D. (2017). Correlates of thymus size and changes during treatment of children with severe acute malnutrition: A cohort study. *BMC Pediatrics, 17*, 70. https://doi.org/10.1186/s12887-017-0821-0

Sahler, C. S., & Greenwald, B. D. (2012). Traumatic brain injury in sports: A review. *Rehabilitation Research & Practice, 2012*, 659652. https://doi.org/10.1155/2012/659652

Schroeder, A. C., & Privalsky, M. L. (2014). Thyroid hormones, T3 and T4, in the brain. *Frontiers in Endocrinology, 5*, 40. https://doi.org/10.3389/fendo.2014.00040

Sell, R., Rothenberg, M. A., & Chapman, C. F. (2018). *Barron's dictionary of medical terms* (7th ed.). Kaplan.

Society for Endocrinology (SFE). (2021). *Melanocyte-stimulating hormone*. You and Your Hormones. Retrieved August 20, 2021, https://www.yourhormones.info/hormones/melanocyte-stimulating-hormone/

Tang, J. C. F., & Anand, B. S. (July 15, 2021). Acute pancreatitis: Practice essentials. *Drug & Diseases: Gastroenterology*. Retrieved August 30, 2022, from https://emedicine.medscape.com/article/181364-overview?reg=1

Taylor, T. (2020). *Endocrine system*. Retrieved August 20, 2021, from https://www.innerbody.com/image/endoov.html

ThyroidUK. (2021). *Thyrotropin-releasing hormone*. Retrieved August 21, 2021, from https://thyroiduk.org/thyrotropin-releasing-hormone

United Nations. (2016). *Witchcraft beliefs trigger attacks against people with albinism, UN expert warns*. Retrieved August 29, 2021, from https://news.un.org/en/story/2016/03/525042-witchcraft-beliefs-trigger-attacks-against-people-albinism-un-expert-warns

Watson, S. (2021). *How insulin works*. WebMD. Retrieved September 18, 2021 from https://www.webmd.com/diabetes/insulin-explained

Wigley, C. B. (2021). Cells, tissues, and systems. In *Gray's anatomy: The anatomical basis of clinical practice* (42nd ed., Ch. 2). Elsevier.

Yadav, D., & Lowenfels, A. B. (2013). The epidemiology of pancreatitis and pancreatic cancer. *Gastroenterology, 144*(6), 1252–1261. https://doi.org/10.1053/j.gastro.2013.01.068

Chapter 4

AIDSinfo. (2020). *Recommendations for the use of antiretroviral drugs in pregnant women with HIV infection and interventions to reduce perinatal HIV transmission in the United States*. Retrieved November 25, 2021, Prenatal Care, Antiretroviral Therapy, and HIV Management in Women with Perinatal HIV Infection | NIH.

Alberts, B., Johnson, A., Lewis, J., Raff, M., Roberts, K., & Walter, P. (2002). *Molecular biology of the cell* (4th ed.). Garland Science. https://www.ncbi.nlm.nih.gov/books/NBK21054/

Ball, A. L. (2007). HIV, injecting drug use and harm reduction: A public health response. *Addiction, 102,* 684–690. https://doi.org/10.1111/j.1360-0443.2007.01761.x

Batchelder, A. W., Lounsbury, D. W., Palma, A., Carrico, A., Pachankis, J., Schoenbaum, E., & Gonzalez, J. S. (2016). Importance of substance use and violence in psychosocial syndemics among women with and at-risk for HIV. *AIDS Care, 28*(10), 1316–1320. https://doi.org/10.1080/09540121.2016.1173637

Beksinska, M., Smit, J., Joanis, C., & Potter, W. (2012). New female condoms in the pipeline. *Reproductive Health Matters, 20*(40), 188–196. https://doi.org/10.1016/S0968-8080(12)40659-0

Blumenreich, M. S. (1990). The white blood cell and differential count. In H. K. Walker, W. D. Hall, & J. W. Hurst (Eds.), *Clinical methods: The history, physical, & laboratory examinations* (3rd ed., pp. 724–727). Butterworths.

Brennan, D. (2021). What are lymphocytes? WebMD Medical Reference. Retrieved November 25, 2021, from https://www.webmd.com/a-to-z-guides/what-are-lymphocytes

Brocato, J., & Wagner, E. E. (2003). Harm reduction: A social work practice model and social justice agenda. *Health & Social Work, 28*(2), 117–125. https://doi.org/10.1093/hsw/28.2.117

Buchacz, K., Baker, R. K., Palella, F. J., Jr., Chmiel, J. S., Lichtenstein, K. A., Novak, R. M., Wood, K. C., Brooks, J. T., & the HOPS Investigators. (2010). AIDS-defining opportunistic illnesses in U.S. patients, 1994–2007: A cohort study. *AIDS, 24,* 1549–1559. https://doi.org/10.1097/QAD.0b013e32833a3967

Cadeddu, M., Garnett, A., Al-Anezi, K., & Farrokhyar, F. (2006). Management of spleen injuries in the adult trauma population: A ten-year experience. *Canadian Journal of Surgery, 49*(6), 386–390.

Campbell, J. (2011a). Lymphatic system. In Campbell's *physiology notes* (pp. 55–64). Lorimer Publications.

Campbell, J. (2011b). Disorders of immunity. In Campbell's *pathophysiology notes* (2nd ed., 2397–2793. Lorimer Publications.

Campbell, J. (2014). Lymphatics *lesson one*: Tissue, *fluid, and afferent lymphatic vessels* [Video]. YouTube. Retrieved November 25, 2021, 2021, from Lymphatics lesson 1, Tissue fluid and afferent lymphatic vessels.

Centers for Disease Control & Prevention (CDC). (1981). Pneumocystis pneumonia—Los Angeles. *Morbidity & Mortality Review, 30*(21), 1–3.

Centers for Disease Control & Prevention (CDC). (1982). Epidemiologic notes and reports possible transfusion—Associated acquired immune deficiency syndrome (AIDS)—California. *Morbidity & Mortality Review, 31*(48), 652–654.

Centers for Disease Control & Prevention (CDC). (1989). Current trends update: Acquired immunodeficiency syndrome associated with intravenous—drug use--United States, 1988. *Morbidity & Mortality Review, 38*(10), 165–170.

Centers for Disease Control & Prevention (CDC). (2020a). *HIV among Pregnant Women, Infants, & Children.* Retrieved November 25, 2021, from https://www.cdc.gov/hiv/group/gender/pregnantwomen/index.html

Centers for Disease Control & Prevention (CDC). (2020b). *HIV in the United States and dependent areas*. HIV Surveillance Report 31. Retrieved August 8, 2021, from https://www.cdc.gov/hiv/statistics/overview/ataglance.html

Centers for Disease Control and Prevention (CDC). (2021). *HIV diagnoses*. Retrieved August 8, 2021, from https://www.cdc.gov/nchs/data/hus/2019/011-508.pdf

Civic, D. (2000). College students' reasons for nonuse of condoms within dating relationships. *Journal of Sex & Marital Therapy, 26*(1), 95–105. doi: 10.1080/009262300278678

Cohen, M. S., Chen, Y. Q., McCauley, M., Gamble, R., Hosseinipour, M. C., Kumarasmy, N., Hakim, J. G., Kumwenda, J., Grinsztejn, B., Pilott, J. H. S., Godbole, S. V., Mehendale, S., Chariyalertsak, S., Santos, B. R., Mayer, K. H., Hoffman, I. F., Eshleman, S. H., Piwowar-Manning, E., Wang, L., Makhema, J., . . . for the HPTN052 Study Team. (2011). Prevention of HIV-1 infection with early antiretroviral therapy. *New England Journal of Medicine, 365*(6), 493–505. https://doi.org/10.1056.NEJMoa1105243

Colbert, B. J., Ankney, J., & Lee, K. T. (2020). The lymphatic and immune systems. In *Anatomy and physiology for health professionals* (4th ed., pp. 319–324). Pearson Publishing.

Dehli, T., Bagenholm, A., Trasti, N. C., Monsen, S. A., & Bartnes, K. (2015). The treatment of spleen injuries: A retrospective study. *Scandinavian Journal of Trauma, Resuscitation and Emergency Medicine, 23*, 85. https://doi.org/10.1186/s13049-015-0163-6

Demetriades, D., Hadjizacharia, P., Constantinou, C., Brown, C., Inaba, K., Rhee, P., & Salim, A. (2006). Selective nonoperative management of penetrating abdominal solid organ injuries. *Annals of Surgery, 244*(4), 620–628. https://doi.org/10.1097/01.sla.000 0237743.22633.01

Des Jarlais, D. C., Arasteh, K., Mcknight, C., Feelemyer, J., Hagan, H., Cooper, H. L. F., & Perlman, D. C. (2014). Combined HIV prevention, the New York City condom distribution program, and the evolution of safer sex behavior among persons who inject drugs in New York City. *AIDS Behavior, 18*, 443–451. https://doi.org/10.1007/s10 461-013-0664-0

Ellis, E. M., Rajagopal, R., & Kiviniemi, M. T. (2018). The interplay between feelings and beliefs about condoms as predictors of their use. *Psychological Health, 33*(2), 176–192. doi:10.1080/08870446.2017.1320797

Fenwick, S. E., Botfield, J. R., Kidman, P., McGeechan, K., & Bateson, D. (2021). Views and experiences of the female condom in Australia: An exploratory cross-sectional survey of cisgender women. *PLoS ONE, 16*(2), e0246664. https://doi. org/10.1371/journal.pone.0246664

Festa, A. (2021). *What does the spleen do?* Retrieved August 6, 2021, from https://www.healthgrades.com/right-care/blood-conditions/what-does-the-spleen-do

Food and Drug Administration. (2019). *The history of the FDA's role in preventing the spread of HIV/AIDS*. Retrieved August 3, 2021, from https://www.fda.gov/about-fda/fda-history-exhibits/history-fdas-role-preventing-spread-hivaids

George, A., & Kishore, L. (2021). Blood, lymphoid tissues, & hemopoiesis. In S. Standring (Ed.), *Gray's anatomy: The anatomical basis of clinical practice* (42nd ed., pp. 71–84). Elsevier.

Korber, B., Muldoon, M., Theiler, J., Gao, F., Gupta R., Lapedes, A., Hahn, B. H., Wolinsky, S., & Bhattacharya, T. (2000). Timing the ancestor of the HIV-1 pandemic strains. *Science, 288*(5472), 1789–1796. https://doi.org/10.1126/science.288.5472.1789

Kozar, R. A., Crandall, M., Shanmuganathan, K., Zarzaur, B. L., Cibyrn, M., Cribari, C., Kaups, K., Schuster, K., Tominaga, G. T., & AAST Patient Assessment Committee. (2018). Organ injury scaling 2018 update: Spleen liver, and kidney. *Journal of Trauma & Acute Care Surgery, 85*(6), 1119–1122. https://doi.org/10.1097/TA.0000000000002058

International Association of Providers of AIDS Care (IAPAC). (2021). *90–90–90.* Retrieved January 24, 2022, https://www.iapac.org/home/advocacy/90-90-90/#:~:text=The%20UNAIDS%2090%2D90%2D90,antiretroviral%20therapy%20achieving%20viral%20suppression

Joint United Nations Program on HIV/AIDS (UNAIDS). (2018). UNAIDS *data* 2018, *state of the epidemic.* Retrieved August 10, 2021, from https://www.unaids.org/sites/default/files/media_asset/unaids-data-2018_en.pdf

Joint United Nations Program on HIV/AIDS (UNAIDS). (2021). *Global HIV Statistics.* Retrieved January 24, 2022, from https://embargo.unaids.org/static/files/uploaded_fi les/UNAIDS_2021_FactSheet_en_em.pdf

Leliefeld, P. H. C., Wessels, C. M., Leenen, L P. H., Koendeman, L., & Pillay, J. (2016). The role of neutrophils in immune dysfunction during severe inflammation. *Critical Care, 20,* 73. https://doi.org/10.1186/s13054-016-1250-4

Malmquist, S., & Prescott, K. (n.d.). Adaptive immunity. In Human biology (Ch 2.7) Retrieved August 8, 2021, from https://open.lib.umn.edu/humanbiology/chapter/2-7-adaptive-immunity/

Masvawure, T. B., Mantell, J. E., Mabude, Z., Ngoloyi, C., Milford, C., Beksinska, M., Smit, J. A. (2014). "It's a different condom, let's see how it works": Young men's reactions to and experiences of female condom use during an intervention trial in South Africa. *Journal of Sex Research, 51*(8), 841–851. doi:10.1080/00224499.2013.814043

Mayo Clinic. (2019). *Female condom.* Patient care and health information. Retrieved November 25, 2021, from https://www.mayoclinic.org/tests-procedures/female-con dom/about/pac-20394129

Naif, H. M. (2013). Pathogenesis of HIV infection. *Infections Disease Reports, 5,* s1e6, 26–30. https://doi.org/10.4081/idr.2013.s1 .e6

National Institute on Allergy & Infectious Disease (NIAID). (2018). *Antiretroviral drug discovery and development.* Retrieved August 8, 2021, from https://www.niaid.nih.gov/diseases-conditions/antiretroviral-drug-development

Newman, T. (2018). *All about the spleen.* Retrieved August 6, 2021, from https://www.medicalnewstoday.com/articles/320698

Ruscelli, P., Gemini, A., Rimini, M., Santella, S., Candelari, R., Rosati, M., Paci, E., Marconi, B., Renzi, C., Commissari, R., Cirocchi, R., Santoro, A., D'Andrea, V., & Parisi, A. (2019). The role of grade of injury in non-operative management of blunt hepatic and splenic trauma. *Medicine, 98*(35), e16746. https://doi.org/10.1097/MD.000000000 0016746

Tinkoff, G., Esposito, T. J., Reed, J., Kilgo, P., Fildes, J., Pasquale, M., & Meredith, J. W. (2008). American Association for the Surgery of Trauma Organ Injury Scale I: Spleen, liver, and kidney, validation based on the National Trauma Data Bank. *Journal of the American College of Surgeons, 207*(5), 646–655. https://doi.org/10.1016/j.jamcolls urg.2008.06.342

Volkov, N. (2012). Drug abuse and HIV. Research report series. National Institute on Drug Abuse. Department of Health and Human Services. National Institutes of Health Publication Number 12-5760. Retrieved November 25, 2021, from https://www.drugabuse.gov/sites/default/files/rrhiv.pdf

Ward, P. J. (2021). Mediastinum. In S. Standring (Ed.), *Gray's anatomy: Anatomical basis of clinical practice* (pp. 1047–1067). Elsevier.

Weeks, M. R., Zhan, J., Li, J., Hilario, H., Abbott, M., & Medina, Z. (2015). Female condom use and adoption among men and women in a general low-income urban U.S. population. *AIDS Behavior, 19(9)*, 1642–1654. doi:10.1007/s10461-015-1052-8.

World Health Organization (WHO). (2008). UNODC, Joint United National Programme on HIV/AIDS: Technical guide for countries to set targets for universal access to HIV prevention, treatment and care for injecting drug users. Geneva. Retrieved on August 9, 2021, from https://www.unodc.org/documents/hiv-aids/publications/People_who_use_drugs/Target_setting_guide2012_eng.pdf

World Health Organization (WHO). (2021). *The global health observatory: HIV/AIDS.* Retrieved August 8, 2021, from https://www.who.int/data/gho/data/themes/hiv-aids

Worobey, M., Watts, T. D., McKay, R. A., Suchard, M. A., Granade, T., Teuwen, D. E., Koblin, B. A., Heneine, W., Lemey, P., & Jaffe, H. W. (2016). 1970s and "Patient 0" HIV-1 genomes illuminate early HIV/AIDS history in North America. *Nature, 539*, 98–115. https://doi.org/10.1038/nature19827

Zarzaur, B. L., & Rozycki, G. S. (2017). An update on nonoperative management of the spleen in adults. *Trauma Surgery & Acute Care Open, 2*, 1–7. https://doi.org/10.1136/tsaco-2017-000075

Chapter 5

Auditory

American Speech-Language-Hearing Association (ASHA). (n.d.). Dizziness and balance. Retrieved June 11, 2021, from https://www.asha.org/public/hearing/dizziness-and-balance/#causes

Campbell, J. (2011). Ears. In *Campbell's physiology notes* (pp. 331–340). Lorimer Publishers.

Centers for Disease Control & Prevention (CDC). (2018). *2018 Demographics: Newborn hearing screening.* Retrieved May 19, 2021, from https://www.cdc.gov/ncbddd/hearingloss/2018-data/15-screening-demographics.html

Centers for Disease Control & Prevention (CDC). (2019). *Meningococcal vaccination: What everyone should know.* Retrieved May 20, 2021, from https://www.cdc.gov/vaccines/vpd/mening/public/index.html

Centers for Disease Control & Prevention (CDC). (2020). *2018 Summary of infants identified with permanent hearing loss enrolled in early intervention (EI) before 6 months of age.* Retrieved May 19, 2021, from https://www.cdc.gov/ncbddd/hearingloss/2018-data/10-early-intervention-by-six-months.html

Cherow, E., Dickman, D. M., & Epstein, S. (1999). Organization resources for families of children with deafness or hearing loss. *Hearing Loss in Children, 46(1)*, 153–162. https://doi.org/10.1016/s0031-3955(05)70088-2

Gondim, F. A. A. (2021). *What is the morbidity and mortality of meningococcal meningitis?* Retrieved May 18, 2021, from https://www.medscape.com/answers/1165557-118297/what-is-the-morbidity-and-mortality-of-meningococcal-meningitis

Healthy People 2030. (2021). *Healthy People 2030: Building a health future for all.* Office of Disease Prevention and Health Promotion. U.S. Department of Health and Human

Services. Retrieved April 27, 2022, from https://health.gov/healthypeople?_ga=
2.147206580.2052394425.1651099816-568907019.1651099816

Hearing Health Foundation. (2021). *Hearing aid use is associated with improved cognitive functioning in hearing-impaired elderly.* Columbia University Medical Center. Retrieved April 27, 2022, from https://hearinghealthfoundation.org/blogs/hearing-aid-use-improved-cognitive-function-in-elderly?rq=dementia

Hearing Loss Association of America. (2021). *Hearing loss basics.* Retrieved April 27, 2022, from https://www.hearingloss.org/hearing-help/hearing-loss-basics/

Jamieson, J. R., Zaidman-Zait, A., & Poon, B. (2011). Family support needs as perceived by parents of preadolescents and adolescents who are dear of hard of hearing. *Deafness & Education International, 13*(3), 110–130. https://doi.org/10.1179/1557069X11Y.000 0000005

Kubler-Ross, E. (1969). *On death and dying.* Scribner Classics.

Mathos, K. K., & Broussard, E. R. (2005). Outlining the concerns of children who have hearing loss and their families. *Journal of the American Academy of Child and Adolescent Psychiatry, 44*(1), 96–100. https://doi.org/10.1097/01.chi.0000145552.03942.40

Meningitis Research Foundation. (2021). *Meningitis research tracker.* Retrieved May 18, 2021, from https://www.meningitis.org/mpt

National Center for Biotechnology Information (NCBI). (2017). *How does our sense of balance work?* Institute for Quality and Efficiency in Health Care. Retrieved June 11, 2021, from https://www.ncbi.nlm.nih.gov/books/NBK279394/

National Institute on Aging (NIA). (2018a). *Age-related hearing loss.* Retrieved May 18, 2021, from https://www.nia.nih.gov/health/hearing-loss-common-problem-older-adults

National Institute on Aging (NIA). (2018b). *Hearing loss: A common problem for older adults.* Retrieved May 18, 2021, from https://www.nia.nih.gov/health/hearing-loss-common-problem-older-adults

Rollop, B. (2019). What are the four levels of deafness? *eLife.* Retrieved May 17, 2021, from https://www.hearingaidknow.com/question/what-are-4-levels-of-deafness#:~:text= Answered%20by%20Steve%20Claridge,%2C%20Moderate%2C%20Severe%20 and%20Profound

Senn, P., Mina, A., Volkenstein, S., Kranebitter, V., Oshima, K., & Heller, S. (2020). Progenitor cells from the adult human inner ear. *Anatomical Record, 303,* 461–470. https://doi.org/10.1002/ar.24228

Singhal, K., Singhal, J., Muzaffar, J., Monksfield, P & Bance, M. (2020). Outcomes of cochlear implantation in patients with post-meningitis deafness: A systematic review and narrative synthesis. *Journal of International Advanced Otology, 16*(3), 395–410. https:// doi.org/10.5152/iao.2020.9040

Stephens, N. M., & Duncan, J. (2020). Caregiver decision-making for school placement of children who are deaf or hard of hearing and children with other disabilities: A global perspective. *Volta Review, 120*(1), 3–20. https://doi.org/10.17955/tvr.120.1.809

Thomas, L. (2019). The ear's sensitivity to sound is controlled by outer hair cells. Retrieved May 15, 2021, from https://www.news-medical.net/news/20190925/The-ears-sensitiv ity-to-sound-is-controlled-by-outer-hair-cells.aspx#:~:text=The%20human%20in ner%20ear%20has,amplify%20sounds%20from%20the%20environment

Tuli, I. P., Pal, I., Sengupta, S., & Bhutia C. (2012). Role of early audiological screening and intervention. *Indian Journal of Otology, 18*(3), 148–153. https://doi.org/10.4103/ 0971-7749.103443

VanOrmer, J. L., Rossetti, K. G., & Zlomke, K. R. (2019). The development of behavioral difficulties in hard-of-hearing and deaf youth. *Child & Family Behavior Therapy*, *41*(4), 179–200. https://doi.org/10.1080/07317107.2019.1659537

Waqas, M., Us-Salam, I., Bibi, Z., Wang, Y., Li, H., Zhu, Z., & He, S. (2020). Stem cell-based therapeutic approaches to restore sensorineural hearing loss in mammals. *Neural Plasticity*, *2020*, 8829660. https://doi.org/10.1155/2020/8829660

Visual System

Allison, K., Patel, D., & Alabi, O. (2020). Epidemiology of glaucoma: The past, present, and predictions for the future. *Cureus*, *12*(11), e11686. https://doi.org/10.7759/cureus.11686

Bambara, J. K., Wadley, V., Owsley, C., Martin, R. C., Porter, C., & Dreer, L. E. (2009). Family functioning and low vision: A systematic review. *Journal of Visual Impairment & Blindness*, *103*(3), 137–149. https://doi.org/10.1177/0145482X0910300303

Beck, A. T., Rush, A. J., Shaw, B. F., & Emery, G. (1979). Specific techniques for the suicidal patient. In *Cognitive therapy of depression* (pp. 215–217). Guilford Press.

Boyd, K., & McKinney, J. K. (2020). *What is glaucoma?* American Association of Ophthalmology. Retrieved May 29, 2021, from https://www.aao.org/eye-health/diseases/what-is-glaucoma

Campbell, J. (2011). Eyes. In *Campbell's physiology notes* (pp. 319–340). Lorimer Publications.

Cockerham, G. C., Goodrich, G. L., Weichel, E. D., Orcutt, J. C., Rizzo, J. F., Bower, K. S., & Schuchard, R. A. (2009). Eye and visual function in traumatic brain injury. *Journal of Rehabilitation Research & Development*, *46*(6), 811–818. https://doi.org/10.1682/JRRD.2008.0109

Colbert, B. J., Ankney, J., & Lee, K. T. (2020). The senses. In Anatomy & *physiology for health professions*: An *interactive journey* (4th ed., pp. 218–235). Pearson.

Federov Restore Vision Clinic. (2021). *Optic nerves*. Retrieved May 23, 2021, from https://www.restorevisionclinic.com/optic-nerve-structure-function-damage-signs-treatment#:~:text=OPTIC%20NERVE%3A%20POSTERIOR%20(E)&text=The%20lens's%20primary%20purpose%20is,visual%20pathway%20to%20the%20brain

Flach, A. J. (2002). Delta-9-tetrahydrocannabinol (THC) in the treatment of end-stage open-angle glaucoma. *Transactions of the American Ophthalmological Society*, *100*, 215–224.

Fong, D. S., Cavellerano, J. D., Aiello, l., Ferris, F. L., III, Gardner, T. W., Klein, R., King, G. L., Blankenship, G., & the American Diabetes Association. (2004). Retinopathy in diabetes. *Diabetes Care*, *27*(Suppl. 1), S84–S87. https://doi.org/10.2337/diacare.27.2007.s84

Land, M. F., & Fernald, R. D. 1992. The evolution of eyes. *Annual Review of Neuroscience*, *15*, 1–29. https://doi.org/10.1146/annurev.ne.15.030192.000245

Khare, S., Rohatgi, J., Bhatia, M. S., & Dhaliwal, U. (2016). Burden and depression in primary caregivers of persons with visual impairment. *Indian Journal of Ophthalmology*, *64*(8), 572–577. https://doi.org/10.4103/0301-4738.191493

Khurana, M., Shoham, N., Cooper, C., & Pitman, A. L. (2021). Association between sensory impairment and suicidal ideation and attempt: A cross-sectional analysis of nationally representative English household data. *BMJ Open*, *11*, e043179. https://doi.org/10.1136/bmjopen-2020-043179

Kim, H.-J., Zhang, K., Moore, L., & Ho, D. (2014). Diamond nanogel-embedded contact lenses mediate lysozyme-dependent therapeutic release. *ACS Nano, 8*(3), 2998–3005. https://doi.org/10.1021/nn5002968

Klumpers, L. E., & Thacker, D. L. (2019). A brief background on cannabis: From plant to medical indications. *Journal of AOAC International, 102*(2), 412–420. https://doi.org/10.5740/jaoacint.18-0208

Lam, B. L., Christ, S. L., Lee, D. J., Zheng, D., & Arheart, K. L. (2008). Reported visual impairment and risk of suicide: The 1986–1996 National Health Interview Surveys. *Archives of Ophthalmology, 126*(7), 975–980. https://doi.org/10.1001/archopht.126.7.975

Marco, J. H., Perez, S., & Garcia-Alandete, J. (2016). Meaning in life buffers the association between risk factors for suicide and hopelessness in participants with mental disorders. *Journal of Clinical Psychology, 72*(7), 689–700. https://doi.org/10.1002/jclp.22285

Mayo Clinic. (2021a). *Farsightedness.* Retrieved May 25, 2021, from https://www.mayoclinic.org/diseases-conditions/farsightedness/symptoms-causes/syc-20372495#:~:text=Overview,objects%20nearby%20may%20be%20blurry

Mayo Clinic. (2021b). Glaucoma. Retrieved May 29, 2021, from Glaucoma—Symptoms and causes—Mayo Clinic.

McIntosh, J. (2015, March). How far away is a cure for blindness? *Medical News Today.* Retrieved May 27, 2021, from https://www.medicalnewstoday.com/articles/291090

Meyer-Rochow, V. B., Hakko, H., Ojamo, M., Uusitalo, H., & Timonen, M. (2015). Suicides in visually impaired persons: A nation-wide register-linked study from Finland based on thirty years of data. *PLoS One, 10*(10), e0141583. https://doi.org/10.1371/journal.pone.0141583

Mick, S., Parfyonov, M., Wittich, W., Phillips, N., & Pichora-Fuller, M. K. (2018). Associations between sensory loss and social networks, participation, support, and loneliness: Analysis of the Canadian Longitudinal Study on Aging, *Canadian Family Physician, 64*, e33–e41.

Miller, S., Daily, L., Leishman, E., Bradshaw, H., & Straiker, A. (2018). Δ^9-Tetrahydrocannabinol and cannabidiol differentially regulate intraocular pressure. *Investigative & Ophthalmology & Visual Science, 59*, 5904–5911. https://doi.org/10.1167/iovs.18-24838

National Aeronautics and Space Administration (NASA). (2010). *Visible light.* Retrieved June 11, 2021, from https://science.nasa.gov/ems/09_visiblelight

National Eye Institute (NEI). (2019a). *Color blindness.* Retrieved June 11, 2021, from https://www.nei.nih.gov/learn-about-eye-health/eye-conditions-and-diseases/color-blindness

National Eye Institute (NEI). (2019b). *Diabetic retinopathy.* Retrieved May 20, 2021, from https://www.nei.nih.gov/learn-about-eye-health/eye-conditions-and-diseases/diabetic-retinopathy

National Eye Institute (NEI). (2019c). *Nearsightedness.* Retrieved May 25, 2021, from http://www.nei.nih.gov/healthyeyes

National Eye Institute (NEI). (2020). *Age-related macular degeneration.* Retrieved May 29, 2021, from https://www.nei.nih.gov/learn-about-eye-health/eye-conditions-and-diseases/age-related-macular-degeneration

Nyman, S. R., Dibb, B., Victor, C. R., & Gosney, M. A. (2012). Emotional well-being and adjustment to vision loss in later life: A meta-synthesis of qualitative studies. *Disability & Rehabilitation, 34*(122), 971–981. https://doi.org/10.3109/09638288.2011.626487

Panahi, Y., Manayi, A., Nikan, M., & Vazirian, M. (2017). The arguments for and against cannabinoids application in glaucomatous retinopathy. *Biomedicine & Pharmacology, 86*, 620–627. https://dx.doi.org/10.1016/j.biopha.2016.11.106

Passani, A., Posarelli, C., Sframeli, A. T., Perciballi, L., Pellegrini, M., Guidi, G., & Figus, M. (2020). Cannabinoids in glaucoma patients: The never-ending story. *Journal of Clinical Medicine, 9*, 3978. https://doi.org/10.3390/jcm9123978

Powell, J. M., & Torgerson, N. G. (2011). Evaluation and treatment of vision and motor dysfunction following acquired brain injury from occupational therapy and neuro-optometry perspectives. In P. S. Suter (Ed.), *Vision rehabilitation: Multidisciplinary care of the patient following brain injury* (Chap. 10). CRC Press.

Radhakrishnan, S., & Iwach, A. (2018). *Glaucoma medication and their side effects.* Glaucoma Research Foundation. Retrieved May 26, 2021, from https://www.glaucoma.org/gleams/glaucoma-medications-and-their-side-effects.php

Reinhardt, J. P. (1996). The importance of friendship and family support in adaptation to chronic vision impairment. *Journals of Gerontology Series B: Psychological Sciences and Social Sciences, 51*(5), P268–P278.

Research!America. (2014). *Attitudinal survey of minority populations on eye and vision health and research.* A Research!America poll conducted by Zogby Analytics & Research to Prevent Blindness & the Alliance for Eye & Vision Research. Retrieved May 29, 2021 from https://www.researchamerica.org/sites/default/files/uploads/AEVRRApoll.pdf

Senra, H., Oliveira, R. A., Leal, I. (2011). From self-awareness to self-identification with visual impairment: A qualitative study with working age adults at a rehabilitation setting. *Clinical Rehabilitation, 25*(12), 1140–1151. https://doi.org/10.1177/0269215511410729

Shah, K., Frank, C. R., & Ehrlich, J. R. (2020). The association between vision impairment and social participation in community-dwelling adults: A systematic review. *Eye, 34*, 290–298. https://doi.org/10.1038/s41433-019-0712-8

Sherbourne, C. D., & Stewart, A. L. (1991). The MOS Social Support Survey. *Social Science and Medicine, 32*(6), 705–714. https://doi.org/10.1016/0277-9536(91)90150-b

Sun, X., Xu, C. S., Chen, A., & Liu, J. (2015). Marijuana for glaucoma: A recipe for disaster or treatment? *Yale Journal of Biology and Medicine, 88*, 265–269.

Tetteh, J., Fordjour, G., Ekem-Ferguson, G., Yawson, A. O., Boima, V., Entsuah-Mensah, K., Biritwum, R., Essuman, A., Mensah, G., & Yawson, A. E. (2020). Visual impairment and social isolation, depression, and life satisfaction among older adults in Ghana: Analysis of the WHO's Study on global AGEing and adult health (SAGE) Wave 2. *BMJ Open Ophthalmology, 5*, e000492. https://doi.org/10.1136/bmjophth-2020-000492

Tham, Y.-C., Li, X., Wong, T. Y., Quigley, H. A., Aung, T., & Chung, C.-Y. (2014). Global prevalence of glaucoma and projections of glaucoma burden through 2040. *Ophthalmology, 121*(11), 2018–2090. https://doi.org/10.1016/j.ophth.2014.05.013

Turbert, D., & Gudgel, D. (2021). *Does marijuana help treat glaucoma or other eye conditions?* American Association of Ophthalmology. Retrieved May 29, 2021, from https://www.aao.org/eye-health/tips-prevention/medical-marijuana-glaucoma-treament

Turbert, D., & Mendoza, O. (2021). *What is color blindness?* American Association of Ophthalmology. Retrieved June 11, 2021, from What Is Color Blindness? American Academy of Ophthalmology (aao.org).

Van Orden, K. A., Witte, T. k., Cukrowicz, K. C., Braithwaite, S., Selby, E. A., Joiner, T. E., Jr. (2010). The interpersonal theory of suicide. *Psychological Review, 117*(2), 575–600. https://doi.org/10.1037/a0018697

Wang, S.-W., & Boerner, K. (2008). Staying connected: Re-establishing social relationships following vision loss. *Clinical Rehabilitation, 22,* 816–824. https://doi.org/10.1177/0269215508091435

Gustatory and Olfactory System

AbScent. (2021). *Assess your sense of smell.* Retrieved June 16, 2021, from https://abscent.org/learn-us/self-assessment

AlJulaih, G. H., & Lasrado, S. (2021). *Anatomy, head and neck, tongue taste buds.* In *StatPearls.* StatPearls Publishing. Retrieved June 2, 2021, from https://www.ncbi.nlm.nih.gov/books/NBK539696/?report=printable

Bartoshuk, L. M., Duffy, V. B., & Miller, I. J. (1994). PTC/PROP tasting: Anatomy, psychophysics, and sex effects. *Physiology & Behavior, 56*(6), 1165–1171. https://doi.org/10.1016/0031-9384(94)90361-1

Borsetto, D., Hopkins, C., Philips, V., Obholzer, R., Tirelli, G., Polesel, J., & Boscolo-Rizzo, P. (2020). Self-reported alteration of sense of smell or taste in patients with COVID-19: A systematic review and meta-analysis on 3563 patients. *Rhinology, 58*(5), 430–436. https://doi.org/10.4193/Rhin20.185

Boscolo-Rizzo, P., Pollesel, J., Spinato, G., Fabbris, C., Calvanese, L., Menegalso, A., Borsetto, D., & Hopkins, C. (2020). Predominance of an altered sense of smell or taste among long-lasting symptoms in patients with mildly symptomatic COVID-19. *Rhinology, 58*(5), 524–526. https://doi.org/10.4193/Rhin20.263

Bruker. (2021). *FoodScreener.* Retrieved on June 9, 2021, from https://www.bruker.com/en/products-and-solutions/mr/nmr-food-solutions/food-screener.html

Butowt, R., & Von Bartheld, C. S. (2020). Anosmia in COVID-19: Underlying mechanisms and assessment of an olfactory route to brain infection. *Neuroscientist, 1,* 22. https://doi.org/10.1177/1073858420956905

Centers for Disease Control and Prevention (CDC). (2021). Symptoms of COVID-19. Retrieved November 11, 2021, from https://www.cdc.gov/coronavirus/2019-ncov/symptoms-testing/symptoms.html

Chen, L., & Thurston, G. (2002). World Trade Center cough. *Lancet, 360*(Suppl.), 37–38. https://doi.org/10.1016/S0140-6736(02)11814-9

Escanilla, O. D., Victor, J. D., & Lorenzo, R. M. (2015). Odor-taste convergence in the nucleus of the solitary tract of the awake freely licking rat. *Journal of Neuroscience, 35*(16), 6284–6297. https://doi.org/10.1523/JNEUROSCI.3526-14.2015

Fandino, A., & Douglas, R. (2021). A historical review of the evolution of nasal lavage systems. *Journal of Laryngology & Otology, 135*(2), 110–116. https://doi.org/10.1017/S002221512100030X

Fifth Sense. (2020). *SmellAbility: Training & testing.* Retrieved June 16, 2021, from https://www.fifthsense.org.uk/smell-training/

Hoffman, M. (2020). *What are sinuses? Pictures of the sinuses.* Human Anatomy. WebMD. Retrieved June14, 2021, from https://www.webmd.com/allergies/picture-of-the-sinuses

Honma, A., Takagi, D., Nakamaru, Y., Homma, A., Suzuki, M., & Fukuda, S. (2016). Reduction of blood eosinophil counts in eosinophilic chronic rhinosinusitis after surgery. *Journal of Laryngology & Otology, 130*, 1147–1152. https://doi.org/10.1017/S0022215116009324

Hou, C., Dong, J., Zhang, G., Lei, Y., Yang, M., Zhang, Y., Liu, Z., Zhang, S., & Huo, D. (2011). Colorimetric artificial tongue for protein identification. *Biosensors & Bioelectronics, 26*, 3981–3986. https://doi.org/10.1016/j.bios.2010.11.025

Krusemark, E. A., Novak, L. R., Gitelman, D. R., & Li, W. (2013). When the sense of smell meets emotion: Anxiety-state-dependent olfactory processing and neural circuitry adaptation. *Journal of Neuroscience, 33*(39). 15324–15332. https://doi.org/10.1523/JNEUROSCI.1835-13.2013

Lavigne, J. J., Savoy, S., Clevenger, M. B., Ritchie, J. E., McDoniel, B., Yoo, S.-J., Anslyn, E. V., McDevitt, J. T., Shear, J. B., & Neikirk, D. (1998). Solution-based analysis of multiple analytes by a sensor array: Toward the development of an "electronic tongue." *Journal of the American Chemical Society, 120*, 6429–6430.

Lechien, J. R., Chiesa-Estomba, C. M., Hans, S., Barillari, M. R., Jouffe, L., & Saussez, S. (2020). Loss of smell and taste in 2013 European patients with mild to moderate COVID-19. *Annals of Internal Medicine, 173*, 672–675. https://doi.org/10.7326/M20-2428

Lechien, J. R., Journe, F., Hans, S., Chiesa-Estomba, C. M., Mustin, V., Beckers, E., Vaira, L. A., DeRiu, G., Hopkins, C., & Saussez, S. (2020). Severity of anosmia as an early symptom of COVID-19 infection may predict lasting loss of smell. *Frontiers in Medicine, 7*. https://doi.org/10.3389/fmed.2020.582802

Lee, M., Jung, J. W., Kim, D., Ahn, Y.-J., Hong, S., & Kwon, H. W. (2015). Discrimination of umami tastants using floating electrode-based bioelectronic tongue mimicking inset taste systems. *ACS Nano, 9*(12), 11728–11736. https://doi.org/10.1021/acsnano.5b03031

Levin, S. M., Herbert, R., Moline, J. M., Todd, A. C., Stevenson, L., Landsbergis, P., Jiang, S., Skloot, G., Baron, S., & Enright, P. (2004). Physical health status of World Trade Center rescue and recovery workers and volunteers—New York City, July 2002–August 2004. *Morbidity & Mortality Weekly Report, 53*, 807–812.

Lim, S. H., Musto, C. J., Park, E., Zhong, W., & Suslick, K. S. (2008). A colorimetric sensor array for detection and identification of sugars. *Organic Letters, 10*(20), 4405–4408. https://doi.org/10.1021/ol801459k

Malmendal, A., Amoresano, C., Trotta R., Lauri, I., De Tito, S., Novellino, E., & Randazzo, A. (2011). NMR spectrometers an "magnetic tongues": Prediction of sensory descriptors in canned tomatoes. *Journal of Agricultural & Food Chemistry, 59*(20), 10831–10838. https://doi.org/10.1021/jf203803q

Manodh, P., Prabhu Shankar, D., Pradeep, D., Santhosh, R., & Murugan, A. (2016). Incidence and patterns of maxillofacial trauma—a retrospective analysis of 3611 patients—an update. *Oral Maxillofacial Surgery, 20*, 377–383. https://doi.org/10.1007/s10006-016-0576-z

Mazzatenta, A., Neri, G., D'Ardes, D., DeLuca, C., Marinari, S., Porreca, E., Cipollone, F., Vecchiet, J., Falcicchia, C., Panichi, V., Origlia, N., & DiGiulio, C. (2020). Smell and taste in severe COVID-19: Self-reported vs. testing. *Frontiers in Medicine, 7*, 589409. https://doi.org/10.3389/fmed.2020.589409

Medical University of South Carolina (MUSC). (n.d.). *Sinusitis.* Retrieved June 14, 2021, from https://muschealth.org/medical-services/ent/sinus-center/sinusitis

Mizuno, K., Mizuno, N., Shinohara, T., & Noda, M. (2004). Mother-infant skin-to-skin contact after delivery results in early recognition of own mother's milk odour. *Acta Paediatrica, 93,* 1640–1645. https://doi.org/10.1080/08035250410023115

National Institute on Deafness and Other Communication Disorders (NIDCD). (2017). *Taste disorders.* National Institutes of Health Publication, No. 14-3231A. Retrieved June 1, 2021, from https://www.nidcd.nih.gov/health/taste-disorders#2

Pinto, J. M. (2011). Olfaction. *Proceedings from the American Thoracic Society, 8,* 46–52. https://doi.org/10.1513/pats.201005-035RN

Prezant, D. J., Weiden, M., Banauch, G. I., McGuinness, G., Rom, W. N., Aldrich, T. K., & Kelly, K. J. (2002). Cough and bronchial responsiveness in firefighters at the World Trade Center site. *New England Journal of Medicine, 347,* 806–815. https://doi.org/10.1056/NEJMoa021300

Sarafoleanu, C., Mella, C., Georgescu, M., & Perederco, C. (2009). The importance of the olfactory sense in the human behavior and evolution. *Journal of Medicine & Life, 2*(2), 196–198.

Savic, I., Berglund, H., Gulyas, B., & Roland, P. (2001). Smelling of odorous sex hormone-like compound causes sex-differentiated hypothalamic activations in humans. *Neuron, 31*(4), 661–668. https://doi.org/10.1016/s0896-6273(01)00390-7

Schaeffer, J. P. (1910). The lateral wall of the cavum nasi in man, with especial reference to the various developmental stages. *Journal of Morphology, 21*(4), 613–702.

Sherman, C. (2019). *The senses: Smell and taste.* Retrieved June 8, 2021, from https://www.dana.org/wp-content/uploads/2019/05/fact-sheet-senses-smell-taste-baw-2020.pdf

Skrandies, W., & Zschieschang, R. (2015). Olfactory and gustatory functions and its relation to body weight. *Physiology & Behavior, 142,* 1–4. https://doi.org/10.1016/j.physbeh.2015.01.024

Spence, C. (2015). Just how much of what we taste derives from the sense of smell? *Flavour, 4,* 30. https://doi.org/10.1186/s13411-015-0040-2

Spinato, G., Fabbris, C., Polesel, J., Cazzador, D., Borsetto, D., Hopkins, C., & Boscolo-Rizzo, P. (2020). Alterations in smell or taste in mildly symptomatic outpatients with SARS-CoV-2 infection. *JAMA, 323*(20), 2089–2090. https://doi.org/10.1001/jama.2020.6771

Toko, K. (2000). Taste sensor. *Sensors & Actuators B, 64,* 205–215. https://doi.org/10.1016/S0925-4005(99)00508-0

Uebi, T., Hariyama, T., Suzuki, K., Kanayama, N., Nagata, Y., Ayabe-Kanamjura, S., Yanase, S., Ohtsubo, Y., & Ozaki, M. (2019). Sampling, identification, and sensory evaluation of odors of a newborn baby's head and amniotic fluid. *Scientific Reports, 9,* 12759. https://doi.org/10.1038/s41598-019-49137-6

Webber, M. P., Glaser, M. S., Weakley, J., Soo, J., Ye, F., Zeig-Owens, R., Weiden, M. D., Nolan, A., Aldrich, T. K., Kelly, K., & Prezant, D. (2011). Physician-diagnosed respiratory conditions and mental health symptoms seven to nine years following the World Trade Center disaster. *American Journal of Industrial Medicine, 54,* 661–671. https://doi.org/10.1002/ajim.20993

Williams, J. A., Bartoshuk, L. M., Fillingim, R. B., & Dotson, C. D. (2016). Exploring ethnic differences in taste perception. *Chemical Senses, 41,* 449–456. https://doi.org/10.1093/chemse/bjw021

Wisnivesky, J. P., Teitelbaum, S. L., Todd, A. C., Boffetta, P., Crane, M., Crowley, L., de la Hoz, R. E., Dellenbaugh, C., Harrison, D., Herbert, R., Kim, H., Jeon, Y., Kaplan, J., Katz, C., Levin, S., Luft, B., Markowitz, S., Moline, J. M., Ozbay, F., Pietrzak, R. H., . . .

Landrigan, P. J. (2011). Persistence of multiple illnesses in World Trade Center rescue and recovery workers: A cohort study. *Lancet, 378,* 888–897. https://doi.org/10.1016/S0140-6736(11)61180-X

Wrobel, B. B., & Leopold, D. A. (2004). Smell and taste disorders. *Facial Plastic Surgery Clinics of North America, 12*(4), 459–468. https://doi.org/10.1016/j.fsc.2004.04.006

Zhang, S., Su, F., Li, J., & Chen, W. (2018). The analgesic effect of maternal milk odor on newborns: A meta-analysis. *Breastfeeding Medicine, 13*(5), 327–334. https://doi.org/10.1089/bfm.2017.0226.

Chapter 6

Advokat, C. D., Comaty, J. E., & Julien, R. M. (2019). *Julien's primer of drug action: A comprehensive guide to the actions, uses, and side effects of psychoactive drugs* (14th ed., pp. 177–216). Worth Publishers, Macmillan Learning.

Alam, M. N., Rizvi, T. H., Alam, M., & Tahir, M. (2018). Ischemic stroke: Frequency and contributing factors of atrial fibrillation in patients with first ischemic stroke. *Professional Medical Journal, 25*(1), 84–89. https://doi.org/10.29309/TPMJ/18.4234

American Association of Neurological Surgeons. (2020). Neurological *conditions and treatments/stroke.* Retrieved November 8, 2021, from https://www.aans.org/en/Patients/Neurosurgical-Conditions-and-Treatments/Stroke

American Health Association. (2021). *Is vaping better than smoking?* Retrieved October 23, 2021, from https://www.heart.org/en/healthy-living/healthy-lifestyle/quit-smoking-tobacco/is-vaping-safer-than-smoking

American Heart Association. (2020a). *Atrial fibrillation medication.* Retrieved November 8, 2021, from https://www.heart.org/en/health-topics/atrial-fibrillation/treatment-and-prevention-of-atrial-fibrillation/atrial-fibrillation-medications

American Heart Association. (2020b). *Cardioversion.* Retrieved November 8, 2021, from https://www.heart.org/en/health-topics/arrhythmia/prevention--treatment-of-arrhythmia/cardioversion

American Heart Association. (2020c) *Understanding blood pressure readings.* Retrieved November 8, 2021, from https://www.heart.org/en/health-topics/high-blood-pressure/understanding-blood-pressure-readings

Campbell, J. (2011). Cardiovascular system. In Campbell's *physiology notes* (pp. 29–54). Lorimar Publishing.

Centers for Disease Control and Prevention (CDC). (2011). *Chemicals in tobacco smoke.* Retrieved January 26, 2022, from https://www.cdc.gov/tobacco/data_statistics/sgr/2010/consumer_booklet/chemicals_smoke/index.htm

Cleveland Clinic. (2020). *Coronary artery disease.* Retrieved December 7, 2020, from https://my.clevelandclinic.org/health/diseases/16898-coronary-artery-disease#:~:text=Coronary%20artery%20disease%20is%20the,called%20plaques)%20inside%20the%20arteries

Cleveland Clinic. (2021). *Pulmonary arteries.* Retrieved from https://my.clevelandclinic.org/health/articles/21486-pulmonary-arteries

Colbert, B. J., Ankney, J., & Lee, K. T. (2020). The cardiovascular system. In *Anatomy and physiology for health professions* (4th ed., pp. 259–289). Pearson Publishing.

Cornelius, M. E., Loretan, C. G., Wang, T. W., Jamal, A., & Homa, D. M. (2022). Tobacco product use among adults: United States, 2020. *Morbidity and Mortality Weekly Report, 71*, 397–405.

Curran, M. A. (2019). *Fetal development.* Retrieved October 23, 2021, from perinatology. com

DiClemente, C. C., & Velasquez, M. M. (2002). Motivational interviewing and the stages of change. In W. R. Miller & S. Rollnick (Eds.), *Motivational interviewing: Preparing people for change* (2nd ed.). Guilford Press. Retrieved November 11, 2021, from https:// www.wellcoach.com/memberships/images/MI_DiClemente_Stages.pdf

Duncan, M. S., Freiberg, M. S., Greevy, R. A., Jr., Kundu, S., Vasan, R. S., Tindle, H. A. (2019). Association of smoking cessation with subsequent risk of cardiovascular disease. *JAMA, 322*(7), 642–650. https://doi.org/10.1001/jama.2019.10298

Educational Fund to Stop Gun Violence and Coalition to Stop Gun Violence (EFSGV). (2021). *A public health crisis decades in the making: A review of 2019 CDC gun mortality data.* Retrieved July 30, 2021, from https://efsgv.org/wp-content/uploads/2019CDCd ata.pdf

Fogoros, R. N. (2020). *Angioplasty surgery: Everything you need to know.* Retrieved October 24, 2021, from https://www.verywellhealth.com/angioplasty-treatment-for-arteries-1745728

Healthy People 2020. (2021). *Tobacco use.* Retrieved October 23, 2021, from https://www. healthypeople.gov/2020/topics-objectives/topic/tobacco-use/national-snapshot

Heron, M. (2019). Deaths: Leading causes for 2017. *National Vital Statistics Reports, 68*(6), 1–77. Retrieved November 11, 2021, from https://www.cdc.gov/nchs/data/nvsr/ nvsr68/nvsr68_06-508.pdf

Hughes, J. R. (1995). Applying harm reduction to smoking. *Tobacco Control, 4,* S33–S38. http://dx.doi.org/10.1136/tc.4.suppl2 .S33

Inaba, D. S., & Cohen, W. E. (2014). The neurochemistry and the physiology of addiction. In *Uppers, downers, all-arounders: Physical and mental effects of psychoactive drugs* (pp. 2.1–2.47). CNS Productions.

Johns Hopkins Medicine. (2020). *Echocardiogram.* Retrieved November 8, 2021, from https://www.hopkinsmedicine.org/health/treatment-tests-and-therapies/echocar diogram

Kahn, M. A. B., Hashim, M. J., Mustafa, H., Baniyas, M. Y., Al Suwaidi, S. K. B. M., Al Katheeri, R., Alblooshi, F. M. K., Almatrooshi, M. E. A. H., Alzaabi, M. E. H., Al Darmaki, R. S., Lootah, S. N. A. H. (2020). Global epidemiology of ischemic heart disease: Results from the Global Burden of Disease Study. *Cureus, 12*(7), e9349. https:// doi.org/10.7759/cureus.9349

Kahn Academy. (n.d.-a). *Components of blood.* Retrieved October 27, 2021, from https:// www.khanacademy.org/science/biology/human-biology/circulatory-pulmonary/a/ components-of-the-blood

Kawall, T., Seecheran, R. V., Seecheran V. K., Persad, S. A., Jagdeo, C.-L., & Seecheran, N. A. (2020). "Shot to the Heart": Case report and concise review of cardiac gunshot injury. *Journal of Investigative Medicine High Impact Case Reports, 8,* 1–4. https://doi.org/ 10.1177/2324709620951652

LaMorte, W. W. (2019). *The transtheoretical model (stages of change).* Retrieved October 22, 2021, from https://sphweb.bumc.bu.edu/otlt/MPH-Modules/SB/BehavioralCha ngeTheories/BehavioralChangeTheories6.html

Locker, A. R., Marks, M. J., Kamens, H. M., & Klein, L. C. (2016). Exposure to nicotine increases nicotinic acetylcholine receptor density in the reward pathway and binge ethanol consumption in C57BL/6J adolescent female mice. *Brain Research Bulletin, 123,* 13–22. https://doi.org/10.1016/j.brainresbull.2015.09.009

Loukas, M. (2021). Heart. In S. Standring (Ed.), *Gray's anatomy: The anatomical basis of clinical practice* (42nd ed., pp. 1068–1096). Elsevier.

Mayo Clinic. (2013). *The heart and the circulatory system: How they work.* Retrieved November 8, 2021, from https://www.youtube.com/watch?v=CWFyxn0qDEU

Mayo Clinic. (2019). Cardiac tests & procedures. Retrieved November 8, 2021, from https://www.mayoclinic.org/tests-procedures/cardiac-catheterization/about/pac-20384695

Mayo Clinic. (2020). Atrial fibrillation. Retrieved November 8, 2021, from https://www.mayoclinic.org/diseases-conditions/atrial-fibrillation/diagnosis-treatment/drc-20350630

Mayo Clinic. (n.d.). Atrial fibrillation. Retrieved from https://www.mayoclinic.org/diseases-conditions/atrial-fibrillation/symptoms-causes/syc-20350624

National Heart, Lung, & Blood Institute, National Institutes of Health. (2019). *Coronary heart disease.* Retrieved November 8, 2021, from https://www.nhlbi.nih.gov/health-topics/coronary-heart-disease

National Institute of Alcohol Abuse and Alcoholism. (2005). *Social work education for the prevention and treatment of alcohol use disorders.* Module 6. National Institutes of Health.

Pappano, A. T., & Wier, W. G. (2019). *Cardiovascular Physiology* (11th ed.). Elsevier. Retrieved November 11, 2021, from https://www.google.com/books/edition/Cardiovascular_Physiology_E_Book/wgpuDwAAQBAJ?hl=en&gbpv=1&dq=Pappano,+A.T.,+%26+Wier,+W.+G.+(2019).+Cardiovascular+Physiology+(11th+ed).+Elsevier.&pg=PP1&printsec=frontcover0

Power, A. E. (2004). Slow-wave sleep, acetylcholine, and memory consolidation. *Proceedings of the National Academic of Sciences of the United States of America, 101*(7), 1795–1796. https://doi.org/10.1073/pnas.0400237101

Shearman, E., Rossi, S., Sershen, H., Hashim, A., & Lajtha, A. (2005). Locally administered low nicotine-induced neurotransmitter changes in areas of cognitive function. *Neurochemical Research, 30*(8), 1055–1066. https://doi.org/10.1007/s11064-005-7132-9

Shrestha, R., Kanchan, T., & Krishan, K. (2021). Gunshot wounds forensic pathology. In StatPearls. StatPearls Publishing.

Singer, S., Rossi, S., Verzosa, S., Hashim, A., Lonow, R., Cooper, T., Sershen, H., & Lajtha, A. (2004). Nicotine-induced changes in neurotransmitter levels in brain areas associated with cognitive function. *Neurochemical Research, 29*(9), 1779–1792. https://doi.org/10.1023/B:NERE.0000035814.45494.15

Tan, C. M. J., & Lewandowski, A. J. (2020). The transitional heart: From early embryonic and fetal development to neonatal life. *Fetal Diagnosis & Therapy, 47*(5), 373–386. https://doi.org/10.1159/000501906

Tuan, T.-C., Chang, S.-L., Tai, C.-T., Lin, Y. J., Hu. Y.-F., Lo, L.-W., Wongcharoen, W., Udyavar, A. R., Chiang, S.-J., Chen, Y.-J., Tsao, H.-M., Ueng, K.-C., & Chen, S.-A. (2008). Impairment of the atrial substrates by chronic cigarette smoking in patients with atrial fibrillation. *Journal of Cardiovascular Electrophysiology, 19,* 259–265. https://doi.org/10.1111/j.1540-8167.2007.01057.x

Healthy People 2030, U.S. Department of Health and Human Services, Office of Disease Prevention and Health Promotion. Retrieved from https://health.gov/healthypeople/ objectives-and-data/social-determinants-health

U.S. Census Bureau. (2020). *National Health Interview Survey (NHIS)*. Retrieved November 8, 2021, from https://www.census.gov/programs-surveys/nhis.html

U.S. Department of Health and Human Services. (2020). *Smoking cessation: A report of the surgeon general—Executive summary* (p. 1). Atlanta, GA: Centers for Disease Control and Prevention, National Center for Chronic Disease Prevention and Health Promotion, Office on Smoking and Health. Retrieved November 8, 2021, from https:// www.hhs.gov/sites/default/files/2020-cessation-sgr-executive-summary.pdf

Wani, M. L., Ahangar, A. G., Wani, S. N., Irshad, I., & Ul-Hassan, N. (2012). Penetrating cardiac injury: A review. *Trauma Monthly, 17,* 230–232.

Ward, J. P. T. (2021). Smooth muscle and the cardiovascular and lymphatic systems. In S. Standring (Ed.), *Gray's anatomy: The anatomical basis of clinical practice* (42nd ed., pp. 127–144). Elsevier.

Watanabe, I. (2018). Smoking and risk of atrial fibrillation. *Journal of Cardiology, 71,* 111–112. https://doi.org/10.1016/j.jjcc.2017.08.001

WebMD. (2021). *How your heart works.* Retrieved October 23, 2021, from https://www. webmd.com/hypertension-high-blood-pressure/hypertension-working-heart

Willacy, H. (2021). *Gunshot injuries.* Retrieved July 30, 2021, from https://patient.info/ doctor/gunshot-injuries

World Health Organization (WHO). (2020). *The top ten causes of death.* Retrieved from https://www.who.int/news-room/fact-sheets/detail/the-top-10-causes-of-death

World Health Organization Commission on Social Determinants of Health. (2008). *Closing the gap in a generation: Health equity through action on the social determinants of health.* https://apps.who.int/iris/bitstream/handle/10665/43943/9789241563703_ eng.pdf?sequence=1

World Population Review. (2021). *Gun deaths by country in 2021.* Retrieved July 30, 2021, from https://worldpopulationreview.com/country-rankings/gun-deaths-by-country

Chapter 7

Anisuzzaman, M., Hosai, S. N., Reza, M. M., Kibria, M. G., & Ferdous, S. (2019). Management of chest trauma in Bangladesh perspective: Experience of a decade. *Cardiovascular Journal, 12*(1), 3–8. https://doi.org/10.3329/cardio.v.12i1.43411

Attia, Y. A., El-Saadony, M. T., Swelum, A. A., Qattan, S. Y. A., Al-qurashi, A. D., Asiry, K. A., Shafi, M. E., Elbestawy, A. R., Gado, A. R., Khafaga, A. F., Hussein, E. O. S., Ba-Awadh, H., Tiwari, R., Dhama, K., Alhussaini, B., Alyileilli, S. R., El-Tarabily, K. A., & El-Hack, M. E. A. (2021). COVID-19: Pathogenesis, advances in treatment and vaccine development and environmental impact—an updated review. *Environmental Science & Pollution Research, 28,* 22241–22264. https://doi.org/10.1007/s11356-021-13018-1

Bernstein, L., & Cha, A. E. (2020). *Doctors keep discovering new ways the coronavirus attacks the body.* Retrieved November 12, 2021, from https://www.washingtonpost. com/health/2020/05/10/coronavirus-attacks-body-symptoms/?arc404=true

Bush, A., & Collins, P. (2021). Development of the lungs, thorax, and respiratory diaphragm. In S. Standring (Ed.), *Gray's anatomy: Anatomical basis of clinical practice* (42nd ed., pp. 314–322). Elsevier.

Bustamante-Marin, X., & Ostrowski, L. E. (2017). Cilia and mucociliary clearance. *Cold Springs Harbor Perspective in Biology, 9*, a028241. https://doi.org/10.1101/cshperspect.a028241

Campbell, J. (2011a). Respiration. In Campbell's *physiology notes* (pp. 85–108). Lorimer Publication.

Campbell, J. (2011b). Disorders of the immune system. In Campbell's *pathophysiology notes* (pp. 2397–2793). Lorimer Publications.

Centers for Disease Control and Prevention (CDC). (2021a). *How COVID-19 spreads.* Retrieved November 14, 2021, from https://www.cdc.gov/coronavirus/2019-ncov/prevent-getting-sick/how-covid-spreads.html

Centers for Disease Control and Prevention (CDC). (2021b). *Myths and facts about COVID-19 vaccines.* Retrieved November 14, 2021, from https://www.cdc.gov/coronavirus/2019-ncov/vaccines/facts.html

Centers for Disease Control and Prevention (CDC). (2021c). *Symptoms of Covid-19.* Retrieved November 13, 2021, from https://www.cdc.gov/coronavirus/2019-ncov/symptoms-testing/symptoms.html

Centers for Disease Control and Prevention (CDC). (2020). *Quarantine and isolation.* Retrieved November 13, 2021, from https://www.cdc.gov/quarantine/quarantineisolation.html

Chaudhry, R., & Bordoni, B. (2019). Anatomy, thorax, lungs. In *StatPearls*. StatPearls Publishing. https://www.ncbi.nlm.nih.gov/books/NBK470197/

Cleveland Clinic. (2020). *Here's the damage coronavirus (Covid-19) can do to your lungs: How the coronavirus causes acute respiratory distress syndrome.* Retrieved November 12, 2021, from https://health.clevelandclinic.org/heres-the-damage-coronavirus-covid-19-can-do-to-your-lungs

Cleveland Clinic. (2021). *Collapsed lung (pneumothorax).* Retrieved November 25, 2021, from https://my.clevelandclinic.org/health/diseases/15304-collapsed-lung-pneumothorax

Colbert, B. J., Ankney, J., & Lee, K. T. (2020a). The cardiovascular system. In *Anatomy and physiology for health professions* (4th ed., pp. 259–280). Pearson Publishing.

Colbert, B. J., Ankney, J., & Lee, K. T. (2020b). Respiration. In *Anatomy and physiology for health professions* (4th ed., pp. 290–318). Pearson Publishing.

Connors, G. J., Carroll, K. M., DiClemente, C. C., Longabaugh, R., & Donavan, D. M. (1997). The therapeutic alliance and its relationship to alcoholism treatment participation and outcome. *Journal of Consulting & Clinical Psychology, 65*(4), 588–598. https://doi.org/10.1037/0022-006X.65.4.588

Dinerstein, C. (2021). *Who are the asymptomatic with COVID-19?* American Council on Science & Health. Retrieved November 13, 2021, from https://www.acsh.org/news/2021/02/09/who-are-asymptomatic-covid-19-15329

Fogg, Q. (2021). Pleura, lungs, trachea, and bronchi. In S. Standring (Ed.), *Gray's anatomy: Anatomical basis of clinical practice* (42nd ed., pp. 1020–1037). Elsevier.

Galiatsatos, P. (2020). *COVID-19: Lung damage.* Retrieved November 12, 2021, from https://www.hopkinsmedicine.org/health/conditions-and-diseases/coronavirus/what-coronavirus-does-to-the-lungs

George, A., & Kishore, U. (2021). Blood, lymphoid tissues, & hemopoiesis. In S. Standring (Ed.). (2021). *Gray's anatomy: The anatomical basis of clinical practice* (42nd ed., pp. 71–84). Elsevier.

Grove, J., & Marsh, M. (2011). The cell biology of receptor-mediated virus entry. *Journal of Cell Biology, 195*(7), 1071–1082. https://doi.org/10.1083/jcb.201108131

Hajjar, W. M., Al-nassar, S. A., Almutair, O. S., Alfahadi, A. H., Aldosari, N. H., & Meo, S. A. (2021). Chest trauma experience: Incidence, associated factors, and outcomes among patients in Saudi Arabia. *Pakistan Journal of Medical Science, 37*(2). https://doi.org/10.12669/pjms.37.2.3842

Hatipoglu, N. (2020). The "new" problem of humanity: New coronavirus (2019-nCoV/COVID-19) disease. *Medical Journal of Bakirkoy, 16*(1), 1–8. https://doi.org/10.5222/BMJ.2020.22931

Ikeda, K., Kawakami, K., Onimaru, H., Okada, Y., Yokota, S., Koshiya, N. Oku, Y., Iizuku, M., & Koizumi, H. (2017). The respiratory control mechanisms in the brainstem and spinal cord: Integrative views of the neuroanatomy and neurophysiology. *Journal of Physiological Science, 67*, 45–62. https://doi.org/10.1007/s12576-016-0475-y

Kahn Academy. (n.d.). *Cellular respiration.* Retrieved November 12, 2021, from https://www.khanacademy.org/science/ap-biology/cellular-energetics/cellular-respiration-ap/a/intro-to-cellular-respiration-and-redox

Last, J. M. (Ed.). (2001). *Dictionary of epidemiology* (4th ed., p. 61). Oxford University Press.

Li, C., Chang, Q., Zhang, J., & Chai, W. (2018). Effects of slow breathing rate on heart rate variability and arterial baroreflex sensitivity in essential hypertension. *Medicine, 97*, 18(e0639). https://doi.org/10.1097/MD.0000000000010639

Mardani, P., Rad, M. M., Paydar, S., Amirian, A., Shahriarirad, R., Erfani, A., & Ranjbar, K. (2021). Evaluation of lung contusions, associated injuries, and outcome in a major trauma center in Shiraz, Southern Iran. *Emergency Medicine International, 2021*, 3789132. https://doi.org/10.1155/2021/3789132

Mayo Foundation for Medical Education and Research (MFMER). (2020). *Infectious diseases.* Symptoms and *causes.* Retrieved May 14, 2020, from https://www.mayoclinic.org/diseases-conditions/infectious-diseases/symptoms-causes/syc-20351173

Naclerio, R. M., Pinto, J., Assanasen, P., & Baroody, F. M. (2007). Observations on the ability of the nose to warm and humidify inspired air. *Rhinology, 45*(2), 102–111.

National Cancer Institute. (2021). *Mortality.* Retrieved November 1, 2021 from https://www.cancer.gov/publications/dictionaries/cancer-terms/def/mortality

National Cancer Institute, SEER Training Modules. (n.d.). *Mechanics of ventilation.* Retrieved November 12, 2021, from https://www.training.seer.cancer.gov/anatomy/respiratory/mechanics.html

National Heart, Lung, & Blood Institute. (n.d.). *Respiratory failure.* Retrieved November 14, 2021, from https://www.nhlbi.nih.gov/health-topics/respiratory-failure

Ochs, M., Nyengaard, J. R., Jung, A., Knudsen, L., Voigt, M., Wahlers, T., Richter, J., & Gundersen, H. J. G. (2004). The number of alveoli in the human lung. *American Journal of Respiratory & Critical Care Medicine, 169*, 120–124. https://doi.org/10.1164/rccm.200308-11070C

Parsons, J. (2020). *How to protect your lungs from lasting COVID-19 damage.* Retrieved November 12, 2021, https://wexnermedical.osu.edu/blog/how-to-protect-your-lungs-from-lasting-covid-19-damage

Powers, K. A., & Dhamoon, A. S. (2021). Physiology, pulmonary ventilation and perfusion. In: *StatPearls.* StatPearls Publishing. Retrieved November 12, 2021, from https://www.ncbi.nlm.nih.gov/books/NBK539907/

SAGE Working Group for Vaccine Hesitancy. (2014). *Report of the SAGE Working Group for Vaccine Hesitancy.* Retrieved November 14, 2021, from https://www.who.int/

immunization/sage/meetings/2014/october/1_Report_WORKING_GROUP_vacc ine_hesitancy_final.pdf

Shastri, M. D., Shukla, S. D., Chong, W. C., KC, R., Dua, K., Patel, R. P., Peterson, G. M., & O'Toole, R. F. (2021). Smoking and COVID-19: What we know so far. *Respiratory Medicine, 176*, 106237. https://doi.org/10.1016/j.rmed.2020.106237

Shelly, M. P., & Nightingale, P. (1999). ABC of intensive care: Respiratory support. *British Medical Journal, 318*, 1674–1677. https://doi.org/10.1136/bmj.318.7199.1674

Singh, R., Kang, A., Luo, X., Jeyanathan, M., Gillgrass, A., Afkhami, S., & Xing, Z. (2021). COVID-19: Current knowledge in clinical features, immunological responses, and vaccine development. *FASEB Journal, 35*(3), e21409. https://doi.org/10.1096/fj.202 002662R

Steckelberg, J. M. (2017). *Bacteria versus viral infections: How do they differ?* Mayo Clinic. Retrieved May 6, 2020 from https://www.mayoclinic.org/diseases-conditions/infecti ous-diseases/expert-answers/infectious-disease/FAQ-20058098

Wang, D., Hu, B., Hu, C., Zhu, F., Liu, X., Zhang, J., Wang, B., Xiang, H., Cheng, Z., Xiong, Y., Zhao, Y., Li, Y., Wang, X., & Peng, Z. (2020). Clinical characteristics of 138 hospitalized patients with 2019 novel coronavirus-infected pneumonia in Wuhan, China. *JAMA, 323*(11), 1061–1069. https://doi.org/10.1001/jama.2020.1585

Wang, K., Zhao, W., Li, J., Shu, W., & Duan, J. (2020). The experience of high-flow nasal cannula in hospitalized patients with 2019 novel coronavirus-infected pneumonia in two hospitals of Chongqing, China. *Annals of Intensive Care, 10*(370), 1–5. https://doi. org/10.1186/s13613-020-00653-z

WebMD. (2021). *Coronavirus incubation period.* WebMD Medical Reference. Retrieved November 13, 2021, from https://www.webmd.com/lung/coronavirus-incubation-per iod?print=true

Weinberger, S. E., Cockrill, B. A., & Mandel, J. (2019). *Principles of pulmonary medicine* (7th ed.). Elsevier.

Wong, N. A., & Saier, M. H., Jr. (2021). The SARS-coronavirus infection cycle: A survey of viral membrane proteins, their functional interactions and pathogenesis. *International Journal of Molecular Sciences, 22*, 1308. https://doi.org/10.3390/ijms22031308World Health Organization (WHO). (2020a). *Clinical management of severe acute respiratory infection (SARI) when COVID-19 disease is suspected: Interim guidance.* WHO/22019-nCoV/clinical/2020.4. Retrieved November 13, 2021, from https://www.who.int/docs/ default-source/coronaviruse/clinical-management-of-novel-cov.pdf

World Health Organization (WHO). (2020b). *Coronavirus disease (COVID-19) weekly ep-idemiological update and weekly operational update.* Retrieved November 1, 2021, from https://www.who.int/emergencies/diseases/novel-coronavirus-2019/situation-reports

World Health Organization (WHO). (2021). *United States of America: WHO coronovirus disease.* Retrieved April 29, 2022, from https://covid19.who.int/region/amro/coun try/us

Zhao, J., Zhao, S., Ou, J., Zhang, J., Lan, W., Guan, W., Wu, X., Yan, Y., Zhao, W., Wu, J., & Chodosh, J. 2020). COVID-19: Coronavirus vaccine development updates. *Frontiers in Immununology,11*, 602256. https://doi.org/10.3389/fimmu.2020.602256Zhou, F., Yu, T., Du, R., Fan, G., Liu, Y., Liu, Z., Xiang, J., Wang, Y., Song, B., Gu, X., Guan, L., Wei, Y., Li, H., Wu, X., Xu, J., Tu, S.,: Zhang, Y., Chen, H., & Cao, B. (2020). Clinical course and risk factors for mortality of adult inpatients with COVID-19 in Wuhan, China: A retrospective cohort study. *Lancet, 395*, 1054–1062. https://doi.org/10.1016/ S0140-6736(20)30566-3

Chapter 8

American Academy of Dermatology (AAD). (2021). *Skin cancer.* Retrieved November 1, 2021, from https://www.aad.org/media/stats-skin-cancer

American Burn Association. (2016). *Burn incidence fact sheet.* Retrieved January 20, 2022, from https://ameriburn.org/who-we-are/media/burn-incidence-fact-sheet/

American Cancer Society. (2020). *Basal and squamous cell skin cancer.* Retrieved January 20, 2022, from https://www.cancer.org/cancer/basal-and-squamous-cell-skin-cancer.html

Blumenthal, E., & Jeffery, S. (2018). Autofluorescence imaging for evaluating debridement in military and trauma wounds. *Military Medicine, 183*(3/4) 429–432. https://doi.org/10.1093/milmed/usx145

Bonsu, K., Kugbey, N., Ayanore, M. A., & Atefoe, E. A. (2019). Mediation effects of depression and anxiety on social support and quality of life among caregivers or persons with severe burns injury. *BMC Research Notes, 12,* 772–778. https://doi.org/10.1186/s13104-019-4761-7

Bruslind, L. (2020). *Bacteria—Surface structures.* LibreTexts, Biology. Retrieved on January 20, 2022, from https://bio.libretexts.org/Bookshelves/Microbiology/Book%3A_Microbiology_(Bruslind)/06%3A_Bacteria_-_Surface_Structures

Campbell, J. (2011a). Skin. In Campbell's *physiology notes* (pp. 241–256). Lorimer Press.

Campbell, J. (2011b). Burns. In Campbell's *pathophysiology notes* (pp. 13224–13525). Lorimer Press.

Cancer.net. (2020). Skin cancer (non-melanoma). Statistics. Retrieved January 20, 2022, from https://www.cancer.net/cancer-types/skin-cancer-non-melanoma/statistics

Centers for Disease Control and Prevention. (2020). *Explosions and blast injuries: A primer for clinicians.* Retrieved January 20, 2022, from https://www.cdc.gov/masstrauma/preparedness/primer.pdf

Christenson, L. J., Borrowman, T. A., Vachon, C. M., et al. (2005). Incidence of basal cell and squamous cell carcinomas in a population younger than 40 years. *JAMA 294*(6), 681–690. doi:10.1001/jama.294.6.681

Christiaens, W., Van de Walle, E., Devresse, S., Van Halewyck, D., Benahmed, N., Paulus, D., & Van den Heede, K. (2015). The view of severely burned patients and healthcare professionals on the blind spots in the aftercare process: a qualitative study. *BMC Health Services Research 15,* 302–313. http://doi.org/10.1186/s12913-015-0973-2

Cleveland Clinic. (2020). *Burns, management and treatment.* Retrieved on January 20, 2022, from https://my.clevelandclinic.org/health/diseases/12063-burns-management-and-treatment

Colbert, B. J., Ankney, J., & Lee, K. (2020). The integumental system. In *Anatomy and physiology for health professions: An interactive journey* (4th ed.), pp. 152–170). Pearson.

Department of Homeland Security. (2020). *IED attack, improvised explosive devices.* Retrieved January 20, 2022, from https://www.dhs.gov/xlibrary/assets/prep_ied_fact_sheet.pdf

Driscoll, I. R., Mann-Salinas, E. A., Boyer, N. L., Pamplin, J. C., Serio-Melvin, M. L., Salinas, J., Borgman, M. A., Sheridan, R L., Melvin, J. J., Peterson, W. C., Graybill, J. C., Rizzo, J. A., King, B. T., Chung, K. K., Cancio, L. C., Renz, E. M., & Stockinger, Z. T. (2018). Burn casualty care in the deployed setting. *Military Medicine, 183*(9/10), 161–167. https://doi.org/10.1093/milmed/usy076

Fijan, S., Frauwallner, A., Langerholc, T., Krebs, B., ter Haar-Younes, J. A., Heschl, A., Turk, D. M., & Rogelj, I. (2019). Efficacy of using probiotics with antagonistic activity against pathogens of wound infections: An integrative review of literature. *Biomedical Research International, 2019*, 1–21. https://doi.org/10.1155/2019/7585486

Frantz, C., Stewart, K. M., & Weaver, V. M. (2010). The extracellular matrix at a glance. *Cell Science at a Glance, 123*(4), 4195–4200. https://doi.org/10.1242/jcs.023820

Griggs, C., Goverman, J. Bittner, E., & Levi, B. (2017). Sedation and pain management in burn patients. *Clinical Plastic Surgery, 44*(3), 535–540. https://doi.org/10.1016/j.cps.2017.02.026

Hla, T. K., Hegarty, M., Russell, P., Drake-Brockman, T. F., Ramgolam, A., & von Ungern-Sternberg, B. S. (2014). Perception of pediatric pain: A comparison of postoperative pain assessments between child, parent, nurse, and independent observer. *Pediatric Anesthesia, 24*, 1127–1131. https://doi.org/10.1111/pan.12484

Hughes, S. L., Giobbie-Hurder, A., Weaver, F. M., Kubal, J. D., & Henderson, W. (1999). Relationship between caregiver burden and health-related quality of life. *Gerontologist, 39*(5), 534–545. https://doi.org/10.1093/geront/39.5.534

Jeschke, G., Pinto, R., Kraft, R., Nathens, A. B., Finnerty, C. C., Gamelli, R. L., Gibran, N. S., Klein, M. B., Arnoldo, B. D., Tompkins, R. G., Herndon, D. N., & the Host Response to Injury Collaborative Research Program. (2015). Morbidity and survival probability in burn patients in modern burn care. *Critical Care Medicine, 43*(4), 808–815. https://doi.org/10.1097/CCM.0000000000000790

Kauvar, D., Cancio, L., Wolf, S., Wade, C., & Holcolm, J. (2006). Comparison of combat and noncombat burns from ongoing U.S. military operations. *Journal of Surgical Research, 132*(2), P195–P200. https://doi.org/10.1016/J.JSS.2006.02.043

Koh, T. J., & DiPietro, L. A. (2013). Inflammation and wound healing: The role of the macrophage. *Expert Review in Molecular Medicine, 13*, e23. https://doi.org?10,1017/S1462399411001943

Kolarsick, P., Kolarsick, M. A., & Goodwin, C. (2011). Anatomy and physiology of the skin. *Journal of the Dermatology Nurses' Association, 3*, 203–213.

Kolarsick, P. A. J., Kolarsick, M. A., & Goodwin, C. (n.d.). *Anatomy & physiology of the skin*, Ch. 1. Retrieved January 28, 2022, from https://www.ons.org/sites/default/files/publication_pdfs/1%20SS%20Skin%20Cancer_chapter%201.pdf

Kowal-Vern, A., & Criswell, B. K. (2005). Burn scar neoplasms: A literature review and statistical analysis. *Burns, 31*, 403–413. https://doi.org/10.1016/j.burns.2005.02.015

Maani, C. V., Hoffman, H G., Fowler, M., Maiers, A. J., Gaylord, K. M., & DeSocio, P. A. (2011). Combining ketamine and virtual reality pain control during severe burn wound care: one military and one civilian patient. *Pain Medicine, 12*, 673–678. https://doi.org/10.1111/j.1526-4637.2011.01091.x

Magnusson, S., Baldursson, B. T., Kjartansson, H., Rolfsson, O., & Sigurjonsson, G. F. (2017). Regenerative and antibacterial properties of acellular fish skin grafts and human amnion/chorion membrane: Implications for tissue preservation in combat casualty care. *Military Medicine, 182*(3/4), 383–388. https://doi.org/10.7205/MILMED-D-16-00142

Mayo Clinic. (2020a) *Bedsores (pressure ulcers)*. Retrieved January 28, 2022, from https://www.mayoclinic.org/diseases-conditions/bed-sores/symptoms-causes/syc-20355893

Mayo Clinic. (2020b). *Burns*. Retrieved January 20, 2022, from https://www.mayoclinic.org/diseases-conditions/burns/diagnosis-treatment/drc-20370545

McDaniel, B., Badri, T., & Steele, R. B. (January 2022). Basal cell carcinoma. In StatPearls [Internet]. Treasure Island: StatPearls Publishing. Retrieved from https://www.ncbi.nlm.nih.gov/books/NBK482439/

McGrath, J. A., & Lai-Cheong, J. E. (2021). Skin and its appendages. In S. Standring (Ed.), *Grey's anatomy: The anatomical basis of clinical practice* (42nd ed., pp. 145–165). Elsevier.

MedlinePlus. (2022). *Aging changes in skin*. MedlinePlus. Retrieved January 28, 2022, from https://medlineplus.gov/ency/article/004014.htm

Mock, C., Peck, M., Peden, M., & Krug, E. (Eds.). (2008). *A WHO plan for burn prevention and care*. World Health Organization.

National Center for Health Statistics (NCHS). (2021). *Ambulatory health care data— NAMCS and NHAMCS web tables*. Retrieved November 1, 2021, from https://www.cdc.gov/nchs/ahcd/web_tables.htm#2011

Patterson, D. R., Hoflund, H., Espey, K., Sharar, S., & Nursing Committee of the International Society for Burn Injuries (NCISBI). (2004). Pain management. *Burns, 30*, A10–A15. https://doi.org/10.1016/j.burns.2004.08.004

Schultz, R., Beach, S. R., Friedman, E. M., Martsolf, G. R., Rodakowski, J., & James, A. E., III. (2018). Changing structures and processes to support family caregivers of seriously ill patients. *Journal of Palliative Medicine, 21*(S2), S-36–S-42. http://doi.org/10.1089/jpm.2017.0437

Shah, A. J., Wadoo, O., & Latoo, J. (2010). Psychological distress in carers of people with mental disorders. *British Journal of Medical Practitioners, 3*(3), a327

Shpichka, A., Butnaru, D., Bezrukov, E. A., Sukhanov, R. B., Atala, A., Burdukovskii, V., Zhang, Y., & Timashev, P. (2019). Skin tissue regeneration for burn injury. *Stem Cell Research & Therapy, 10*, 94–110. https://doi.org/10.1186/s13287-019-1203-3

Singh, G., & Archana, G. (2008). Unraveling the mystery of vernix caseosa. *Indian Journal of Dermatology, 53*(2), 54–60. https://doi.org/10.4103/0019-5154.41645

Slominski, A. T., Zmijewski, M. A., Skobowiat, C., Zbytek, B., Slominski, R. M., & Steketee, J. D. (2012). Sensing the environment: Regulation of local and global homeostasis by the neuroendocrine system. *Advances in Anatomy, Embryology, & Cell Biology, 212*, v-115

Souto, E. B., Ribeiro, A. F., Ferreira, M. I., Teixeira, M. C., Shimojo, A. A. M., Soriano, J. L., Naveros, B., Durazzo, A., Lucarini, M., Souto, S. B., & Santini, A. (2020). New nanotechnologies for the treatment and repair of skin burns infections. *International Journal of Molecular Sciences, 21*, 393–411. https://doi.org/10.3390/ijms21020393

Strayer, S. M., & Reynolds, P. (2003). Diagnosing skin malignancy: Assessment of predictive clinical criteria and risk factors. *Journal of Family Practice, 52*(3), 210–218.

Wallace, A. B. (1951). The exposure treatment of burns. *Lancet, 257*(6653), 501–504. https://doi.org/10.1016/s0140-6736(51)91975-7

Wallace, H. A., Basehore, B. M., & Zito, P. M. (2020). *Wound healing process*. In StatPearls. StatPearls Publishing.

Walton, M. K. (2011). Communicating with family caregivers. *American Journal of Nursing, 111*(12), 47–53. https://doi.org/10.1097/01.NAJ.0000408186.67511.b9

Warby, R., & Maani, C. (2021). Burn classification. In StatPearls. StatPearls Publishing. Retrieved January 28, 2022, from https://www.statpearls.com/articlelibrary/viewarticle/18714/

World Health Organization. (2018). *Burns*. Retrieved January 20, 2022, from https://www.who.int/news-room/fact-sheets/detail/burns

Xiang, F., Song, H.-P., & Huang, Y.-S. (2019). Clinical features and treatment of 140 cases of Marjolin's ulcer at a major burn center in southwest China. *Experimental and Therapeutic Medicine, 17,* 3403–3410. https://doi.org/10.3892/etm.2019.7364

Yu, N., Long, X., Lujan-Hernandez, J. R., Hassan, K. Z., Bai, M., Wang, Y., Wang, X., & Zhao, R. (2013). Marjolin's ulcer: A preventable malignancy arising from scars. *World Journal of Surgical Oncology, 11,* 313–331. https://doi.org/10.1186/1477-7819-11-313

Zhang, J.-M., & An, J. (2007). Cytokines, inflammation, and pain. *International Anesthesiologists Clinics,* 45(2), 27–37. https://doi.org/10.1097/AIA.0b013e318 034194e

Chapter 9

Adams, M. A. (2021). Functional anatomy of the musculoskeletal system. In S. Standring (Ed.), *Grey's anatomy: The anatomical analysis of clinical practice* (42nd ed., pp. 85–126). Elsevier.

ALS Association. (2022). https://www.als.org/understanding-als

Anderson, B. W., Kortz, M. W., & Al Kharazi, K. A. (2021). Anatomy, Head, Neck, Skull. In StatPearls. StatPearls Publishing. Retrieved November 17, 2021, from https://www.ncbi.nlm.nih.gov/books/NBK499834/?report=printable

Association of Professors of Medicine (Washington, D.C.) Consensus Development Conference. (1991). Prophylaxis and treatment of osteoporosis. *American Journal of Medicine,* 90(1), 107–110. https://doi.org/10.1016/0002-9343(91)90512-v

Beukelman, D., Fager, S., & Nordness, A. (2011). Communication support for people with ALS. Neurology *Research International, 2011,* 714693. https://doi.org/10.1155/2011/714693

Bhandari, M., Dosanjh, S., Tornetta, P., & Matthews, D. (2006). Musculoskeletal manifestations of physical abuse after intimate partner violence. *Journal of Trauma: Injury, Infection, & Critical Care,* 61(6), 1473–1479. https://doi.org/10.1097/01.ta.0000196419.36019.5a

Blackhall, L. J. (2012). Amyotrophic lateral sclerosis and palliative care: Where we are, and the road ahead. *Muscle Nerve 45,* 311–318. https://doi.org/10.1002/mus.22305

Bongioanni, P. (2012). Communication impairment in ALS patients: Assessment and treatment. In M. Maurer (Ed.), *Amyotrophic lateral sclerosis.* IntechOpen. https://doi.org/10.5772/30426

Brauer, C. A., Coca-Perraillon, M., Cutler, D. M., & Rosen, A. B. (2009). Incidence and mortality of hip fractures in the United States. *Journal of the American Medical Association,* 302(14), 1573–1579. https://doi.org/10.1001/jama.2009.1462

Britton, S. (2018). *Understanding skeletal muscles: An introduction to origin, insertion and, action.* Retrieved April 18, 2021, from https://www.youtube.com/watch?v=OeCA2mn9mNc

Burge, R., Dawson-Hughes, B., Solomon, D. H., Wong, J. B., King, A., & Tosteson, A. (2007). Incidence and economic burden of osteoporosis-related fractures in the United States, 2005–2025. *Journal of Bone and Mineral Research,* 22(3), 465–475. https://doi.org/10.1359/JBMR.061113

Campagne, D. (2021). *Overview of sprains and other soft-tissue injuries.* Merck Manual Professional Version. Retrieved July 19, 2021, from https://www.merckmanuals.com/

professional/injuries-poisoning/sprains-and-other-soft-tissue-injuries/overview-of-sprains-and-other-soft-tissue-injuries

Campbell, J. (2011). *Campbell's physiology notes* (pp. 271–290). Lorimer Press.

Cancer.net. (n.d.). *Long-term side effects of cancer treatment.* Retrieved July 19, 2021, from https://www.cancer.net/survivorship/long-term-side-effects-cancer-treatment

Centers for Disease Control and Prevention. (2021a). *Global Polio Eradication Initiative.* Retrieved November 10, 2021, from https://www.cdc.gov/polio/gpei/index.htm

Centers for Disease Control and Prevention (2021b). *Our progress against polio.* Retrieved November 10, 2021, from https://www.cdc.gov/polio/progress/index.htm

Centers for Disease Control and Prevention. (2021c). *Osteoporosis or low bone mass in older adults: United States, 2017–2018.* Retrieved November 10, 2021, from https://www.cdc.gov/nchs/data/databriefs/db405-H.pdf

Center for Medicare & Medicaid Services (CMS). (2021). *Hospice.* Retrieved July 19, 2021, from https://www.cms.gov/Medicare/Medicare-Fee-for-Service-Payment/Hospice

Chen, L.-R., Ko, N.-Y., & Chen, K.-H. (2019). Medical treatment for osteoporosis. From molecular to clinical opinions. *International Journal of Molecular Science, 20,* 2213. https://doi.org/10.3390/ijms20092213

Clarke, B. (2008). Normal bone anatomy and physiology. *Clinical Journal of American Society of Nephrology, 3*(Suppl. 3), C131–S139. https://doi.org/10.2215/CJN.04151206

Clemente, C. D. (1985). Muscles and fasciae. In Gray's *anatomy* (30th ed., pp. 429–590). Lee & Febiger Publisher.

Colbert, B. J., Ankey, J., & Lee, K. T. (2020). The muscular system. In Anatomy and *physiology for health professionals*: An *interactive journey* (4th ed., pp. 129–151). Pearson Publishing.

Conger, K. (2018). *Study identifies stem cell that gives rise to new bone, cartilage in humans.* Stanford School of Medicine, News Center. Retrieved June 27, 2021, from https://med.stanford.edu/news/all-news/2018/09/study-identifies-stem-cell-that-gives-rise-to-new-bone-cartilage.html

Daly, R. M. (2017). Exercise and nutritional approaches to prevent frail bones, falls and fractures: An update. *Climacteric, 20*(2), 119–124.

Davis, H. D., Shook, M., & Varacallo, M. (2020). Anatomy, skeletal muscle. In *StatPearls.* StatPearls Publishing. https://www.ncbi.nlm.nih.gov/books/NBK537236/

Foster, L. A., & Salajegheh, M. K. (2019). Motor neuron disease: Pathophysiology, diagnosis, and management. *American Journal of Medicine, 132,* 32–37. https://www.doi.org/10.1016/j.amjmed.2018.07.012

Fox, M. (2018, March 15,). *Stephen Hawking had ALS for 55 years; how did he do it?* CBS News. Retrieved May 8, 2021, from https://www.nbcnews.com/health/health-care/stephen-hawking-had-als-55-years-how-did-he-do-n857006

Gourley, S. L., Espitia, J. W., Sanacora, G., & Taylor, J. R. (2012). Antidepressant-like properties of oral riluzole and utility of incentive disengagement models of depression in mice. *Psychopharmacology, 219*(3), 805–814. https://doi.org/10.1007/s00213-011-2403-4

Gosangi, B., Park, H., Thomas, R., Gujrathi, R., Bay, C. P., Raja, A. S., Seltzer, S. E., Balcom, M. C., McDonald, M. L., Orgill, D. P., Harris, M. B., Boland, G. W., Rexrode, K., & Khurana, B. (2021). Exacerbation of physical intimate partner violence during COVID-19 lockdown. *Radiology, 298*(1), E38–E45. https://doi.org/10.1148/radiol.2020202866

Han, S. D., & Mosqueda, L. (2020). Elder abuse in the Covid-19 era. *Journal of American Geriatrics Society*, 68(7), 1386–1387. https://doi.org/10.1111/jgs.16496

Haver, E. V. (2021). *Muscle injuries*. Physiopedia. Retrieved April 15, 2021, from https://www.physio-pedia.com/index.php?title=Muscle_Injuries&oldid=270510

Health Resources & Services Administration (HRSA). (2021a). *Donation and transplantation statistics*. Retrieved July 4, 2021, from https://bloodstemcell.hrsa.gov/data/donation-and-transplantation-statistics

Health Resources & Services Administration (HRSA). (2021b). *Number transplants, summary table by cell source, Table 13*. Retrieved July 4, 2021, from https://bloodstemcell.hrsa.gov/sites/default/files/bloodstemcell/data/transplant-activity/transplants-year-cell-source.xlsx

Hernlund, E., Svedbom, A., Ivergard, M., Comptson, J., Cooper, C., Stenmark, J., McCloskey, E. B., Jonsson, B., & Kanis, J. A. (2013). Osteoporosis in the European Union: Medical management, epidemiology, and economic burden. *Archives of Osteoporosis 9*, 136. https://doi.org/10.1007/s11657-013-0136-1

Hogle, J. M. (2002). Poliovirus cell entry: Common structural themes in viral cell entry pathways. *Annual Review of Microbiology*. 56, 677–702. Retrieved May 8, 2021, from https://www.ncbi.nlm.nih.gov/pmc/articles/PMC1500891/pdf/nihms-10773.pdf

Hwang, C.-S., Weng, H.-H., Wang, L.-F., Tsai, C.-H., & Chang, H.-T. (2014). An eye-tracking assistive device improves the quality of life for ALS patients and reduces the caregivers' burden, *Journal of Motor Behavior*, 46(4), 233–238. https://doi.org/10.1080/00222895.2014.891970

Kahn Academy. (2012). *The eleven major muscle groups*. Retrieved April 18, 2021, from https://www.youtube.com/watch?v=rKE63BBouP8&list=TLPQMTgwNDIwMjEwco33_UPSGA&index=2

Kanis, J. A., Melton, L. J., III, Christiansen, C., Johnston, C. C., & Khaltaev, N. (1994). The diagnosis of osteoporosis. *Journal of Bone and Mineral Research*, 9(8), 1137–1141.

Koromila, T., Georgoulias, P., Dailiana, Z., Ntzani, E. E., Samara, S., Chassanidis, C., Aleporou-Marinou, V., & Kollia, P. (2013). CER1 gene variations associated with bone mineral density, bone markers, and early menopause in postmenopausal women. *Human Genomics, 7*, 21. https://doi.org/10.1186/1479-7364-7-21

Lillo, P., Moshi, E., & Hodges, J. R. (2012). Caregiver burden in amyotrophic lateral sclerosis is not dependent on patients' behavioral changes than physical disability: A comparative study. *BMC Neurology*, 12, 156–162. https://doi.org/10.1186/1471-2377-12-156

Majmudar, S., Wu, J., & Paganoni, S. (2014). Rehabilitation in amyotrophic lateral sclerosis: Why it matters. *Muscle Nerve*, 50(1), 4–13. https://www.doi.org/10.1002/mus.24202

Makaroun, L. K., Bachrach, R. L., & Rosland, A.-M. (2020). Elder abuse in the time of Covid-19—Increased risks for older adults and their caregivers. *American Journal of Geriatric Psychiatry*, 28(8), 876–880. https://doi.org/10.1016/j.jagp.2020.05.017

McCombe, P. A., & Henderson, R. D. (2010). Effects of gender in amyotrophic lateral sclerosis. *Gender Medicine*, 7(6), 557–570. https://doi.org/10.1016/j.genm.2010.11.010

Motor Neurone Disease Association (MNDA). (2018). *What is MND?* Retrieved April 18, 2021, from https://www.youtube.com/watch?v=tq0MO2x31NA

Mugnier, B., Daumas, A., Couderc, A.-L., Mizzi, B., Gonzalez, T., Amrani, A., Leveque, P., Aymes, B., Argenson, J.-N., & Villani, P. (2019). Clinical effectiveness of osteoporosis treatment in older patients: A fracture liaison service-based prospective study. *Journal of Women & Aging, 31*(6), 553–565. https://doi.org/10.1080/08952841.2018.1529473

Myelodysplastic Syndromes Foundation (MDS). (2014). *What does my blood marrow do?* Retrieved June 27, 2021, from https://www.mds-foundation.org/wp-content/uploads/2019/05/Blood-Marrow-Booklet_English_Online_5.8.19.pdf

National Cancer Institute. (n.d.). SEER *training modules, introduction to the muscular system.* U.S. National Institutes of Health. Retrieved July 18, 2021, from Introduction to the Muscular System | SEER Training (cancer.gov).

National Center for Biotechnology Information. (2021). *PubChem compound summary for CID 5070, riluzole.* Retrieved April 25, 2021, from https://pubchem.ncbi.nlm.nih.gov/compound/Riluzole

National Health Service. (2016). *Guidance for commissioning AAC services and equipment.* Retrieved May 8, 2021, from https://www.england.nhs.uk/commissioning/wp-content/uploads/sites/12/2016/03/guid-comms-aac.pdf

National Institute on Neurological Disorders and Strokes (NINDS). (2021). *Motonneuron disease, fact sheet.* Treatment. National Institutes of Health. Retrieved April 28, 2021, from https://www.ninds.nih.gov/Disorders/All-Disorders/Amyotrophic-Lateral-Sclerosis-ALS-Information-Page

National Institute on Neurological Disorders and Strokes (NINDS). (2022). https://www.ninds.nih.gov/motor-neuron-diseases-fact-sheet

National Osteoporosis Guideline Group (NOGG). (2017). *Clinical guideline for the prevention and treatment of osteoporosis.* Retrieved June 26, 2021, from https://www.nogg.org.uk/ (sheffield.ac.uk).

Ong, T., Kantachuvesiri, P., Sahota, O., & Gladman, J. R. F. (2018). Characteristics and outcomes of hospitalized patients with vertebral fragility fractures: A systematic review. *Age & Ageing, 47*(1), 17–25. https://doi.org/10.1093/ageing/afx079

Oshinsky, D. M. (2005). *Breaking the back of polio. Yale School of Medicine Magazine.* Retrieved on April 11, 2020, from https://medicine.yale.edu/news/yale-medicine-magazine/breaking-the-back-of-polio/

Paganoni, S., Karam, C., Joyce, N., Bedlack, R., & Carter, G. T. (2015). Comprehensive rehabilitative care across the spectrum of amyotrophic lateral sclerosis. *NeuroRehabilitation, 37*(1), 53–68. https://www.doi.org/10.3233/NRE-151240

Pagnini, F., Rossi, G., Lunetta, C., Banfi, P., Castelnuovo, G., Corbo, M., & Molinari, E. (2010). Burden, depression, and anxiety in caregivers of people with amyotrophic lateral sclerosis. *Psychology, Health & Medicine, 15*(6), 685–693. https://doi.org/10.1080/13548506.2010.507773

Passweg, J. R., Baldomero, H., Bader, P., Bonini, C., Cesaro, S., Dreger, P., Duarte, R. F., Dufour, C., Kuball, J., Farge-Bandel, D., Gennery, A., Kroger, N., Lanza, F., Nagler, A., Surenda, A., & Mohty, M., for the European Society for Blood and Marrow Transplantation (EBMT). (2016). Hematopoietic stem cell transplantation in Europe 2014: More than 40,000 transplants annually. *Bone Marrow Transplantation, 51,* 786–792. https://doi.org/10.1038/bmt.2016.20

Paspaliaris, V., & Kolios, G. (2019). Stem cells in osteoporosis: From biology to new therapeutic approaches. *Stem Cells International, 2019,* 1730978. https://doi.org/10.1155/2019/1730978

Policy Advice. (2021). *Fitness industry statistics 2021.* Retrieved July 18, 2021, from https://policyadvice.net/insurance/insights/fitness-industry-statistics/

Roberts, A. L., Johnson, N. J., Chen, J. T., Cudkowicz, M. E., & Weisskopf, M. G. (2016). Race/ethnicity, socioeconomic status, and ALS mortality in the United States. *American Academy of Neurology*, *8*(22), 2300–2308. https://www.doi.org/10.1212/WNL.0000000000003298

Saladi-Schulman, J. (2018). *What is bone marrow and what does it do?* Retrieved June 27, 2021, from https://www.healthline.com/health/function-of-bone-marrow

Santos, A. J., Nunes, B., Kislaya, I., Gil, A. B., & Ribeiro, O. (2019). Elder abuse victimization patterns: Latent class analysis using perpetrators and abusive behaviours. *BMC Geriatrics*, *19*, 117. https://doi.org/10.1186/s12877-019-1111-5

Sarafrazi, N., Embogo, E. A., & Shepherd, J. A. (2021, March). Osteoporosis or low bone mass in older adults: United States, 2017–2018. NCHS Data Brief No. 405. https://www.cdc.gov/nchs/data/databriefs/db405-H.pdf

Scala, R., & Pisani, L. (2018). Noninvasive ventilation in acute respiratory failure: Which recipe for success? *European Respiratory Review*, *27*, 180029, https://www.doi.org/10.1183/16000617.0029-2018

Sharma, D., Larriera, AI., Palacio-Mancheno, P. E., Gatti, V., Fritton, J. C., Bromage, T. G., Cardoso, L., Doty, S. B., & Fritton, S. P. (2018). The effects of estrogen deficiency on cortical bone microporosity and mineralization. *Bone*, *110*, 1–10. https://doi.org/10.1016/j.bone.2018.01.019

Svedbom, A., Hernlund, E., Ivergard, M., Compston, J., Cooper, C., Stenmark, J., McCloskey, E. V., Jonsson, B., Kanis, J. A., & the EU review panel of the IOF. (2013). Osteoporosis in the European Union: A compendium of country-specific reports. *Archives of Osteroporosis*, *8*, 137.

Tajeu, G. S., Delzell, E., Smith, W., Arora, T., Curtis, J. R., Saag, K. G., Morrisey, M. A., Yun, H., & Kilgore, M. L. (2014). Death, debility, and destitution following hip fracture. *Journal of Gerontology Series A: Biological Sciences and Medical Sciences*, *69*(3), 346–353. https://doi.org/10.1093/gerona/glt105

Turner, M. R., Parton, M. J., Shaw, C. E., Leigh, P. N., & Al-Chalabi, A. (2003). Prolonged survival in motor neuron disease: A descriptive study of the King's database 1990–2002. *Journal of Neurology, Neurosurgery, and Psychiatry*, *74*, 995–997. https://www.doi.org/10.1136/jnnp.74.7.995

Westbrook, K. E., Nessel, T. A., & Varacallo, M. (2020). Anatomy, head and neck, facial muscles. In StatPearls. StatPearls Publishing. Retrieved December 30, 2020, from https://www.ncbi.nlm.nih.gov/books/NBK493209/?report=printable

Wick, J. Y. (2009). Spontaneous fracture: Multiple causes. *Consultant Pharmacist*, *24*(7), 100–112. https://doi.org//10.4140/tcp.n.2009.100

Wolf, G. (2008). Energy regulation by the skeleton. *Nutrition Reviews*, *66*(4), 229–233. https://doi.org/10.1111/j.1753-4887.2008.00027.x

World Health Organization (WHO). (2007). *WHO Scientific Group on the Assessment of Osteoporosis at Primary Health Care Level*. Retrieved June 26, 2021, from https://www.who.int/chp/topics/Osteoporosis.pdf

World Health Organization (WHO). (2020). *Polio: Global Eradication Initiative*. Retrieved April 30, 2022, from https://apps.who.int/iris/bitstream/handle/10665/344329/9789240030763-eng.pdf?sequence=1

World Health Organization (WHO). (2021a). *Violence against women. Fact sheet*. Retrieved June 26, 2021, from https://www.who.int/news-room/fact-sheets/detail/violence-against-women

World Health Organization (WHO). (2021b). *Violence against women*. Health *impact*. Retrieved June 26, 2021, from https://www.who.int/reproductivehealth/publications/violence/VAW_health_impact.jpeg?ua=1

World Health Organization (WHO). (2021c). *Violence against women. Key facts*. Retrieved June 26, 2021, from https://www.who.int/news-room/fact-sheets/detail/violence-against-women

Wu, L., & Lewis, M. W. (2015). Disabilities among veterans and civilians and their utilization of healthcare. *Health and Social Care in the Community, 3*(1), 296–314. https://www.doi.org/10.1080/21642850.2015.1089176

Yang, C., Ren, J., Li, B., Jin, C., Ma, C., Cheng, C., Sun, Y., & Shi, X. (2019). Identification of gene biomarkers in patients with postmenopausal osteoporosis. *Molecular Medicine Reports, 19*, 1065–1073l https://doi.org/10.3892/mmr.2018.9752

Zhao, R., Xu, Z., & Zhao, M. (2015). Antiresorptive agents increase the effects of exercise on preventing postmenopausal bone loss in women: A meta-analysis. *PLoS One, 10*(1), e0116729. https://doi.org/10.1371/journal.pone.0116729

Chapter 10

Aby, J. (2020). Neuro/*reflexes*. Stanford University, Lucille Packard Children's Hospital/Stanford Medicine. Retrieved November 8, 2021, from https://med.stanford.edu/newborns/professional-education/photo-gallery/neuro-reflexes.html#sucking_reflex

American Cancer Society (ACS). (2020). *What is colorectal cancer?* Retrieved November 7, 2021, from https://www.cancer.org/content/dam/CRC/PDF/Public/8604.00.pdf

American Diabetes Association. (2013). Diagnosis and classification of diabetes mellitus. *Diabetes Care, 36*(Suppl. 1), S67–S74.

American Society for Metabolic & Bariatric Surgery (ASMBS). (2020). *Bariatric surgery procedures*. Retrieved November 7, 2021, from https://asmbs.org/patients/bariatric-surgery-procedures#bypass

Ballou, S., & Keefer, L. (2017). Psychological interventions for irritable bowel syndrome and inflammatory bowel diseases. *Clinical and Translational Gastroenterology, 8*, e214. https://doi.org/10.1038/ctg.2016.69

Berkovitz, B. K. B. (2021). Mouth. In S. Standring (Ed.), *Gray's anatomy: The anatomical basis of clinical practice* (42nd ed., pp. 636–663). Elsevier.

Bird, Y., Lemstra, M., Rogers, M., & Moraros, J. (2015). The relationship between socioeconomic status/income and prevalence of diabetes and associated conditions: A cross-sectional population-based study in Saskatchewan, Canada. *International Journal of Equity in Health, 14*, 93. http://doi.org/10.1186/s12939-015-0237-0

Campbell, J. (2011). Digestive system. In Campbell's *physiology notes* (pp. 167–196). Lorimer Publications.

Cancer Research, UK. (2020). *Coping with cancer*. Retrieved November 7, 2021, https://www.cancerresearchuk.org/about-cancer/coping/physically/diet-problems/managing/drip-or-tube-feeding/types

Centers for Disease Control and Prevention (CDC). (2013). *NCD burden of disease*. Retrieved January 21, 2022, from https://www.cdc.gov/globalhealth/healthprotection/fetp/training_modules/2/NCD-Burden-of-Disease_FG_Final_09252013.pdf

Centers for Disease Control and Prevention (CDC). (2019). *Childhood obesity facts*. Retrieved January 21, 2022, from https://www.cdc.gov/obesity/data/childhood.html

Centers for Disease Control and Prevention (CDC). (2020a). *Adult obesity, causes and consequences.* Retrieved on November 7, 2021, from https://www.cdc.gov/obesity/adult/causes.html

Centers for Disease Control and Prevention (CDC). (2020b). *Adult obesity facts.* Retrieved January 21, 2022, from https://www.cdc.gov/obesity/data/adult.html

Center for Disease Control and Prevention (CDC). (2020c). *Facts about cleft lip and cleft palate.* Retrieved November 7, 2021, https://www.cdc.gov/ncbddd/birthdefects/cleft lip.html

Centers for Disease Control and Prevention (CDC). (2020d). *Health and economic costs of chronic diseases.* Retrieved January 21, 2022, from https://www.cdc.gov/chronicdise ase/about/costs/index.htm

Centers for Disease Control and Prevention (CDC). (2022). *Consequences of obesity.* Retrieved from https://www.cdc.gov/obesity/basics/consequences.html

Cleft Lip & Palate Association (CALPA) (UK). (2020). *Feeding.* Retrieved November 7, 2021, https://www.clapa.com/treatment/feeding/

Clemente, C. D. (1985). The digestive system. In Gray's *anatomy* (30th ed., pp. 1402–1514). Lea & Fibiger.

Cobb, L. K., Appel, L. J., Franco, M., Jones-Smith, J. C., Nur, A., & Anderson, C. A. M. (2015). The relationship of the local food environment with obesity: A systematic review of methods, study quality, and results. *Obesity, 23*(7), 1331–1344. http://doi.org/10.1002/oby.21118

Colbert, B. J., Ankney, J., & Lee, K. T. (2020). The gastrointestinal system. In Anatomy & *physiology for health professions*: An *interactive journey* (4th ed., pp. 346–372). Pearson.

Collins, P. (2021). Development of the peritoneal cavity, gastrointestinal tract and its adnexae. In S. Standring (Ed.), *Gray's anatomy: The anatomical basis of clinical practice* (42nd ed., pp. 323–340). Elsevier.

Conrad, C. (2021). Pancreas. In S. Standring (Ed.), *Gray's anatomy: The anatomical basis of clinical practice* (42nd ed., pp. 1223–1231). Elsevier.

Corsetti, M., Tack, J., Attara, G., & Sewel, M. (2018). *IBS Global Impact Report 2018.* Retrieved November 7, 2021, file:///C:/Users/maril/Documents/IBS-Global-Impact-Report%20(1).pdf

Corwin, R. L. (2011). The face of uncertainty eats. *Current Drug Abuse Review, 4*(3), 174–181. https://doi.org/10.2174/1874473711104030174

Corwin, R. L., & Wojnicki, F. H. (2009). Baclofen, raclopride, and naltrexone differentially affect intake of fat and sucrose under limited access conditions. *Behavioural Pharmacology, 20*(5-6), 537–548. https://doi.org/10.1097/FBP.0b013e3283313168

Costacou, T., & Mayer-Davis, E. J. (2003). Nutrition and prevention of type 2 diabetes. *Annual Review of Nutrition, 23*, 147–170. http://doi.org/10.1146/annurev.nutr.23.011 702.073027

Danese, A., & Tan, M. (2014). Childhood maltreatment and obesity: systematic review and meta-analysis. *Molecular Psychiatry, 19*, 544–554. https://doi.org/10.1038/mp.2013.54

Faresjo, A., Walter, S., Norlin, A.-K., Faresjo, T., & Jones, M. P. (2016). Gastrointestinal symptoms—An illness burden that affects daily work in patients with IBS. *Health and Quality of Life Outcomes, 17*, 113. https://doi.org/10.1186/s12955-019-1174-1

Farooqi, S., & O'Rahilly, S. (2006). Genetics of obesity in humans. *Endocrine Reviews, 27*(7), 710–718. https://doi.org/10.1210/er.2006-0040

Fuhrman, J. (2018). The hidden dangers of fast and processed food. *American Journal of Lifestyle Medicine*, *12*(5), 375–381. https://doi.org/10.1177/1559827618766483

Galvez, M. P., Pearl, M., & Yen, I. H. (2010). Childhood obesity and the built environment: A review of the literature from 2008–2009. *Current Opinions in Pediatrics*, *22*(2), 202–207. https://doi.org/10.1097/MOP.0b013e328336eb6f

Garland, E. L., Gaylord, S. A., Palsson, O., Faurot, K., Mann, J. D., Whitehead, W. E. (2012). Therapeutic mechanisms of a mindfulness-based treatment for IBS: Effects on visceral sensitivity, catastrophizing, and affective processing of pain sensations. *Journal of Behavioral Medicine*, *35*(6), 591–602. https://doi.org/10.1007/s10865-011-9391-z

Gaylord, S. A., Palsson, O. S., Garland, E. L., Faurot, K. R., Coble, R. S., Mann, J. D., Frey, W., Leniek, K., & Whitehead, W. E. (2011). Mindfulness training reduces the severity of irritable bowel syndrome in women: Results of a randomized controlled trial. *American Journal of Gastroenterology*, *106*(9), 1678–1688. http://doi.org/10.1038/ajg.2011.184

Going, J. J., Ballantyne, S., MacDonald, A., & Forshaw, M. J. (2021). Abdominal oesophagus and stomach. In S. Standring (Ed.), *Gray's anatomy: The anatomical basis of clinical practice* (42nd ed., pp. 1160–1172). Elsevier.

Hanyuda, A., Cao, Y., Hamada, T., Nowak, J. A., Qian, Z. R., Masugi, Y., da Silva, A., Liu, L., Kosumi, K., Soong, T. R., Jhun, I., Wu, K., Zhang, X., Song, M., Meyerhardt, J. A., Chan, A. T., Fuchs, C. S., Giovannucci, E. L., Ogino, S., & Nishihara, R. (2017). Body mass index and risk of colorectal carcinoma subtypes classified by tumor differentiation status. *European Journal of Epidemiology*, *32*, 393–407. https://doi.org/10.1007/s10654-017-0254-y

Hopkins, C. (2021). Nose, nasal cavity and paranasal sinuses. In S. Standring (Ed.), *Gray's anatomy: The anatomical basis of clinical practice* (42nd ed., pp. 686–701). Elsevier.

Johns Hopkins Medicine. (2020). *Gallbladder disease.* Retrieved November 7, 2021, https://www.hopkinsmedicine.org/health/conditions-and-diseases/gallbladder-disease

Maleckas, A., Gudaityte, R., Petereit, R., Venclauskas, L., & Velickiene, D. (2016). Weight regain after gastric bypass: Etiology and treatment options. *Gland Surgery*, *5*(6), 617–624. http://doi.org/10.21037/gs.2016.12.02

Mayo Clinic. (2020). *Irritable bowel syndrome.* Retrieved November 7, 2021, https://www.mayoclinic.org/diseases-conditions/irritable-bowel-syndrome/symptoms-causes/syc-20360016

Mishra, M. (2017). Mindfulness and well-being. *Indian Journal of Health and Wellbeing*, *8*(10), 1121–1123. http://www.iahrw.com/index.php/home/journal_detail/19#list

Narayanaswami, V., & Dwoskin, L. P. (2017). Obesity: Current and potential pharmacotherapeutics and targets. *Pharmacology & Therapeutics*, *170*, 116–147. https://doi.org/10.1016/j.pharmthera.2016.10.015

National Institute of Dental and Craniofacial Research (NIDCR). (n.d.). *Saliva and salivary gland disorders.* Retrieved November 10, 2021, from https://www.nidcr.nih.gov/health-info/saliva-salivary-gland-disorders

National Institute of Diabetes and Digestive & Kidney Disorders (NIDDKD). (2017). *Your digestive system and how it works.* Retrieved November 10, 2021, from https://www.niddk.nih.gov/health-information/digestive-diseases/digestive-system-how-it-works

Shonin, E., & Kabat-Zinn, J. (2016). This is not McMindfulness by any stretch of the imagination. *Psychologist*, *29*(2), 124–125. Retrieved November 7, 2021, https://thepsychologist.bps.org.uk/not-mcmindfulness-any-stretch-imagination

Stunkard A. J., Harris J. R., Pedersen N. L., & McClearn, G. E. (1990). The body-mass index of twins who have been reared apart. *New England Journal of Medicine, 322,* 1483–1487. https://doi.org/10.1056/NEJM199005243222102

T. H. Chan School of Public Health. (2020). *Obesity prevention source.* Retrieved November 7, 2021, https://www.hsph.harvard.edu/obesity-prevention-source/obesity-trends/obesity-rates-worldwide/

Trowbridge, K., Lawson, L. M., Andrews, S. M., Pecora, J., & Boyd, S. (2017). Preliminary investigation of workplace-provided compressed mindfulness-based stress reduction with pediatric medical social workers. *Health and Social Work, 42*(4), 207–214. https://doi.org/10.1093/hsw/hlx038

U.S. Cancer Statistics Working Group. (2020). *U.S. cancer statistics data visualizations tool, based on 2019 submission data (1999–2017).* U.S. Department of Health and Human Services, Centers for Disease Control and Prevention and National Cancer Institute. Retrieved November 7, 2021, from https://gis.cdc.gov/Cancer/USCS/DataViz.html

Volkov, N. D., Wang, G.- J., Tomasi, D., & Baler, R. D. (2013). Obesity and addiction: Neurological overlaps. *Obesity Reviews, 14,* 2–18. https://doi.org/10.1111/j.1467-789x.2012.01031.x

Chapter 11

Aatsha, P. A., & Kewal, K. (2021). Embryology, sexual development. In StatPearls. StatPearls Publishing. Retrieved December 23, 2021, from https://www.ncbi.nlm.nih.gov/books/NBK557601/

Allison, S. J., & Gibson, W. (2018). Mirabegron, alone and in combination, in the treatment of overactive bladder: Real-world evidence and experience. *Therapeutic Advances in Urology, 10*(12), 411–419. https://doi.org/10.1177/1756287218801282

American Psychological Association (APA). (2015). Guidelines for psychological practice with transgender and gender non-conforming people. *American Psychologist, 70*(9), 832–864. http://dx.doi.org/10.1037/a0039906

Amerman, E. C. (2019). The urinary system. In Human *anatomy and physiology* (2nd ed., pp. 941–984). Pearson Publishing. Retrieved December 5, 2021, from https://www.pearson.com/content/dam/one-dot-com/one-dot-com/us/en/higher-ed/en/products-services/course-products/amerman-1e-info/pdf/amerman-sample-chapter24.pdf

Aoki, Y., Brown, H. W., Brubaker, L., Cornu, J. N., Daly, J. O., & Cartwright, R. (2017). Urinary incontinence in women. *Nature Reviews Disease Primers, 3,* 17042. https://www.doi.org/10.1038/nrdp.2017.42

Bagga, H. S., Fisher, P. B., Tasian, G. E., Blaschko, S. D., McCulloch, C. E., McAninch, J. W., & Breyer, B. N. (2015). Sports-related genitourinary injuries presenting to United States emergency departments. *Urology, 85*(1), 239–244. https://doi.org/10.1016/j.urology.2014.07.075

Bowling, J., Vercruysse, C., Bello-Ogunu, F., Krinner, L. M., Greene, T., Webster, C., & Dahl, A. A. (2020). "It's the nature of the beast": Community resilience among gender diverse individuals. *Journal of Community Psychology, 48,* 2191–2207. https://doi.org/10.1002/jcop.22371

Bulletti, C., Coccia, M. E., Battistoni, S., & Borini, A. (2010). Endometriosis and infertility. *Journal of Assisted Reproduction & Genetics, 27,* 441–447. https://doi.org/10.1007/s10815-010-9436-1

Caldwell, P. H. Y., Sureshkumar, P., & Wong, W. D. F. (2016). Tricyclic and related drugs for nocturnal enuresis in children. *Cochrane Database of Systematic Reviews, 1,* CD002117. https://doi.org/10.1002/14651858.CD002117.pub2

Campbell, A. (2021). Preimplantation development. In S. Standring (Ed.), *Grey's anatomy: The anatomical basis of clinical practice* (42nd ed., pp. 170–177). Elsevier.

Campbell, J. (2011a). The renal and urinary systems. In Campbell's *physiology notes* (pp. 211–239). Lorimer Press.

Campbell, J. (2011b). Renal disorders. In Campbell's *pathophysiology notes* (Chap. 23). Lorimer Press.

Campbell, J. (2014). *Renal system I, urinary system and kidneys.* Retrieved November 19, 2021, from https://www.youtube.com/watch?v=YqDykFdZJts

Centers for Disease Control and Prevention (CDC). (2016). U.S. selected practice recommendations for contraceptive use. *Morbidity & Mortality Weekly Report, 65*(RR-4), 1–66.

Centers for Disease Control and Prevention (CDC). (2018). *Sexually transmitted disease surveillance, 2017.* Division of STD Prevention. Retrieved April 30, 2022, from https://www.cdc.gov/std/stats17/2017-STD-Surveillance-Report_CDC-clearance-9.10.18.pdf

Centers for Disease Control and Prevention (CDC). (2019a). *Infertility.* Retrieved April 30, 2022, from https://www.cdc.gov/nchs/fastats/infertility.htm

Centers for Disease Control and Prevention (CDC). (2019b). *Parasites: Pubic lice.* Retrieved January 7, 2022, from https://www.cdc.gov/parasites/lice/pubic/index.html

Centers for Disease Control and Prevention (CDC). (2020a). *Chronic kidney disease surveillance system—Prevalence of CKD stages 1–4 by year.* Retrieved April 30, 2022, from https://nccd.cdc.gov/ckd/detail.aspx?Qnum=Q372

Centers for Disease Control and Prevention (CDC). (2020b). *Chronic kidney disease surveillance system—Prevalence of treated end-stage renal disease (ESRD) per million U.S. residents.* Retrieved April 30, 2022, from https://nccd.cdc.gov/ckd/detail.aspx?Qnum=Q67

Centers for Disease Control and Prevention (CDC). (2020c). *Current contraceptive status among women aged 15–49: United States, 2017–2019.* Retrieved April 30, 2022, from https://www.cdc.gov/nchs/products/databriefs/db388.htm

Centers for Disease Control and Prevention (CDC). (2021a). *Chronic kidney disease basics.* Retrieved April 30, 2022, from https://www.cdc.gov/kidneydisease/basics.html

Centers for Disease Control and Prevention (CDC). (2021b). *Chronic kidney disease in the United States, 2021.* Retrieved April 30, 2022, from https://www.cdc.gov/kidneydisease/publications-resources/ckd-national-facts.html

Centers for Disease Control and Prevention (CDC). (2021c). Trichomoniasis: CDC *fact sheet.* Retrieved January 7, 2022, from https://www.cdc.gov/std/trichomonas/stdfact-trichomoniasis.htm

Children's Minnesota. (2015). *Chlamydia in newborns.* Retrieved January 7, 2022, from https://www.childrensmn.org/educationmaterials/childrensmn/article/15339/chlamydia-in-newborns

Cleveland Clinic. (2020). *Fetal development: Stages of growth.* Retrieved January 14, 2022, from https://my.clevelandclinic.org/health/articles/7247-fetal-development-stages-of-growth

Colbert, B. J., Ankney, J., & Lee, K. T. (2020). The reproductive system. In *Anatomy & physiology for health professions: An interactive journey* (4th ed., pp. 394–423). Pearson.

Collins, P. (2021). The urogenital system. In S. Standring (Ed.), *Grey's anatomy: The anatomical basis of clinical practice* (42nd ed., pp. 341–364). Elsevier.

Collins, P., Hall, M. A., & Brown, K. (2021). Pre- and postnatal growth and the neonate. In S. Standring (Ed.), *Grey's anatomy: The anatomical basis of clinical practice* (42nd ed., pp. 365–381). Elsevier.

Colvin, E. G. H., Tobon, J. I., Jeffs, L., & Veltmen, A. (2019). Transgender clients at a youth mental health care clinic: Transcending barriers to access. *Canadian Journal of Human Sexuality, 28*(3), 272–276. https://doi.org/10.3138/cjhs.2019-0004

Curran, M. A. (2019). *Fetal development.* Retrieved January 14, 2022, from https://perinatology.com/Reference/Fetal%20development.htm

Das, B. B., Ronda, J., & Trent, M. (2016). Pelvic inflammatory disease: Improving awareness, prevention, and treatment. *Infection & Drug Resistance, 9*, 191–197. https://doi.org/10.2147/IDR.S91260

Davis, C. P. (2021). *Medical definition of glomerulus.* MediciNet. Retrieved November 21, 2021, from https://www.medicinenet.com/glomerulus/definition.htm

De Meersman, R. E., & Wilkerson, J. E. (1982). Judo nephropathy: Trauma versus nontrauma. *Journal of Trauma, 22*(2), 150–152.

Erlich, T., & Kitrey, N. D. (2018). Renal trauma: The current best practice. *Therapeutic Advances in Urology, 10*(10), 295–303. https://doi.org/10.1177/1756287218785828

Eunice Kennedy Shriver National Institute of Child Health and Human Development. (2018). *Uterine fibroids.* Retrieved January 4, 2022, from https://www.nichd.nih.gov/health/topics/uterine

Evans, M. (2021). *Failing kidneys and different treatment options* [Video]. Retrieved December 8, 2021, from Failing Kidneys and Different Treatment Options - YouTube.

Flores, A. R. (2019). *Social acceptance of LGBT people in 174 countries, 1981–2017.* Williams Institute. Retrieved January 10, 2022, from Global-Acceptance-Index-LGBT-Oct-2019.pdf (ucla.edu).

Friedman, B.-C., Friedman, B., & Goldman, R. D. (2011). Oxybutynin for treatment of nocturnal enuresis in children. *Canadian Family Physician, 57*(May), 559–561.

Furton, E. J. (2017). A critique of "gender dysphoria" in *DSM-5. Ethics and Medics, 421*(7), 1–4.

Gomella, L. G., & Chung, P. H. (2021). Bladder, prostate and urethra. In S. Standring (Ed.), *Grey's anatomy: The anatomical basis of clinical practice* (42nd ed., pp. 1276–1291). Elsevier.

Gormley, E. A., Lightner, D. J., Burgio, K. L., Chai, T. C., Clemens, J. Q., Culkin, D. J., Das, A. K., Forster, H. E., Jr., Scarpero, H. M., Tessier, C. D., & Vasavada, S. P. (2012). Diagnosis and treatment of overactive bladder (non-neurogenic) in adults: AUA/SUFU guideline. *Journal of Urology, 188*, 2455–2463. https://dx.doi.org/10.1016/j.juro.2012.09.079

Greenstein, M., Turley, R. K., & Turley, R., Jr. (2020). *Anatomy and function of the urinary system.* Brigham & Women's Hospital. Retrieved December 5, 2021, from https://healthlibrary.brighamandwomens.org/conditions/heart/newsrecent/85,P01468

Grondahl, M. L., Christiansen, S. L., Kesmodel, U.S., Agerholm, I. E., Lemmen, J. G., Lundstrom, P., Bogstad, J., Raaschou-Jensen, M., & Ladelund, S. (2017). Effect of women's age on embryo morphology, cleavage rate and competence—A multicenter cohort study. *PLoS One, 12*(4), 30172456. https://doi.org/10.1371/journal.pone.0172456

Heinze, S. (2019a). *Female reproductive system.* Science with Susanna. Retrieved January 2, 2022, from Female Reproductive System - YouTube.

Heinze, S. (2019b). *Male reproductive system*. Science with Susanna. Retrieved January 2, 2022, from Male Reproductive System - YouTube.

Hisrich, H. (2021). *Nephron, part 1: Glomerulus filtration and urine production*. Retrieved November 21, 2021, from https://video.search.yahoo.com/yhs/search;_ylt=AwrC5 pZmc5phYBEAGss0nIlQ;_ylu=c2VjA3NlYXJjaAR2dGlkAw--;_ylc=X1MDMTM1 MTE5NTcwMARfcgMyBGFjdG4DY2xrBGNzcmNwdmlkA2hDLlFuakV3TGpHej BrY3lYOXBwdEFPNU1qWXdNQUFBQUFEN1lQclAEZnIDeWhzLWluZm9zcGFj ZS0wMDQEZnIyA3NhLWdwBGdwcmlkA0dWbEp0NU1PU25PV1hxZFFE5MGxM WkEEb19yc2x0A3ZYwBG5fc3VnZwMxMARvcmlnaW4W4DdmlkZW8uc2VhcmNoLnlh aG9vLmNvbQRwb3M3MDMMARwcXN0cgMgMEcHFzdHJsAwRxc3RybAMxMARxdWVyeQNnbG9tZXJ1bHVzBHRfc3RtcAMxNjMzNTEyMTA0?p=glomerulus&ei=UTF-8&fr2=p%3As%2Cv%3Av%2Cm%3Asa&fr=yhs-infospace-004&hsimp= yhs-004&hspart=infospace&type=ud-c-us--s-p-eowd3oqj--exp-none--subid- none#action=view&id=3&vid=b0fddc3f3c24d98e41ddfc730f46d62b

Horowitz, C. R., & Jackson, J. C. (1997). Female "circumcision": African women confront American medicine. *Journal of General Internal Medicine, 12*, 491–499. https://doi.org/ 10.1046/j.1525-1497.1997.00088.x

Horrocks, S., Somerset, M., Stoddart, H., & Peters, T. J. (2004). What prevents older people from seeking treatment for urinary incontinence? A qualitative exploration of barriers to the use of community continence services. *Family Practice, 21*(6), 689–696. https://doi.org/10.1093/fampra/cmh622

Hubert, J. (2019). *Anatomy & physiology of the urinary tract*. Academy of Neurologic Physical Therapy. Retrieved December 7, 2021, from https://www.neuropt.org/docs/ default-source/sci-sig/fact-sheets/sci-sig-fact-sheet-urinary-tract-anatomy-physiol ogy.pdf?sfvrsn=6da25343_2&sfvrsn=6da25343_2

Hull, M. G., Glazener, C. M., Kelly, N. J., Conway, D. I., Foster, P. A., Hinton, R. A., Coulson, C., Lambert, P. A., Watt, E. M., & Desai, K. M. (1985). Population study of causes, treatment, and outcome of infertility. *British Medical Journal (Clinical Research ed.), 291*(6510), 1693–1697. https://doi.org/10.1136/bmj.291.6510.1693

Itagaki, M. W., & Knight, N. B. (2004). Kidney trauma in martial arts: A case report of kidney contusion in jujitsu. *American Journal of Sports Medicine, 32*(2), 522–524. https://doi.org/10.1177/0363546503258879

Iwanaga, J. (2021). Kidney & ureter. In S. Standring (Ed.), *Grey's anatomy: The anatomical basis of clinical practice* (42nd ed., pp. 1259–1275). Elsevier.

Jauniaux, E., & Burton, G. J. (2021). Implantation and placentation. In S. Standring (Ed.), *Grey's anatomy: The anatomical basis of clinical practice* (42 ed., pp. 178–187). Elsevier.

Khan, S. R., Pearle, M. S., Robertson, W. G., Gambaro, G., Canales, B. K. Doizi, S., Traxer, O., & Tiselius, H.-G. (2017). Kidney stones. *Nature Reviews Disease Primers, 2*, 16008. https://www.doi.org/10.1038/nrdp.2016.8

Kirli, E. A., Turk, S., & Kirli, S. (2021). The burden of urinary incontinence on caregivers and evaluation of its impact on their emotional status. *Alpha Psychiatry, 22*(1), 43–48. https://doi.org/10.5455/apd.119660

Lai, W.-H., Rau, C.-S., Wu, S.-C., Chen, Y.-C., Kuo, P.-J., Hsu, S.-Y., Hsieh, C.-H., & Hsieh, H.-Y. (2016). Post-traumatic acute kidney injury: A cross-sectional study of trauma patients. *Scandinavian Journal of Trauma, Resuscitation and Emergency Medicine, 24*, 136. https://doi.org/10.1186/s13049-016-0330-4

Leung, F. W., & Schnelle, J. F. (2008). Urinary and fecal incontinence in nursing home residents. *Gastroenterology Clinics of North America, 37*(3), 697–707. https://doi.org/10.1016/j.gtc.2008.06.005

Lewis, M. W. (2008). The interactional model of maternal-fetal attachment: An empirical analysis. *Journal of Prenatal & Perinatal Psychology & Health, 23*(1), 49–65.

Litwin, M. S., & Saigal, C. S. (Eds.). (2012). Urinary tract stones. In Urologic *diseases in America* (pp. 313–345). U.S. Department of Health & Human Services. Retrieved November 20, 2021, from file:///C:/Users/maril/Downloads/Trackstar-Urologic%20Diseases%20Chap%2009.pdf).

Maternik, M., Krzeminska, K., & Zurowska, A. (2015). The management of childhood urinary incontinence. *Pediatric Nephrology, 30,* 41–50. https://doi.org/10.1007/s00467-014-2791-x

Mayo Clinic. (2021). *Male circumcision.* Retrieved January 12, 2022, from https://www.mayoclinic.org/tests-procedures/circumcision/about/pac-20393550?p=1

McDowell, D. T., Noone, D., Tareen, F., Waldron, M., & Quinn, F. (2012). Urinary incontinence in children: Botulinum toxin is a safe and effective treatment option. *Pediatric Surgery International, 28,* 315–320. https://doi.org/10.1007/s00383-011-3039-5

MedlinePlus. (2021). Urinary incontinence. Retrieved November 20, 2021, from https://medlineplus.gov/urinaryincontinence.html#

Mendonca, S., Bhardwaj, S., Sreenivasan, S., & Gupta, D. (2021). Is twice-weekly maintenance hemodialysis justified? *Indian Journal of Nephrology, 31,* 27–32. https://doi.org/10.4103/ijn.ijn_338_19

Murray, I., & Paolini, M. A. (2021). Histology, kidney, and glomerulus. In StatPearls. StatPearls Publishing. Retrieved November 21, 2021, from Histology, Kidney and Glomerulus - StatPearls - NCBI Bookshelf (nih.gov).

Narayan, R. (n.d.). *How do your kidneys work?* Retrieved November 20, 2021, from https://www.khanacademy.org/test-prep/mcat/organ-systems/the-renal-system/v/how-do-our-kidneys-work

National Center on Biotechnology Information. (2021). Circumcision by *country, 2021.* Retrieved December 28, 2021, from https://www.ncbi.nlm.nih.gov/pmc/articles/PMC4772313/table/Tab1/?report=objectonly

National Institute of Diabetes and Digestive and Kidney Diseases (NIDDKD). (2017). *Symptoms & causes of kidney stones.* Retrieved November 20, 2021, from https://www.niddk.nih.gov/health-information/urologic-diseases/kidney-stones/symptoms-causes

National Institute on Diabetes & Digestive Kidney Diseases (NIDDKD). (2018). *Your kidneys & how they work.* Retrieved November 20, 2021, from https://www.niddk.nih.gov/health-information/kidney-disease/kidneys-how-they-work

National Kidney Foundation (NKF). (2021a). *How your kidneys work.* Retrieved November 20, 2021, from https://www.kidney.org/kidneydisease/howkidneyswrk

National Kidney Foundation (NKF). (2021b). *Dialysis.* Retrieved December 8, 2021, from https://www.kidney.org/atoz/content/dialysisinfo#what-does-dialysis-do

Nitti, V. W. (2001). The prevalence of urinary incontinence. *Reviews in Urology, 3 Suppl 1*(Suppl 1), S2–S6. Retrieved from https://www.ncbi.nlm.nih.gov/pmc/articles/PMC1476070/#:~:text=In%20men%2C%20the%20prevalence%20of%2C%20trauma%2C%20or%20neurological%20injury

Office on Women's Health (OWH). (2019a). Birth *control methods*. U.S. Department of Health and Human Services. Retrieved December 29, 2021, from www.womenshealth. gov/a-z-topics/birth-control-methods

Office on Women's Health (OWH). (2019b). Stages of *pregnancy*. U.S. Department of Health and Human Services. Retrieved January 13, 2022, from https://www.women shealth.gov/pregnancy/youre-pregnant-now-what/stages-pregnancy

Ogobuiro, I., & Tuma, F. (2021). Physiology, renal. In *StatPearls*. StatPearls Publishing.

O'Hare, A. M., Tamura, M. K., Lavalle, D. C., Vig, E. K., Taylor, J. S., Hall, Y. N., Katz, R., Curtis, R., & Engelberg, R. A. (2019). Assessment of self-reported prognostic expectations of people undergoing dialysis United States Renal Data System Study of Treatment Preferences (USTATE). *Journal of the American Medication Association Internal Medicine, 179*(10), 1325–1333. https://doi.org/10.1001/jamainternmed.2019.2879

Osterberg, E. C., Awad, M. A., Gaither, T. W., Sanford, T., Alwaal, A., Hampson, L. A., Yoo, J., McAninch, J. W., & Breyer, B. N. (2017). Major genitourinary-related bicycle trauma: Results from 20 years at a level-1 trauma center. *Injury, 48*(1), 153–157. https://doi.org/10.1016/j.injury.2016.07.006

Pansota, M. S., Iftikhar, A., Ahmed, A., Ahmad, I., Tariq, H. M., & Saleem, M. S. (2019). Factors for urinary incontinence in females presenting in tertiary care hospital. *Journal of University Medical & Dental College, 10*(3), 9–13.

Patel, D. P., Redshaw, J. D., Breyer, B. N., Smith, T. G., Erickson, B. A., Majercik, S. D., Gaither, T. W., Craig, J. R., Gardner, S., Presson, A. P., Zhang, C., Hotaling, J. M., Brant, W. O., & Myers, J. B. (2015). High-grade renal injuries are often isolated in sports-related trauma. *Injury, 46*(7), 1245–1249. https://doi.org/10.1016/j.injury.2015.02.008

Peabody, A. M. (2015). *The different types of female genital mutilation*. https://globalw omanpeacefoundation.org/2015/07/29/the-different-types-of-female-genital-mut ilation

Planned Parenthood. (n.d.). https://www.plannedparenthood.org/learn/stds-hiv-safer-sex/chlamydia/chlamydia-symptoms

Pollak, M. R., Quaggin, S. E., Hoenig, M. P., & Dworkin, L. D. (2014). The glomerulus: The sphere of influence. *Clinical Journal of American Society of Nephrology, 9*(8), 1461–1469. https://doi.org/10.2215/CJN.09400913

Prior, R. (2013). Reproductive system. In Biology 12 *study guide—BC curriculum* (6th ed.) Prior Educational Resources. Retrieved December 20, 2021, from www.Biology-Study-Guides.com

Rosato, E., Farris, M., & Bastianelli, C. (2016). Mechanism of action of ulipristal acetate for emergency contraception: A systematic review. *Frontiers in Pharmacology, 6*, 315. https://doi.org/10.3389/fphar.2015.00315

Schiavi, M. C., D'Oria, O., Aleksa, N., Vena, F., Prata, G., Di Tucci, C., Savone, D., Sciuga, V., Giannini, A., Meggiorini, M. L., Monti, M., Zullo, M. A., Muzii, L., & Panici, P. B. (2018). Usefulness of ospemifene in the treatment of urgency in menopausal patients affected by mixed urinary incontinence who underwent mid-urethral sling surgery. *Gynecological Endocrinology, 35*(2), 155–159. https://doi.org/10.1080/09513 590.2018.1500534

Schober, J. (2021). Male reproductive system. In S. Standring (Ed.), *Grey's anatomy: The anatomical basis of clinical practice* (42 ed., pp. 1292–1306). Elsevier.

Simbar, M., Nazarpour, Mirzababaie, M., Hadi, M. A., E., Tehrani, F., R., & Majd, H. A. (2018). Quality of life and body image of individuals with gender dysphoria.

Journal of Sex & Marital Therapy, 44(6), 523–532. https://doi.org/10.1080/00926 23X.2017.1419392

Stanton, M. C., Ali, S., & Chaudhuri, S. (2017). Individual, social and community-level predictors of wellbeing in a U.S. sample of transgender and gender non-conforming individuals. Culture, *Health, & Sexuality, 19*(1), 32–49. https://doi.org/10.1080/13691 058.2016.1189596

Stewart, E. A., Nicholson, W. K., Bradley, L., & Borah, B. J. (2013). The burden of uterine fibroids for African-American women: Results of a national survey. *Journal of Women's Health, 22*(10), 807–816. https://doi.org/10.1089/jwh.2013.4334

Stover, A. C., Dunlap, G., & Neff, B. (2008). The effects of a contingency contracting program on the nocturnal enuresis of three children. *Research on Social Work Practice, 18*(5), 421–428. https://doi.org/10.1177/1049731507314007

Swanson, J. G., Kaczorowski, J., Skelly, J., & Finkelstein, M. (2005). Urinary incontinence: Common problem among women over 45. *Canadian Family Physician, 51*(1), 84–85.

Talley, K. M. C., Davis, N. J., & Wyman, J. F. (2017). Determining a treatment plan for urinary incontinence in an older adult: Application of the four-topic approach to ethical decision-making. *Urologic Nursing, 37*(4), 181–119. https://doi.org/10.7257/ 1053-816X.2017.37.4.181

Tinder. (n.d.). *Non-binary people explain what "non-binary" means to them.* https://www. youtube.com/watch?v=kVe8wpmH_IU&t=96s

Trussell, J., Aiken, A. R. A., Micks, E., & Guthrie, K. A. (2018). Efficacy, safety, and personal considerations. In R. A. Hatcher, A. L. Nelson, J. Trussell, C. Cwiak, P. Cason, M. S. Policar, A. Edelman, A. R. A. Aiken, J. Marrazzo, & D. Kowal (Eds.), *Contraceptive technology* (21st ed.). Ayer Company Publishers.

United States Renal Data system (USRDS). (2020). 2020 USRDS *annual data report*: Epidemiology *of kidney disease* in the United States (Table 9, p. 31). https://www. usrds.org/media/2371/2019-executive-summary.pdf. Retrieved December 9, 2021, from 2019-executive-summary.pdf (usrds.org).

Vande Walle, J., Rittig, S., Bauer, S., Eggert, P., Marschall-Kehrel, D., & Tekgul, S. (2012). Practical consensus guidelines for the management of enuresis. *European Journal of Pediatrics, 171*, 971–983. https://doi.org/10.1007/s00431-012-1687-7

Voelzke, B. B., & Leddy, L. (2014). The epidemiology of renal trauma. *Translational Andrology & Urology, 3*(2), 143–149. https://doi.org/10.3978/j.issn.2223-4683.2014.04.11

Wiggins, R. C. (2007). The spectrum of podocytopathies: A unifying view of glomerular diseases. *Kidney International, 71*, 1205–1214. https://doi.org/10.1038/sj.ki.5002222

Wilson, B. D. M., & Meyer, I. H. (2021). *Nonbinary LGBTQ adults in the United States.* Retrieved January 10, 2022, from Publications – Williams Institute (ucla.edu)

Woodman, P. J. (2021). Female reproductive system. In S. Standring (Ed.), Grey's anatomy: *The anatomical basis of clinical practice* (42 ed., pp. 1307–1330). Elsevier.

World Health Organization (WHO). (2020). Female *genital mutilation*. Retrieved January 2, 2022, from https://www.who.int/news-room/fact-sheets/detail/female-genital-mutilation

World Health Organization (WHO). (2021). *Sexually transmitted infections (STIs).* Retrieved January 7, 2022, from https://www.who.int/news-room/fact-sheets/detail/ sexually-transmitted-infections-stis

Yan, J., Wu, K., Tang, R., Ding, L., & Chen, A.-J. (2012). Effect of maternal age on the outcomes of in vitro fertilization and embryo transfer (IVF-ET). *Science China: Life Sciences, 55,* 694–698. https://doi.org/10.1007/s11427-012-4357-0

Yoshida, M., Takeda, M., Gotoh, M., Yokoyama, O., Kakizaki, H., Takahashi, S., Masumori, N., Nagai, S., & Minemura, K. (2020). Efficacy of vibegron, a novel beta3-adrenoreceptor agonist, on severe urgency urinary incontinence related to overactive bladder: Post hoc analysis of a randomized, placebo-controlled, double-blind, comparative phase 3 study. *British Journal of Urology International, 125,* 709–717. https://doi.org/10.1111/bju.15020

Index

For the benefit of digital users, indexed terms that span two pages (e.g., 52–53) may, on occasion, appear on only one of those pages.
Figures and boxes are indicated by *f* and *b* following the page number

urinary system, 166–70
in vitro fertilization, 185–86
uterus, 170–72
UV light. *See* ultraviolet (UV) light

vaccines
COVID-19, 107*f*, 107–8, 110–12
human papillomavirus (HPV), 180–81
meningitis, 56–57
poliomyelitis, 143
vagina, 170–71
vas deferens, 176
vasopressin (desmopressin), 187
ventilation, 106
viral load, 44, 46, 48–49, 53
visual system
aqueous humor, 61–62, 80–81
astigmatism, 66, 80–81
choroid, 61–62, 80–81
ciliary muscles, 66
color blindness, 62–63
cones, 62–63
cornea, 61–62, 66, 80–81
diabetic retinopathy, 67–68, 68*f*, 80–81
DNE contact lens, 67
eyeglasses, 66–67
function of, 62–63
glaucoma, 63–64, 80–81
hyperopia, 65–66, 66*f*
injuries, 65
intraocular pressure, 64, 67, 80–81
iris, 61–62, 80–81
myopia, 65–66, 66*f*, 80–81
normal vision, 65–66, 66*f*

online resources, 82
overview, 61
pupil, 61–63, 80–81
sclera, 61–62, 66, 80–81
structure of, 61–62, 62*f*
vision loss and mental health, 69–70
vitreous humor, 61–62, 80–81
vitreous humor, 61–62, 80–81
Von Bartheld, C. S., 77–78
vulva, 172, 198

Wagner, E. E., 51–52
Wallace "rule of nines," 119
Watson, S., 28–29
Westbrook, K. E., 133
white blood cells (WBCs), 40, 41, 42–44, 46–47, 52
white matter, 10–11
Wick, J. Y., 140–41
World Health Organization (WHO), 199
circumcision data, 183
HIV data, 50
osteoporosis, 140
Worobey, M., 44–45
Wrobel, B. B., 74

yolk stalk, 175

Zarzaur, B. L., 46–47
Zhang, S., 74
Zhao, J., 108
Zhao, R., 144
zidovudine (AZT), 48–49
Zschieschang, R., 72
zygote, 172